T0264007

Surgical Complications and Management Strategies

Guest Editor

LAURIE R. GOODRICH, DVM, MS, PhD

VETERINARY CLINICS OF NORTH AMERICA: EQUINE PRACTICE

www.vetequine.theclinics.com

Consulting Editor
A. SIMON TURNER, BVSc, MS

December 2008 • Volume 24 • Number 3

SAUNDERS an imprint of ELSEVIER, Inc.

W.B. SAUNDERS COMPANY

A Division of Elsevier Inc.

1600 John F. Kennedy Boulevard • Suite 1800 • Philadelphia, Pennsylvania 19103

http://www.vetequine.theclinics.com

VETERINARY CLINICS OF NORTH AMERICA: EQUINE PRACTICE Volume 24, Number 3
December 2008 ISSN 0749-0739, ISBN-13: 978-1-4160-6369-8, ISBN-10: 1-4160-6369-2

Editor: John Vassallo; j.vassallo@elsevier.com

© 2009 Elsevier ■ All rights reserved.

This journal and the individual contributions contained in it are protected under copyright by Elsevier, and the following terms and conditions apply to their use:

Photocopying

Single photocopies of single articles may be made for personal use as allowed by national copyright laws. Permission of the Publisher and payment of a fee is required for all other photocopying, including multiple or systematic copying, copying for advertising or promotional purposes, resale, and all forms of document delivery. Special rates are available for educational institutions that wish to make photocopies for non-profit educational classroom use. For information on how to seek permission visit www.elsevier.com/permissions or call: (+44) 1865 843830 (UK)/(+1) 215 239 3804 (USA).

Derivative Works

Subscribers may reproduce tables of contents or prepare lists of articles including abstracts for internal circulation within their institutions. Permission of the Publisher is required for resale or distribution outside the institution. Permission of the Publisher is required for all other derivative works, including compilations and translations (please consult www.elsevier.com/permissions).

Electronic Storage or Usage

Permission of the Publisher is required to store or use electronically any material contained in this journal, including any article or part of an article (please consult www.elsevier.com/permissions). Except as outlined above, no part of this publication may be reproduced, stored in a retrieval system or transmitted in any form or by any means, electronic, mechanical, photocopying, recording or otherwise, without prior written permission of the Publisher.

Notice

No responsibility is assumed by the Publisher for any injury and/or damage to persons or property as a matter of products liability, negligence or otherwise, or from any use or operation of any methods, products, instructions or ideas contained in the material herein. Because of rapid advances in the medical sciences, in particular, independent verification of diagnoses and drug dosages should be made.

Although all advertising material is expected to conform to ethical (medical) standards, inclusion in this publication does not constitute a guarantee or endorsement of the quality or value of such product or of the claims made of it by its manufacturer.

Veterinary Clinics of North America: Equine Practice (ISSN 0749-0739) is published in April, August, and December by Elsevier Inc., 360 Park Avenue South, New York, NY 10010-1710. Business and Editorial Offices: 1600 John F. Kennedy Blvd., Suite 1800, Philadelphia, PA 19103-2899. Customer Service office: 11830 Westline Industrial Drive, St. Louis, MO 63146. Subscription prices are $200.00 per year (domestic individuals), $332.00 per year (domestic institutions), $100.00 per year (domestic students/residents), $233.00 per year (Canadian individuals), $415.00 per year (Canadian institutions), $269.00 per year (international individuals), $415.00 per year (international institutions), and $136.00 per year (international and Canadian students/residents). To receive student/resident rate, orders must be accompanied by name of affiliated institution, date of term, and the signature of program/residency coordinator on institution letterhead. Orders will be billed at individual rate until proof of status is received. Foreign air speed delivery is included in all *Clinics* subscription prices. All prices are subject to change without notice. **POSTMASTER:** Send address changes to *Veterinary Clinics of North America: Equine Practice,* 11830 Westline Industrial Drive, St. Louis, MO 63146. Customer Service (orders, claims, online, change of address): Elsevier Periodicals Customer Service, 11830 Westline Industrial Drive, St. Louis, MO 63146. Tel: 1-800-654-2452 (U.S. and Canada); 314-453-7041 (outside U.S. and Canada). Fax: 314-523-5170. E-mail: journalscustomerservice-usa@elsevier.com (for print support); journalsonlinesupport-usa@elsevier (for online support).

Reprints. For copies of 100 or more of articles in this publication, please contact the Commercial Reprints Department, Elsevier Inc., 360 Park Avenue South, New York, NY 10010-1710. Tel.: 212-633-3812; Fax: 212-462-1935; E-mail: reprints@elsevier.com.

Veterinary Clinics of North America: Equine Practice is covered in *MEDLINE/PubMed (Index Medicus), Excerpta Medica, Current Contents/Agriculture, Biology and Environmental Sciences,* and *ISI.*

Printed and bound in the United Kingdom
Transferred to Digital Print 2011

Contributors

CONSULTING EDITOR

A. SIMON TURNER, BVSc, MS
Diplomate, American College of Veterinary Surgeons; Professor, Department of Clinical Sciences, College of Veterinary Medicine and Biomedical Sciences, Colorado State University, Fort Collins, Colorado

GUEST EDITOR

LAURIE R. GOODRICH, DVM, MS, PhD
Diplomate, American College of Veterinary Surgeons; Assistant Professor of Equine Surgery and Lameness, Department of Clinical Sciences, College of Veterinary Medicine and Biomedical Sciences, Colorado State University, Fort Collins, Colorado

AUTHORS

BENJAMIN J. AHERN, BVSc
Member, Australian College of Veterinary Scientists; Resident in Large Animal Surgery, New Bolton Center, University of Pennsylvania, Kennett Square, Pennsylvania

GARY M. BAXTER, VMD, MS
Professor of Surgery; and Assistant Department Head; and Equine Section Head, Department of Clinical Sciences, James L. Voss Veterinary Teaching Hospital, Colorado State University, Fort Collins, Colorado

DENNIS E. BROOKS, DVM, PhD
Diplomate, American College of Veterinary Ophthalmologists; Professor of Ophthalmology, Department of Large Animal Clinical Sciences, College of Veterinary Medicine, University of Florida, Gainesville, Florida

PADRAIC M. DIXON, MVB, PhD, MRCVS
Professor of Equine Surgery, Division of Veterinary Clinical Studies, Easter Bush Veterinary Centre; Department of Clinical Science, University of Edinburgh, Royal (Dick) School of Veterinary Studies, Midlothian, Scotland, United Kingdom

SARAH DUKTI, DVM
Diplomate, American College of Veterinary Surgeons; Clinical Assistant Professor, Department of Emergency Medicine and Surgery, Marion duPont Scott Equine Medical Center, Virginia-Maryland Regional College of Veterinary Medicine, Leesburg, Virginia

ROLF M. EMBERTSON, DVM
Diplomate, American College of Veterinary Surgeons; Rood and Riddle Equine Hospital, Lexington, Kentucky

DAVID E. FREEMAN, MVB, PhD
Diplomate, American College of Veterinary Surgeons; Professor and Associate Chief of Staff, Department of Large Animal Clinical Sciences, College of Veterinary Medicine, University of Florida, Gainesville, Florida

LAURIE R. GOODRICH, DVM, MS, PhD
Diplomate, American College of Veterinary Surgeons; Assistant Professor of Equine Surgery and Lameness, Department of Clinical Sciences, College of Veterinary Medicine and Biomedical Sciences, Colorado State University, Fort Collins, Colorado

EILEEN SULLIVAN HACKETT, DVM, MS
Assistant Professor of Equine Surgery and Critical Care, Department of Clinical Sciences, Colorado State University, Fort Collins, Colorado

R. REID HANSON, DVM
Diplomate, American College of Veterinary Surgeons; Diplomate, American College of Veterinary Emergency and Critical Care; Professor of Equine Surgery, Department of Clinical Sciences, College of Veterinary Medicine, Auburn University, Auburn, Alabama

DIANA M. HASSEL, DVM, PhD
Assistant Professor of Equine Surgery and Critical Care, Department of Clinical Sciences, Colorado State University, Fort Collins, Colorado

CLAIRE HAWKES, BVSc, MRCVS
Horserace Betting Levy Board Resident in Equine Respiratory Medicine and Surgery, Division of Veterinary Clinical Studies, Easter Bush Veterinary Centre, Midlothian, Scotland, United Kingdom

DEAN A. HENDRICKSON, DVM, MS
Diplomate, American College of Veterinary Surgeons; Professor of Surgery, Department of Clinical Sciences, James L. Voss Veterinary Teaching Hospital, College of Veterinary Medicine and Biomedical Sciences, Colorado State University, Fort Collins, Colorado

C. WAYNE McILWRAITH, MS, PhD
Diplomate, American College of Veterinary Surgeons; Professor of Surgery; and Director, Orthopedic Research Center; and Barbara Cox Anthony University Endowed Chair, Department of Clinical Sciences, Colorado State University, Fort Collins, Colorado

SCOTT MORRISON, DVM
Rood and Riddle Equine Hospital, Lexington, Kentucky

ERIC J. PARENTE, DVM
Diplomate, American College of Veterinary Surgeons; Associate Professor of Surgery, New Bolton Center, University of Pennsylvania, Kennett Square, Pennsylvania

DEAN W. RICHARDSON, DVM
Diplomate, American College of Veterinary Surgeons; Charles W. Raker Professor of Surgery; and Chief of Large Animal Surgery, New Bolton Center School of Veterinary Medicine, University of Pennsylvania, Kennett Square, Pennsylvania

NEIL TOWNSEND, BSc, BVSc, MRCVS
Horse Trust Resident in Equine Surgery, Division of Veterinary Clinical Studies, Easter Bush Veterinary Centre, Midlothian, Scotland, United Kingdom

ANN E. WAGNER, DVM, MS
Diplomate, American College of Veterinary Pathologists; Diplomate, American College of Veterinary Anesthesiologists; Professor, Anesthesiology, Department of Clinical Sciences, Colorado State University, Fort Collins, Colorado

NATHANIEL WHITE, DVM
Diplomate, American College of Veterinary Surgeons; Jean Ellen Shehan Professor and Director, Department of Emergency Medicine and Surgery, Marion duPont Scott Equine Medical Center, Virginia-Maryland Regional College of Veterinary Medicine, Leesburg, Virginia

Contents

medical management. This article addresses some of the most common surgical complications of abdominal surgery for colic to help prevent, recognize, and treat these complications.

Colic is a serious disease of the horse and may require surgical correction. Postoperative complications may result in an increase in short-term morbidity and mortality. Commonly encountered nonsurgical complications are detailed. Anticipation and timely treatment of common postoperative complications after colic surgery may improve overall survival.

This article describes surgical complications associated with laparoscopy, how to avoid them, how to recognize them if they do happen, and how to deal with them in the most expedient method possible. Complications of sedation, anesthesia, positioning, the general surgical approach, and complications associated with specific surgical procedures are examined. The best defense against surgical complications is a thorough training program and an understanding of anatomy that will help the surgeon work in the three-dimensional environment while being limited to two dimensions on the monitor. The author concludes that it is critical to be able to convert the surgery to an open procedure if there are problems with the equipment or the patient.

Arthroscopic complications are infrequent but when they occur can cause significant morbidity in the equine patient. This article reviews intraoperative and postoperative complications along with ways to avoid them. Additionally, therapeutic methods of managing these complications also are discussed.

Complications are a price all surgeons eventually pay. Experience and increasing skill will decrease many of them but certainly not all. The most important thing is for the surgeon to react correctly to a complication. Acknowledge the mistake (or bad luck) quickly and take whatever steps you can to correct the problem. Because so many equine orthopaedic cases have the potential for complications, recognizing and responding properly to these complications are imperative for successful outcomes. Discussion of the most common complications, their prevention and corrections, is presented.

Corneal transplantation, amniotic membrane transplantation, phacoemulsification cataract extraction, and laser glaucoma therapy are routine ophthalmic surgical procedures in horses. This article discusses the indications, techniques, and postoperative complications of these and other ophthalmic surgical procedures in horses. Meticulous and accurate anatomic repair can minimize postoperative complications to maintain positive visual outcomes in ophthalmic surgery of the horse.

General anesthesia of horses entails considerable risk of morbidity and mortality. A large-scale, multicenter study reported that the death rate from non–colic-related anesthetics was 0.9%, while the perianesthetic mortality rate at a single, busy equine surgical practice was somewhat more favorable, at 0.12%. While any perianesthetic death is devastating, mortality figures alone do not reflect the overall morbidity of equine anesthesia in terms of nonterminal events or injuries related to recovery. In some circumstances, recognition of perianesthetic complications may allow appropriate intervention to prevent the complication from worsening or progressing to mortality. This article describes some of the complications that may occur during and after general anesthesia of horses, and suggests ways to prevent or mitigate them.

RELATED INTEREST

Veterinary Clinics of North America: Food Animal Practice (Vol. 24, No. 2)
Field Surgery of Cattle, Part I
David E. Anderson, DVM, MS and Matt D. Miesner, DVM, MS, *Guest Editors*

Veterinary Clinics of North America: Food Animal Practice (Vol. 24, No. 3)
Field Surgery of Cattle, Part II
David E. Anderson, DVM, MS and Matt D. Miesner, DVM, MS, *Guest Editors*

THE CLINICS ARE NOW AVAILABLE ONLINE!

Access your subscription at:
www.theclinics.com

Preface

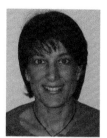

Laurie R. Goodrich, DVM, MS, PhD
Guest Editor

Many of the wisest and most experienced clinicians will say they have learned more from the things that have gone wrong with their cases than the things that have gone right. The patients we treat—those who are admitted to the hospital, have successful surgical procedures performed, and go home without incident—are the ones we covet. These cases bring great satisfaction to our work lives and frequently result in happy clients, and because unanticipated costs usually are not involved, the business aspect of these cases typically is straightforward. We often take credit for the good things associated with these cases, because they represent the long hours of training and practice that we have invested in our specialty and the goal most of us strive towards: surgical success without incident. But the patients in which complications occur are the ones that great doctors are made of. They are the patients that we worry over until their complications resolve, check on in the middle of the night, research the reasons why things are not going as planned, and self-examine and critique the decisions we have made. Regardless of the result, cases fraught with complications make us reconsider the course of treatment or surgical decisions we have chosen, perhaps seek better methods to avoid future complications, and, most importantly, instill humility to our innermost egos.

As an intern, surgical resident, clinical instructor, and then assistant professor, I have gone through the ranks of neophyte, to neophyte with some training, to clinician that sometimes still feels like a neophyte at many things. In the field of veterinary surgery, we do not experience the numbers of cases that our human counterparts often do. In most hospitals, this requires us to be "a jack of all trades." We still are not at the point where our profession is specialized enough to warrant subspecialties, and we may never be at a point where economics justify such specialization. Therefore, most of us will be expected to attain surgical skills based on much smaller numbers than surgeons in the human field. We know that repetition is the best teacher, and, in an ideal world, we would have done several surgical procedures in training before we went forward on our own. In most situations, this is not the case, and we will perform surgeries that we have never completed before on live patients. Hopefully, broad training and board certification in surgery we receive gives us the knowledge, skills,

doi:10.1016/j.cveq.2008.11.002
0749-0739/08/$ – see front matter © 2009 Elsevier Inc. All rights reserved.

and confidence to navigate through uncharted territory we encounter. However, we will find ourselves dealing with complications and managing their after effects if we do enough cases.

I was a clinical instructor at Cornell University after completing my surgical residency. For many, this can be a "fragile" time of transition when one goes from being trained, to training others when barely confident with one's own skills. My mentors used to tell me "if you ain't got anything going wrong, you probably ain't doing anything." I often was irritated by that statement, believing they were just trying to make me feel better about a case that did not go particularly well. I now realize they had acquired the wisdom and the realistic rhetoric that accompanies the quote "good judgment comes from experience and experience often comes from bad judgment."

Training surgical residents is one of my favorite aspects of being a surgeon at a teaching hospital. It brings me great satisfaction to watch them grow, gain the confidence to perform procedures with increasing surgical prowess, and become confident and competent surgeons. It is interesting to observe the wide degree of eagerness among residents to perform certain procedures depending on their personalities, experiences, and training. As I reflect on my training and the many great mentors I had, I believe I have learned the most from those who were willing to tell me about all of the things that could go wrong before teaching me how to perform the surgery and manage the case right. I believe the wisest and most humble clinicians are the best teachers and surgeons, because they have gained the insight into the many complications that can occur even with the most experienced surgeons.

I am proud to say that this edition of *Veterinary Clinics of North America: Equine Practice* is the first of its kind in veterinary medicine: perhaps a long time coming. The goal of this issue is to bring to light some of the most common and perhaps some of the uncommon complications associated with many of the surgical procedures we will be expected to perform in our careers. It certainly is not meant to be a substitute for those great mentors who train and educate us first hand on complications, but it is meant to help clinicians manage complications when they occur and educate clinicians to avoid those pitfalls; the ones that, had the knowledge been available that they could happen beforehand, a different strategy might have been taken. Most importantly, when you read the articles by the experienced authors of this issue, you will realize that the experts have gained much of their insights from dealing with complicated cases, and, regardless of how much or little experience the surgeon has, "checking the ego at the scrub room" is an integral part of successful case management.

The authors of the articles are experts in their fields and subspecialties. Many of them have developed significant advances in the specialty they have written about. I am incredibly grateful to them for willingly sharing their years of experiences, great photos, and wisdom they have gained by managing complications. There is no substitute for experience. It has been stated that "we learn wisdom from failure much more than success" and I believe the authors reflect that paradigm.

Because most surgeries are performed under general anesthesia, I have included an article on the complications associated with anesthesia (written by Dr. Ann Wagner, a talented and experienced anesthesiologist). I also have included an article on pain management of orthopedic pain, because if it is not controlled, it becomes a major complication that results in great morbidity and sometimes the demise of the patient because of support-limb laminitis. Because preventing and managing support-limb laminitis is also crucial to the success of orthopedic procedures, I have included an informative and superbly written article by Drs. Baxter and Morrison, who have extensively researched and managed these cases.

I thank Dr. Simon Turner and John Vassallo for giving me the honor of editing this issue and the editorial staff at Elsevier for their patience and accurate editorial skills.

Finally, I dedicate this book to my late, beloved father, Dr. Gordon M. Goodrich; a skilled and humble dentist for many decades, he led his life by example and impressed upon me how a life dedicated to helping others can make a difference in so many lives.

Laurie R. Goodrich, DVM, MS, PhD
Department of Clinical Sciences
College of Veterinary Medicine and Biomedical Sciences
Colorado State University
300 West Drake Road
Fort Collins, CO 80523, USA

E-mail address:
laurie.goodrich@colostate.edu (L.R. Goodrich)

Surgical Complications of the Equine Upper Respiratory Tract

Benjamin J. Ahern, BVSc, Eric J. Parente, DVM*

KEYWORDS

- Upper respiratory • Sinus • Laryngeal
- Epiglottis • Laser • Palate

LARYNGEAL SURGERY

Laryngoplasty

Laryngeal hemiplegia has been recognized as a performance-limiting disease process in horses since the 1800s.[1] Treatment by laryngoplasty was first performed by Cadiot,[2] who transcutaneously sutured the paralyzed arytenoid to the thyroid cartilage. With remarkably little variation, the technique described by Marks and colleagues[3] in 1970 is still accepted as the treatment of choice, despite the limited success and host of possible complications. The reported success rate of the modern laryngoplasty procedure ranges from 5% to 95%.[4–9] Of interest, there has not been a marked improvement in reported success rates chronologically.[4,7,10–12] Furthermore, reported successful results vary depending on the outcome variable evaluated (eg, degree of abduction or return to racing) and on the breed of the surgical population. Thoroughbred racehorses have a lower success rate (48% or 66%, respectively) compared to breeds not intended for racing (90% or 95%, respectively).[5,11] In one study looking at postoperative racing success involving Thoroughbred racehorses, approximately 60% of horses won at least one start after surgery.[10]

The limited success and complications reported are not reflective of a procedure infrequently performed. The reported incidence of clinical disease ranges from 2.6% to 8.3%.[6–8,12] The following section presents the authors' current understanding of laryngoplasty complications. These complications have been separated into three time periods corresponding to when they occur.

Intraoperative complications

The likelihood of intraoperative complications is significantly reduced with increasing surgical laryngoplasty experience. A thorough knowledge of surgical anatomy and an

New Bolton Center, University of Pennsylvania, 382 West Street Road, Kennett Square, PA 19348, USA
* Corresponding author.
E-mail address: ejp@vet.upenn.edu (E.J. Parente).

Vet Clin Equine 24 (2009) 465–484
doi:10.1016/j.cveq.2008.10.004
0749-0739/08/$ – see front matter

© 2009 Elsevier Inc. All rights reserved.

understanding of the mechanical forces involved are essential for maximizing the probability of successful abduction.

Hemorrhage Intraoperative hemorrhage can obstruct visualization, can make suture placement difficult, and can increase the risk of incisional complications; this is particularly true in the region of the caudal aspect of the cricoid cartilage. The cranial thyroid artery crosses the cricoid at this region, and needle penetration results in some hemorrhage. When inadvertent damage to vascular structures in this region causes obstruction of the surgical field, tightening of the laryngoplasty suture often serves to reduce the bleeding without any further treatment.

Suture placement Suture penetration to the laryngeal lumen is extremely rare with experience but can cause significant postoperative infections when not addressed. Intraoperative endoscopic assessment can prevent suture penetration from occurring, or at least allow the surgeon to address it immediately. Intubation with a slightly smaller (18–20 mm endotracheal tube) allows for ample tracheal access to evaluate for inadvertently placed sutures (**Fig. 1**). When tracheal penetration occurs, the suture should be cut at the caudal cricoid to minimize the amount of suture that is dragged through during its removal. A new suture can be inserted to replace it without difficulty.

Needle bending or breakage is another problem encountered during laryngoplasty procedures[8,13] and depends on the size and type of the needle being used and on surgeon experience. Passing the needle through the caudal cricoid cartilage is the most likely situation for excessive stress on the needle, and broken needles can be difficult to locate and remove from this region. As surgical incisions become smaller, the temptation is to place the needle in such a way that it is necessary to utilize excessive force when passing the needle through the cartilage. An adequate incision, given the surgeon's experience and good retraction by assistants, helps to allow for optimal access for suture placement and to avoid this complication.

Rarely, cartilage fracture during suture placement is encountered, and muscular process fracture has been reported during prosthesis placement.[9] Repositioning of

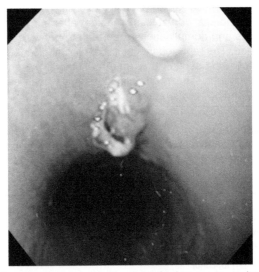

Fig. 1. Endoscopic view of suture penetration into the lumen. An endoscope was not used intraoperatively to check for suture penetration.

the suture to obtain a larger bite of the cartilage in a different plane to the fracture line and the use of caution during tightening of the prosthesis are advisable in this situation.

Early postoperative complications

General surgical complications Racehorses and draft breeds are the two most common breeds of horses requiring laryngoplasty procedures. For draft breeds, general surgical complications such as neuropathies and myopathies are more common, likely due to their heavier frames. Specifically for laryngoplasty surgeries, postanesthetic complications have been reported as being 7% in draft breeds compared with 1.2% in lighter-breed horses.[9] Serious complications in the postoperative period requiring tracheostomy have been reported to be as high as 19% in draft breeds[14] compared with only 0% to 0.4%[7-9] in other breeds. Experienced anesthetic management for these higher-risk patients minimizes these potential complications, and the availability of a sling for recovery and emergency tracheostomy equipment when performing laryngoplasty surgery on draft breeds is advisable.

Immediate postoperative respiratory obstruction Rarely, horses undergoing anesthesia can wake up with complete laryngeal paralysis.[15] The specific cause is unknown, but it is suspected that a recurrent laryngeal neuropathy can develop that is associated with the horse's position on the surgery table and possibly with hypoxia. If a horse recovers from anesthesia without the ability to attain and maintain abduction of one or both arytenoids, it could experience a complete upper respiratory obstruction. It is advised to recover horses with a nasotracheal tube to ensure a patent airway during recovery and to remove it after the animal is standing and stable. When a horse develops right-sided recurrent laryngeal neuropathy associated with surgery, the animal should be kept in a stall with limited risk of exertion and reevaluated at 1- to 2-month intervals. It is likely that the neuropathy will resolve over several months.

Immediate postoperative dysphagia and excessive abduction Dysphagia is considered by many to be related to degree of abduction of the arytenoid. Nine percent to 16% of horses that underwent laryngoplasty procedures have been reported to have some degree of nasal discharge in the immediate postoperative period.[7,16] Although marked dysphagia was associated exclusively with high amounts of abduction in one article,[8] the present authors and other investigators do not believe this association has a direct linear correlation.[10] Intraoperative endoscopic assessment should prevent excessive abduction and help ameliorate this complication. Rates of intraoperative target abduction vary depending on the study and have been reported to be 60% to 70%,[8,9,17] 70% to 90%,[9] and 50% to 80%.[8] Furthermore, one study reported that abduction above resting position did not improve performance but increased the rate of complications.[6] Laryngoplasty procedures result in airway contamination over normal or hemiplegic states.[18] When excessive abduction is observed postoperatively and combined with significant coughing and dysphagia, a second surgery to remove, replace, or loosen the prosthesis should be delayed for 2 to 3 weeks to determine whether it resolves spontaneously (**Fig. 2**). This resolution may be related to loss of abduction or to "settling" of the arytenoids, which commonly occurs postoperatively.[8]

Another likely associated postoperative complication is coughing, which may or may not have a significant effect on performance.[19] It has been reported to occur in 13% of draft breeds,[9] in 18% and 33% of mixed breeds,[6,15] and in 26%, 40%, and 43% of racehorses[4,7] undergoing laryngoplasty. In some cases, coughing may solely be a manifestation of overabduction of the arytenoid, but it is more likely due to altered pharyngeal function[20] whose origin is not yet fully understood. Given that the most

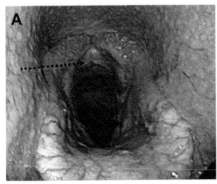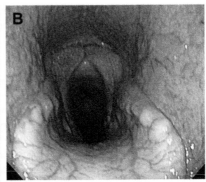

Fig. 2. (*A*) Endoscopic view of a horse with excessive abduction of the left arytenoid 1 day postoperatively. Note thin rim of mucous (*arrow*) commonly seen on the dorsal rim of the glottis with excessive abduction. (*B*) Note the mild loss of abduction over several weeks and the lack of any signs of dysphagia.

common cause for postoperative coughing is aspiration of feed material, most management procedures are aimed at reducing this complication by reducing aspiration. Options include muzzling of patients in the postoperative period for 2 to 4 hours (ie, until completely recovered from anesthesia), feeding from the ground, reducing dust in the environment, and washing any feed material from the mouth before exercise.[4,7,9,19,21]

Incisional swelling (seroma) Seroma formation is generally related to surgical experience with the procedure. A thorough understanding of anatomy and adherence to surgical principles helps to reduce this complication. Even in the hands of experienced surgeons, seroma formation can occur, with reported rates of 1% to 7%.[4,7,8] Assessment of seroma formation is easily performed by determining whether the vertical ramus of the mandible is not well defined. When this is the case, there is a surprisingly large amount of fluid over the larynx that may cause dysphagia postoperatively.[8] An effective therapy for draining these seromas involves removing two to three skin sutures and expressing the fluid twice a day until resolution.[9] Repeat surgery with placement of Penrose drains has been performed[8] but is rarely warranted because seromas often resolve with less aggressive therapy.

Infection A wide range of postoperative infection rates (0%, 2%, and 4%–17%) has been reported for laryngoplasty procedures.[5,6,8,9,12] An infection rate as high as 33% has been reported for draft horses; however, some of the procedures in this study were performed on standing horses, and the infection rate is significantly higher due to the increased procedural difficulty.[14] The variability in reported postoperative infection rates is probably related in part to the many variations of the procedure that are performed. Variations such as the use of widely different suture materials— ranging from wire[8] to nonabsorbable[9] and even absorbable suture material in one report[22]—may play a role in the rate of infection. The formation of sinus tracts from the prosthesis to the skin or even into the larynx can occur,[8,19] which may require removal for resolution to occur.[10] The addition of a laryngotomy to perform a ventriculectomy may also result in increased reported infection rates. Most laryngoplasty infections, when noted early in the postoperative period, can be effectively treated with the establishment of drainage and appropriate antimicrobials based on culture and sensitivity patterns and without suture removal.[7,8] A persistent draining tract that is not responsive to such treatment warrants suture removal and endoscopic reevaluations to ensure that a chondropathy does not follow.

Loss of abduction—early Spontaneous decrease in the degree of abduction or settling in the immediate postoperative period is a well-recognized phenomenon and occurs mostly in the first 7 days.[4,8] Intraoperative endoscopy during suture placement allows for the degree of abduction to be carefully controlled. Reported optimal intraoperative abduction ranges from 60%[23] to (more recently) 70% to 90% of maximal abduction.[9] Although greater abduction has been associated with higher rates of complications,[6] it has also been associated with a greater likelihood to return to work and improved performance.[19] As a result, the optimal degree of abduction appears to be a balance of many factors and should likely be decided on a case-by-case basis. For example, for horses performing at submaximal levels (eg, jumpers, draft horses), the concern is more often with reduction in noise and not necessarily maximal airflow. Hence, laryngoplasty at a lower percentage of maximal abduction may be sufficient for their purpose and may not have as many postoperative complications. In contrast, racehorses require maximal airway dilation to allow them to compete and, as a result, may require more aggressively abducted laryngoplasty procedures.

Strand and colleagues[10] reported almost 6% (3/52) of horses that underwent laryngoplasty procedures had failure due to suture cut-through or loosening during surgery or in the immediate postoperative period. This failure has been attributed to failure at the muscular process[13] and the cricoid.[8] Satisfactory abduction at 9 days postoperatively was achieved in 77% of laryngoplasty surgery, with failures mostly attributable to suture cutting through the laryngeal cartilages.[4] These failures occurred in two 2-year-olds and a 3-year-old, leading Strand and colleagues[10] to hypothesize that the cartilage of young horses was weaker and more prone to failure compared with older horses. This claim was refuted, however, in an in vitro study determining pull-through forces that indicated no difference related to age.[24] Furthermore, the density of the cricoid cartilage has been found to be unrelated to age,[25] suggesting that failure is independent of this factor.

After inadequate abduction postoperatively is definitive, repeated operation is required and can be performed at any time, but it is probably easiest in the early postoperative period before the formation of mature fibrous tissue. Of 200 laryngoplasty surgeries performed in one study, 5% had repeated surgery to tighten or replace prostheses within 7 days postoperatively.[8] During the repeat operation, it is important to cut the previous sutures, removing them from the muscular process and freeing any fibrous tissue binding it to the wing of the thyroid. After this is done, movement of the arytenoid should be observed with the endoscope by finger manipulation of the muscular process. When the muscular process is free of adhesions, adequate abduction should be obtained with the new suture placement.

Late postoperative complications
Loss of abduction—long term Long-term loss of abduction is a commonly reported failure of laryngoplasty surgery. It is often extremely difficult to determine the exact reason for this failure. Complications such as prosthesis or cartilage failure are two commonly postulated reasons. Efforts to determine the reason for these long-term failures have been attempted. Suggested factors include acute mechanical cartilage failure, cyclic cartilage failure resulting in gradual prosthesis loosening, improper prosthesis placement resulting in biomechanical disadvantage, and any disease state rendering cartilage weaker than normal.[19] Efforts to reduce acute mechanical pull-out using novel prosthesis systems have been performed but have not gained

widespread acceptance.[26] Recurrent laryngeal neurectomy to abolish any residual adductor muscle activity that may contribute to continued cyclic forces acting on the prosthesis was not effective in improving postoperative racing performance.[19] Grade III laryngeal hemiplegic horses commonly have a greater amount of cricoarytenoideus dorsalis muscle mass present at surgery compared with those with grade IV. Because the muscle is somewhat interposed between the cartilage and suture, atrophy of the cricoarytenoideus muscle over time may contribute to long-term prosthesis loosening. Improper placement of the prosthesis overly lateral on the cricoid results in loss of mechanical advantage and decreased abduction. Recent research focusing on the conformation of the caudal aspect of the cricoid has revealed significant variability (J. Dahlberg and E.J. Parente, unpublished data, 2008). This variability may allow the prosthesis to migrate ventrally along the caudal aspect of the cricoid, allowing for progressive abduction failure. Attention to placement of the prosthesis, close to the midline, helps to ameliorate this complication.

A further attempt to prevent long-term loss of abduction by the author has been to surgically fuse the cricoarytenoid articulation. This procedure only minimally increases surgical time with experience and results in a strong articular fusion (E.J. Parente, unpublished data), which should assist in maintaining abduction of the arytenoid long-term. Care should be taken, however, in horses that have had this procedure and are dysphagic or cough excessively in the immediate postoperative period because repeat operation to reduce the degree of abduction should be performed before formation of a mature fusion.

Arytenoid granulation tissue The formation of focal granulation tissuelike projections from the axial surface above the vocal process with some thickening of the cartilage (chondritis) is an unusual surgical complication. It has been reported to occur in 1% of horses in a large retrospective study.[8] The formation of excessive arytenoid granulation may form in relation to a laser vocal cordectomy procedure when performed concurrently with a laryngoplasty.[27] Removal of the granulation tissue with standing laser surgery and appropriate antimicrobials should prevent the problem from worsening and can still result in a good airway. If the disease progresses, then arytenoidectomy may be necessary.

Late-term coughing and dysphagia Coughing and chronic aspiration pneumonia are common complications reported by owners and trainers at a rate varying between 5% and 43%.[6–8,10,23] A correlation between the degree of abduction and these complications is not readily apparent in many cases.[10] Often, this coughing is associated with eating.[8] Subclinical aspiration can occur even without coughing many years postoperatively. The author has seen several cases of pneumonia secondary to aspiration months after laryngoplasty, without an early history of coughing/dysphagia. Endoscopic examination often does not reveal overabducted arytenoid position (**Fig. 3**). Why this complication develops at this stage is not clear, but resolution of the pneumonia without surgical intervention has not been successful. Mobilization of the muscular process is required to resolve the pneumonia, but the horse often no longer has an adequate glottic opening for performance.

Epiglottic Entrapment

Entrapment of the epiglottis in a fold of subepiglottic tissue is a common abnormal finding in racehorses.[11,28,29] It is, however, less common than laryngeal hemiplegia or dorsal displacement of the soft palate (DDSP),[30] making up approximately 3% of all upper respiratory obstructive lesions.[31] Diagnosis of persistent epiglottic

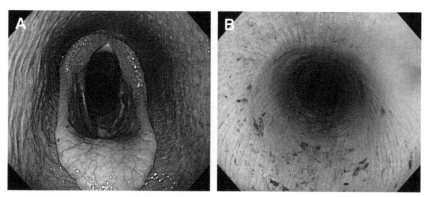

Fig. 3. (*A*) Endoscopic view of a horse that underwent a laryngoplasty more than a year ago and recently demonstrated dysphagia. (*B*) Note the feed material within the trachea despite the limited degree of abduction.

entrapment (EE) is readily confirmed by way of endoscopic examination. Intermittent entrapment can be more difficult to diagnose. Most entrapments are uncomplicated, with a small number being excessively thickened or ulcerated.[32] EE is commonly an acquired condition that is associated with the onset of hard work.[31,33] Uncomplicated cases of EE result in significantly less airway obstruction than does laryngeal hemiplegia[34] but can provoke DDSP and thus more significant airway obstruction in some cases.[35] Correction of EE is indicated in horses to reduce respiratory noise and improve racing success;[36–38] however, instances of horses racing adequately with diagnosed and untreated EE have been reported.[39,40]

Axial division of the entrapping tissue without subepiglottic resection is currently advocated.[6] Laryngotomy and excision of redundant tissue, which has been performed historically, should be avoided in uncomplicated cases of EE due to a lower postoperative prognosis for racing successfully (27%) in comparison to axial division.[28,29] A more minimalistic approach is recommended to preserve tissue, minimize scarring, and reduce the likelihood of complications such as DDSP. The division of the entrapping tissue is commonly performed using laser (Nd:YAG or diode) or a hooked bistoury knife. The use of transendoscopic electrosurgical division had a very high complication rate, with 40% re-entrapment, and as such, has fallen out of use.[41]

Laser division

Standing transendoscopic axial division of the entrapping fold using a laser per nasum is commonly performed as outpatient surgery. This procedure has proved to be a safe method to treat EE, with a low (4%) rate of recurrence.[32,42] Experience with the handling of endoscopically guided lasers, to minimize the amount of energy used, is important. The use of these lasers helps to avoid inadvertent tissue damage that may result in excessive scarring and possibly lead to DDSP. Currently, the rate of DDSP ranges from 10% to 15% using this technique.[32] Transendoscopic laser surgery also offers the option and advantage of debulking excessively thickened and ulcerated subepiglottic tissue while in its normal anatomic position rather than retroverting it caudally to access the tissue through a laryngotomy.

Thermal damage to the dorsal surface of the epiglottis can occur with this method of treatment, particularly in less-experienced hands (**Fig. 4**). Care should be taken to lightly cut through the membrane in sequential layers rather than a single layer, and to only cut the tissue under greatest tension. When a small area of the dorsal

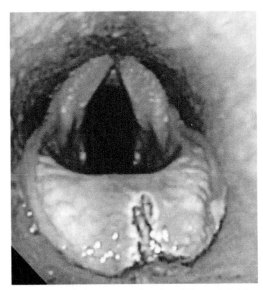

Fig. 4. Moderately severe thermal damage to the tip of the epiglottis after laser axial division of an EE. Care was not taken to cut through the membrane in layers of tissue that were under tension.

membrane incurs thermal damage, granulation tissue may develop but should resolve over several weeks with continued medical treatment.

Bistoury hook

The use of a curved bistoury hook to divide the entrapping fold has a similar success rate for the correction of the entrapment as a laser.[30] This technique may be performed by way of the oral or nasal cavity and in standing or anesthetized patients. Only an oral approach in an anesthetized patient may be performed without requiring endoscopic guidance.[31] These procedures do not require any other specialized equipment and, when done standing to avoid general anesthesia, can be cost-effective. Transnasal and transoral divisions are associated with re-entrapment rates of 5% to 15% and 10%, respectively.[33,36,41,43] Both approaches are associated with a postoperative rate of DDSP of approximately 10%.[29,36,43] Although not reported in the literature, there is anectodotal evidence of trauma to the tip of the epiglottis (because the tip cannot be visualized under the entrapping membrane). The tip is often rolled up caudally in entrapments when there is distortion of the normal shape preoperatively (**Fig. 5**).

Utilization of a transnasal approach in the standing horse has resulted in serious complications involving accidental division of the soft palate or laceration of the epiglottis and pharynx.[44,45] As a result, this procedure is not recommended by many clinicians. The likelihood of lacerating the soft palate can be reduced by performing the procedure with the horse anesthetized.[46]

A transoral approach replaces the possibility of inadvertent laceration of the soft palate with that of laceration of the oropharynx, tongue, and oral cavity.[38] Such lacerations did not occur in a small number of standing horses, and it was contended that if they were to occur, laceration of these structures would be of significantly less consequence compared with lacerations of the soft palate.[38] In the standing horse, damage

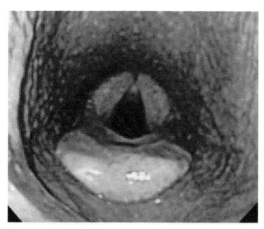

Fig. 5. The epiglottis is entrapped. The membrane is not thick or ulcerated, but more significant is that the epiglottis does not have the normal triangular appearance to the tip under
the membrane. It is deformed underneath the entrapping membrane.

to the endoscope could be a costly complication.[31] A transoral approach under general anesthesia is the alternative.[43] This option decreases the likelihood of inadvertent
laceration and removes any difficulty relating to the tractability of the horse during the
procedure. Of technical note for these oral procedures is the requirement of the surgeon's hand to reach the caudal aspect of the oral cavity. This may be problematic for
surgeons who have large hands (ie, glove size 8 or greater) and for horses that have
narrow oral cavities.[31]

Arytenoidectomy

Arytenoidectomy is performed most commonly for treatment of arytenoid chondropathy or less frequently for failed laryngoplasty. It is now well accepted that a partial arytenoidectomy is the preferred form of arytenoidectomy, with varying descriptions of
the technique and varying results.[18,47–51] Success rates in racehorses range from 60%
to 80%.[50,51] Experimental evidence shows that partial arytenoidectomy closely
restores most, but not all, respiratory mechanics to normal.[18,52]

Intraoperative complications are uncommon. The most likely complication is poor
visualization (due to limited light and hemorrhage) inhibiting the precision of the
surgery. Lighting can be enhanced by a headlamp and by light supplemented from
a videoendoscope placed within the orpharynx. Using the videoendoscope is also
advantageous because it provides a different, valuable view of the larynx that cannot
be appreciated through a laryngotomy. Hemorrhage can be minimized by using a contact laser technique to perform the initial mucosal incisions and by performing blunt
dissection of the muscle off the lateral side of the arytenoid.[51]

Postoperative complications are more common and will likely result in poor postoperative performance. Poor postoperative performance can be secondary to an inadequate airway and, to a lesser extent, some degree of lower airway inflammation from
dysphagia. The amount of lower airway inflammation has been reported in almost all
cases on a microscopic basis.[18] One report documented 36% of horses with evidence
of gross dysphagia (feed material at the nares).[47] Although there is not adequate experimental evidence to support this assertion, it should be presumed that the technique with which the arytenoidectomy is performed will have a major impact on the

ability of the horse to swallow appropriately and that minimizing the amount of damage to adjacent soft tissue will minimize the degree of dysphagia.

Preserving a mucosal flap for a partial primary closure when performing an arytenoidectomy is controversial. Previous reports have noted postoperative complications associated with hematoma under the mucosal flap, resulting in a severely restricted airway.[48] To avoid the complications of a narrowed airway in the immediate postoperative period, some investigators advocate not preserving a flap.[50] Although preserving a mucosal flap may increase the likelihood of postoperative complications, it can be performed successfully by experienced surgeons and appears to improve the percentage of horses that have improved performance.[51] Care taken to minimize hemorrhage intraoperatively and leaving the ventral edge of the flap open to drain if necessary minimize any fluid accumulation behind the mucosal flap.[51]

Another factor that could adversely affect the airway is the presence of intralaryngeal granulation tissue. Horses should be evaluated 30 to 45 days postoperatively, and any intralaryngeal granulation tissue may be removed by transendoscopic laser surgery at that time. Delay in removing any tissue that is present may result in a more cartilaginous mass that is difficult to remove at a later date. In one study in which a mucosal flap was employed, 17% of the horses had intralaryngeal granulation tissue that warranted laser resection.[51]

The final postoperative complication that should be considered is noise. In the one article commenting on noise in the postarytenoidectomy patient, abnormal noise was reported in most.[49] Given that the airway no longer has normal contour, even in the best-case scenario, it is not surprising that abnormal respiratory noise is present in the exercising horse. Clearly, when there is extraneous soft tissue that can dynamically deviate into the airway on inspiration, the noise will be worse, but it is possible that the horse can sound abnormal but still perform without significant airway obstruction.

SINUS SURGERY

Many complications associated with sinus surgery can be avoided or at least minimized by a thorough understanding of the anatomy and by good surgical planning. Too frequently, sinus surgery is approached as a seek and destroy mission that can result in much more extensive tissue damage than is required to achieve whatever the primary goal may have been. With improved diagnostic imaging and earlier intervention, a more precise surgical plan can be developed that minimizes the risk of complications. Complications can be divided into those associated with the surgical approach, general intraoperative complications, and those associated with the primary disease entity.

Surgical Approach

Although some sinus disease can be managed medically or with sinoscopy, much is still treated by frontonasal sinus flap osteotomy or maxillary flap osteotomy.[53] More recently, a modification to the frontonasal flap that is performed on the standing horse has been described.[54] Postoperative incisional drainage occurs in approximately 10% of all sinusotomies, and infrequently, a sequestrum can be found as the inciting factor at an edge of the osteotomy.[55] Considering that sinus surgery is often not a clean surgery, a low percentage of incisional drainage is not surprising. Close inspection of the osteotomy intraoperatively to remove any devascularized areas of bone can minimize the possibility of sequestrum development. When incisional drainage occurs, symptomatic treatment and the use of antimicrobials based on culture results are usually sufficient. More prolonged or unresponsive drainage can be better assessed by ultrasound and may require standing local surgical debridement for resolution of a focal septic osteitis.

Poor cosmetic outcomes can occur after sinusotomy. Suture periostitis is an uncommon postoperative development of large, firm swellings on the operated side and occasionally on the contralateral side not directly associated with the surgical incisions (**Fig. 6**). The swellings occur infrequently, are more associated with frontal bone approaches,[55] and are thought to be exuberant periosteal reactions at the junctions of the facial bone plates. In the acute phase, they can be mildly painful to palpation and result in obvious lacrimation from obstruction of the lacrimal ducts. Generally, these swellings resolve without treatment over several months.

Although some clinicians advocate discarding the bone of the sinusotomy flap, maintaining the bone of the flap generally results in an excellent cosmetic appearance. In a more recently described retrospective study in which a modified frontonasal flap was employed and the bone discarded, only 58% of the horses had a good cosmetic appearance, 29% had an appearance that was considered fair, and 13% had an appearance that was considered poor.[54] Sinocutaneous fistulas are extremely rare complications. Unrecognized trauma to the flap during the surgery can result in loss of vascular supply and subsequent necrosis of part or all of the flap. Care should be exercised to maintain contact between the bony flap, periosteum, and overlying soft tissues. Effective treatment is extremely difficult.

General Intraoperative Complications

Uncontrolled or large-volume hemorrhage is a serious complication that clinicians should be concerned about with sinus surgery. Although the intraoperative hemorrhage is unlikely to be so severe that it cannot be controlled, the loss could have a negative impact on visualization of the surgical field and on the anesthetic recovery. Poor recoveries could be associated with hypoxemia and low blood pressures. Monitoring blood loss during surgery and controlling fluid loading decrease the risk of recovery problems.

There is little in the literature regarding the volume of blood loss during surgery and the percentage of patients receiving transfusions. Furthermore, the degree with which

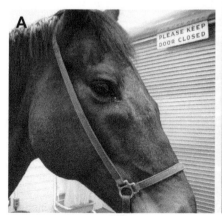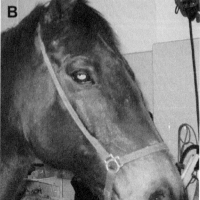

Fig. 6. (A) A horse that underwent a frontal sinusotomy several months earlier for treatment of a progressive ethmoid hematoma. The swellings developed without any signs of drainage or infection. (B) The same horse 6 months later without any treatment.

blood loss is monitored is extremely variable among hospitals, and the trigger point for transfusion is variable among anesthesiologists. Blood loss can be estimated by collecting the blood with a large bucket under the surgery table and by weighing the bucket to calculate the volume. The patient can then be treated accordingly. Hemorrhage associated with the surgical approach itself and the exploration of the sinuses is minimal. Care should be taken to not induce significant bleeding early in the surgical procedure because hemorrhage early in the surgical exploration can inhibit thorough exploration of the sinus and complete excision of the primary problem. It is only when the highly vascularized turbinate structures are disrupted that hemorrhage is severe, and thus any disruption of the turbinates should be left as the last part of the surgical procedure when possible. The use of phenylephrine in lavage solutions can decrease hemorrhage during surgery, and blood donors should be available if needed.

Complications associated with the packing can also occur. Packing the sinus and nasal passage after establishing a large fistula into the nasal passage and just prior to recovery is fairly routine. If the packing enters the nasal passage from a fistula in the caudal region, there is a possibility that the packing would be pushed too far caudally and ventrally through the fistula onto the soft palate and that it could loosen postoperatively. The packing would be mobilized by the horse's pharyngeal action to the point at which it could be swallowed into the esophagus (**Fig. 7**). Horses that are observed to be swallowing more than normal should have an endoscopic examination performed to determine whether they are swallowing unrecognized bleeding caudal to the packing or are attempting to swallow the packing itself. When part of the packing is in the esophagus, the entire packing can be removed nasally, or the packing can be grasped endoscopically and pulled out of the unpacked nostril and sutured in place for later complete removal. A temporary tracheostomy would be warranted to ensure an adequate airway. This complication can be easily prevented by using a sterile

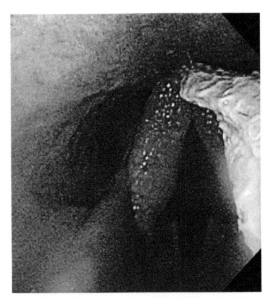

Fig. 7. Endoscopic view of the nasopharynx from the right nostril. The packing was placed within the left nasal passage at the end of a left sinus surgery and the packing is now within rostral esophagus above the larynx.

stockinette to act as a sleeve when the packing is performed.[56] The packing is placed within the stockinette, preventing independent loose loops from being dislodged.

Primary Disease

Probably the most common complication in the treatment of sinus disease is incomplete resolution of the primary problem being treated. Inadequate exposure or planning can result in inadequate debridement or extirpation and subsequent recurrence. A second surgery can be performed through the original site if necessary, but this increases the likelihood of incisional complications.

Treatment of primary sinusitis has one of the highest success rates (84%).[57] Early mild sinusitis can be effectively treated with antimicrobials with or without lavage, whereas more sustained sinusitis often has a thick abscesslike lining within the sinus that should be removed surgically to enhance resolution. A sinonasal fistula is often recommended to provide longer-term drainage and direct access to the sinus by way of endoscopy postoperatively. The need for this fistula, which can close prematurely, is questionable.[57] If it closes prematurely, it can be reopened by transendoscopic laser surgery; however, creating a large opening by removing the caudal aspect of the dorsal turbinate usually maintains access to the sinus and is unlikely to completely close (**Fig. 8**).

Paranasal sinus cysts also have a high success rate (82%–93%) for complete resolution.[55,57] Complete extirpation of the entire cyst lining is ideal, but a recent report suggests that it is not always necessary for resolution.[55] Although complete extirpation may not be necessary for resolution, a high percentage of horses without complete extirpation have prolonged or persistent nasal discharge.[55] This finding suggests that there is still a secretory lining present or that the structural changes in the nasal cavity are resulting in increased inflammatory conditions.

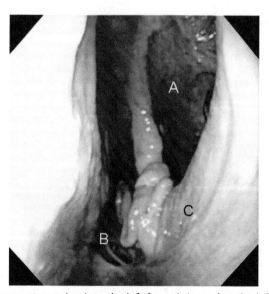

Fig. 8. A large permanent opening into the left frontal sinus after the left dorsal turbinate had been removed during a sinusotomy. (A) The opening. (B) The ethmoid recess. (C) The ventral turbinate.

Large masses, such as paranasal sinus cysts or neoplasia, can also result in significant facial deformity, nasal cavity deformity, or infraorbital nerve trauma. The superficial bony deformities often resolve with resolution of the primary disease process. Damage to the infraorbital canal within the sinus can result in a neuritis, in unilateral hypalgesia, and rarely in self-mutilation of the muzzle.[55,57] Although the hypalgesia may be present prior to surgery, the self-mutilation is more commonly a postoperative problem likely associated with surgical trauma to the nerve or increased inflammation around the nerve. Resolution of the inflammation within the sinus cavity can resolve the self-mutilation, and treatment with medication such as gabapentin can also be beneficial.

Progressive ethmoidal hematomas are common. There are multiple approaches to treatment, each with specific complications. The most common complication is recurrence or incomplete resolution (**Fig. 9**). The range of reported recurrence is wide partly

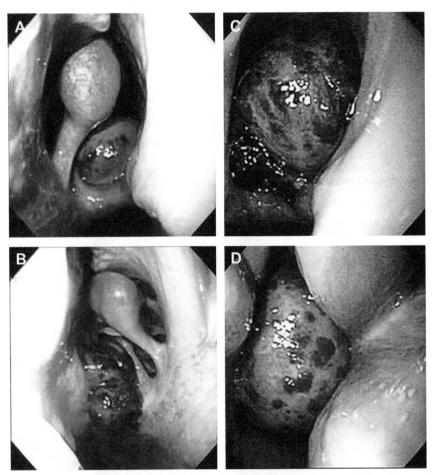

Fig. 9. (*A, B*) The ethmoid recess of the right and left nasal passage, respectively, with a small progressive ethmoid hematoma. (*C, D*) Endoscopic views of the same horse 3 years later, despite multiple treatments with intralesional formalin and no evidence of clinical signs for 3 years.

because of the different methods of follow-up evaluation.[58–60] Despite what has been reported, many clinicians believe that the true recurrence rate is much higher when horses are evaluated endoscopically and radiographically beyond just 1 or 2 years. Any horse prevented with small-volume epistaxis should be evaluated endoscopically and radiographically. It is common to have sinus involvement with endoscopically apparent nasal pathology. Concurrent treatment of both sites is warranted.

Intralesional formalin treatment for the nasal ethmoid hematomas is inexpensive, is minimally invasive, and can be very effective for the short duration. Serial treatments are required, with limited complications reported. Infrequently, with large hematomas that are injected within the nasal passage transendoscopically, there is an episode several days after treatment of moderate epistaxis from a small portion of the hematoma sloughing off. It is self-limiting and requires no treatment, but the owner should be warned of this possible occurrence. There has also been one report of brain damage from extension of the formalin into the cranial vault,[61] which necessitated euthanasia.

Surgical treatment entails laser ablation or mechanical debridement, most commonly under general anesthesia. Although not specifically reported, laser ablation can lead to adjacent thermal injury. Surgical debridement can result in incomplete excision or excessive intraoperative hemorrhage because of the extensive vascular bed at the origin of the lesion.

Treatment of sinus neoplasia has the highest (88%) rate of incomplete resolution or recurrence. There are infrequent cases of benign tumors that can be responsive to surgical debridement and to some adjunctive therapy, but biopsy should be considered for any presumed tumor before a sinusotomy is performed unless the owner wants to pursue treatment regardless of the prognosis.

INTERMITTENT DORSAL DISPLACEMENT OF THE SOFT PALATE

The number of different treatments for intermittent DDSP symbolizes the difficulty in diagnosis and treatment. Having an ineffective treatment is the most common complication. The ineffectiveness can be a result of incorrect diagnosis (and thus inappropriate treatment) or just the inherent difficulty in treating a dynamic, intermittent abnormality. Failure rates range from 10% to 50%.[35,62–68] It is not unusual for horses to undergo multiple surgeries for displacement of the soft palate because of the perceived continued poor performance after an initial surgery, even when a definitive diagnosis is not determined.

Laser palatoplasty and thermal cautery of the palate[63,65] are treatments aimed at increasing the stability of the caudal margin of the soft palate to prevent displacement by inducing fibrosis and collagen contracture. Although not published, there are anecdotal reports of excessive thermal injury resulting in fistula formation between the naso and orpharynx through the palate.

Staphylectomy is a surgical procedure that has been recommended for many years but is less commonly performed presently. Only a small margin of the free edge of the palate should be resected. A large resection can result in permanent dysphagia or aspiration and cannot be treated effectively.

The tie-forward procedure requires a larger surgical approach, leaving foreign material (suture) and requiring greater surgical manipulation of the larynx/hyoid, and not surprisingly, can have some complications. The rate of complications is less than 8%, and most cases do not require treatment.[64] Suture breakage or cartilage failure can return the larynx to its original position, and when this occurs, surgery can be repeated. An ultrasound examination is the most precise way to determine whether there is surgical failure. Incisional seroma is the most common complication and typically does not require treatment. Difficulty swallowing or swelling associated with the stylohyoid bones is extremely rare. Suture removal, reported in less than 1%, can be performed when management changes do not improve the condition of the patient.[64]

LASER SURGERY

Although incorporating the laser into upper respiratory surgery has brought great benefits, it has also brought another set of potential complications. In most situations, it obviates the need for a skin incision, yet the cost is working in a smaller area with fewer surgical instruments, which in turn creates greater difficulty in manipulating tissues, clearing any hemorrhage, and adversely affects visualization.

Almost uniformly, a diode or Nd:YAG laser is used transendoscopically. The wavelengths of these lasers can travel down a long optical fiber without attenuation of the energy. The fiber tip is sharp and can cut the lining of the biopsy channel of the videoendoscope, causing irreparable damage to the endoscope. Some type of small-diameter polyethelene tubing should be placed along the length of the biopsy channel to protect the inner lining, or a small piece of tubing should be placed over the tip of the fiber to pass through the endoscope and then removed after the fiber exits the channel.

Collateral thermal damage is the most common complication that can have a long-term effect on the surgical outcome. Treatment of collateral thermal damage consists of time and anti-inflammatory medications. This treatment may resolve the problem when there are minimal changes but may be incompletely effective with more severe problems. The best treatment is prevention. Prevention is best achieved by using the minimum energy needed to complete the procedure. Cutting effectiveness is improved the most by keeping the tissue under tension (one must ensure that the tissue being cut is under greater tension than the adjacent tissue) and by maintaining contact with the laser fiber.

Hemorrhage is the second most common complication. The laser decreases bleeding by coagulating smaller adjacent vessels but will not affect larger vessels. The bleeding is not so excessive that it requires treatment, but it can prohibit visualization and absorb laser energy, significantly decreasing the cutting capacity of the laser fiber. Hemorrhage can be stopped in most cases by applying the laser to the soft tissue around the vessel to create a diffusion of energy to the vessel and by compressing the vessel with the swelling of the apposing soft tissues.

TRACHEAL DISORDERS

Because surgery on the trachea is uncommon, little information exists about complications associated with tracheal surgery. Generally, it is believed that surgery on the trachea is limited because of the limited amount of soft tissue and the tension on the tissue. Surgical resection of tracheal rings can be performed successfully when necessary but should be limited to three rings.[69]

Tracheostomies for treatment of upper airway obstructions are the most common tracheal surgeries performed. They are easily performed in the standing horse and have limited complications. The most common complication is partial dehiscence of the stoma, which can occur in almost 10% of patients in the immediate postoperative period, but tracheostomy rarely (<3%) requires a revision surgery for stenosis or narrowing of the site to maintain a patent airway.[70]

Tracheal collapse is being diagnosed more commonly, and attempts to resolve the collapse have been approached using intraluminal and extraluminal stents.[71]

Extraluminal stenting can be successful and requires appropriate planning to ensure adequate prosthesis size before surgery. The primary complication is causing a recurrent laryngeal neuropathy because of the nerve's close association to the trachea, particularly at the thoracic inlet. This neuropathy is unlikely to resolve but, when unilateral, may be of no clinical consequence in a pet. Intraluminal stenting has been performed, but apparently has even more complications,[71] including stent migration and excessive growth of intraluminal granulation tissue, which in itself can be obstructive.

REFERENCES

1. Fleming G. Laryngismus paralytica ("roaring"). Vet J Ann Comp Pathol 1882;14: 1–12.
2. Cadiot PJ. Roaring in horses, its pathology and treatment. In: Cadiot PJ, Almy J, editors. A treatise on surgical therapeutics of domestic animals. London: Swan Somnnenschein & Co.; 1893. p. 15–78.
3. Marks D, Mackay-Smith M, Cushing L, et al. Use of a prosthetic device for surgical correction of laryngeal hemiplegia in horses. J Am Vet Med Assoc 1970; 157(2):157–63.
4. Goulden BE, Anderson LG. Equine laryngeal hemiplegia. III. Treatment by laryngoplasty. N Z Vet J 1982;30(1–2):1–5.
5. Kidd JA, Slone DE. Treatment of laryngeal hemiplegia in horses by prosthetic laryngoplasty, ventriculectomy and vocal cordectomy. Vet Rec 2002;150(15):481–4.
6. Russell AP, Slone DE. Performance analysis after prosthetic laryngoplasty and bilateral ventriculectomy for laryngeal hemiplegia in horses: 70 cases (1986–1991). J Am Vet Med Assoc 1994;204(8):1235–41.
7. Hawkins JF, Tulleners EP, Ross MW, et al. Laryngoplasty with or without ventriculectomy for treatment of left laryngeal hemiplegia in 230 racehorses. Vet Surg 1997;26(6):484–91.
8. Dixon RM, McGorum BC, Railton DI, et al. Long-term survey of laryngoplasty and ventriculocordectomy in an older, mixed-breed population of 200 horses. Part 1: maintenance of surgical arytenoid abduction and complications of surgery. Equine Vet J 2003;35(4):389–96 [erratum appears in Equine Vet J 2003 Sep;35(6):619].
9. Kraus BM, Parente EJ, Tulleners EP. Laryngoplasty with ventriculectomy or ventriculocordectomy in 104 draft horses (1992–2000). Vet Surg 2003;32(6):530–8.
10. Strand E, Martin GS, Haynes PF, et al. Career racing performance in Thoroughbreds treated with prosthetic laryngoplasty for laryngeal neuropathy: 52 cases (1981–1989). J Am Vet Med Assoc 2000;217(11):1689–96.
11. Davenport-Goodall CL, Parente EJ. Disorders of the larynx. Vet Clin North Am Equine Pract 2003;19(1):169–87.
12. Speirs VC, Bourke JM, Anderson GA. Assessment of the efficacy of an abductor muscle prosthesis for treatment of laryngeal hemiplegia in horses. Aust Vet J 1983;60(10):294–9.
13. Scherzer S, Hainisch EK. Evaluation of a canine cranial cruciate ligament repair system for use in equine laryngoplasty. Vet Surg 2005;34(6):548–53.
14. Bohanon TC, Beard WL, Robertson JT. Laryngeal hemiplegia in draft horses. A review of 27 cases. Vet Surg 1990;19(6):456–9.
15. McGorum BC. Laryngeal paralysis with known and suspected causes. In: McGorum BC, Dixon PM, Robinson NE, Schumacher J, editors. Equine respiratory medicine and surgery. Philadelphia: Elsevier; 2007. p. 479–82.

16. Abeele K, van den Steenhaut M, Martens A, et al. Results of laryngoplasty combined with ventriculectomy in equine laryngeal hemiplegia: a review of 105 cases. Vlaams Diergeneeskundig Tijdschrift 1997;66(6):298–302.

17. Ducharme NG, Hackett RP, Fubini SL, et al. The reliability of endoscopic examination in assessment of arytenoid cartilage movement in horses. Part II. Influence of side of examination, reexamination, and sedation. Vet Surg 1991;20(3):180–4.

18. Radcliffe CH, Woodie JB, Hackett RP, et al. A comparison of laryngoplasty and modified partial arytenoidectomy as treatments for laryngeal hemiplegia in exercising horses. Vet Surg 2006;35(7):643–52.

19. Davenport CL, Tulleners EP, Parente EJ. The effect of recurrent laryngeal neurectomy in conjunction with laryngoplasty and unilateral ventriculocordectomy in Thoroughbred racehorses. Vet Surg 2001;30(5):417–21.

20. Greet TR, Baker GJ, Lee R. The effect of laryngoplasty on pharyngeal function in the horse. Equine Vet J 1979;11(3):153–8.

21. Dixon PM, McGorum BC, Railton DI, et al. Long-term survey of laryngoplasty and ventriculocordectomy in an older, mixed-breed population of 200 horses. Part 2: owners' assessment of the value of surgery. Equine Vet J 2003;35(4):397–401.

22. Nameth F. Technique and results of the surgical treatment of roaring in 398 horses, using a modified Mackay-Smith method. Pferdeheilkunde 1987;3(1): 27–31.

23. Ducharme NG, Hackett RP. The value of surgical treatment of laryngeal hemiplegia in horses. Compend Contin Educ Pract Vet 1991;13(3):473–5.

24. Dean PW, Nelson JK, Schumacher J. Effects of age and prosthesis material on in vitro cartilage retention of laryngoplasty prostheses in horses. Am J Vet Res 1990; 51(1):114–7.

25. Behrens E, Poteet B, Cohen N. Equine cricoid cartilage densitometry. Can J Vet Res 1993;57(4):307–8.

26. Schumacher J, Wilson AM, Pardoe C, et al. In vitro evaluation of a novel prosthesis for laryngoplasty of horses with recurrent laryngeal neuropathy. Equine Vet J 2000;32(1):43–6.

27. Brown JA, Derksen FJ, Stick JA, et al. Laser vocal cordectomy fails to effectively reduce respiratory noise in horses with laryngeal hemiplegia. Vet Surg 2005; 34(3):247–52.

28. Boles C, Raker C, Wheat J. Epiglottic entrapment by arytenoepiglottic folds in the horse. J Am Vet Med Assoc 1978;172:338–42.

29. Lumsden J, Stick J, Caron J, et al. Surgical treatment for epiglottic entrapment in horses: 51 cases (1981–1992). J Am Vet Med Assoc 1994;205:729–35.

30. Beard W, Waxman S. Evidence-based equine upper respiratory surgery. Vet Clin North Am Equine Pract 2007;23:229–42.

31. Russell T, Wainscott M. Treatment in the field of 27 horses with epiglottic entrapment. Vet Rec 2007;161:187–9.

32. Auer J, Stick J. Equine surgery. 3rd edition. Philadelphia: Saunders Elsevier; 2006.

33. Honnas C, Wheat J. Epiglottic entrapment. A transnasal surgical approach to divide the aryepiglottic fold axially in the standing horse. Vet Surg 1988;17:246–51.

34. Williams J, Meagher D, Pascoe J, et al. Upper airway function during maximal exercise in horses with obstructive upper airway lesions. Effect of surgical treatment. Vet Surg 1990;19:142–7.

35. Parente E, Martin B, Tulleners E, et al. Dorsal displacement of the soft palate in 92 horses during high-speed treadmill examination (1993–1998). Vet Surg 2002;31:507–12.

36. Greet T. Experiences in treatment of epiglottal entrapment using a hook knife per nasum. Equine Vet J 1995;27:122–6.

37. Martin BJ, Reef V, Parente E, et al. Causes of poor performance of horses during training, racing, or showing: 348 cases (1992–1996). J Am Vet Med Assoc 2000; 216:554–8.
38. Perkins J, Hughes T, Brain B. Endoscope-guided, transoral axial division of an entrapping epiglottic fold in fifteen standing horses. Vet Surg 2007;36:800–3.
39. Raphel C. Endoscopic findings in the upper respiratory tract of 479 horses. J Am Vet Med Assoc 1982;181:470–3.
40. Brown J, Hinchcliff K, Jackson M, et al. Prevalence of pharyngeal and laryngeal abnormalities in Thoroughbreds racing in Australia, and their association with performance. Equine Vet J 2005;37:397–401.
41. Jann H, Cook W. Transendoscopic electrosurgery for epiglottal entrapment in the horse. J Am Vet Med Assoc 1985;187:484–92.
42. Tulleners E. Transendoscopic contact neodymium:yttrium aluminum garnet laser correction of epiglottic entrapment in standing horses. J Am Vet Med Assoc 1990; 196:1971–80.
43. Ross M, Gentile D, Evans L. Transoral axial division, under endoscopic guidance, for correction of epiglottic entrapment in horses. J Am Vet Med Assoc 1993;203: 416–20.
44. Holcombe S, Robertson J, Richardson L. Surgical repair of iatrogenic soft palate defects in two horses. J Am Vet Med Assoc 1994;205:1315–7.
45. Epstein K, Parente E. Epiglottic fold entrapment. In: McGorum B, Dixon P, Robinson N, et al, editors. Equine respiratory medicine and surgery. Philadelphia: Saunders Elsevier; 2007. p. 459–67.
46. Mee A, Cripps P, Jones R. A retrospective study of mortality associated with general anaesthesia in horses: elective procedures. Vet Rec 1998;142:275–6.
47. Speirs VC. Partial arytenoidectomy in horses. Vet Surg 1986;15:316–20.
48. Dean PW, Cohen ND. Arytenoidectomy for advanced unilateral chondropathy with accompanying lesions. Vet Surg 1990;19:364–70.
49. Tulleners EP, Harrison IW, Raker CW. Management of arytenoid chondropathy and failed laryngoplasty in horses: 75 cases (1979–1985). J Am Vet Med Assoc 1988;192:670–5.
50. Barnes AJ, Slone DE, Lynch TM. Performance after partial arytenoidectomy without mucosal closure in 27 Thoroughbred racehorses. Vet Surg 2004;33:398–403.
51. Parente EJ, Tulleners EP, Southwood LL. Long-term study of partial arytenoidectomy with primary mucosal closure in 76 thoroughbred racehorses (1992–2006). Equine Vet J 2008;40(3):214–8.
52. Lumsden JM, Derksen FJ, Stick JA, et al. Evaluation of partial arytenoidectomy as a treatment for equine laryngeal hemiplegia. Equine Vet J 1994;26:125–9.
53. Freeman DE, Orsini PG, Ross MW, et al. A large frontonasal bone flap for sinus surgery in the horse. Vet Surg 1990;19(2):122–30.
54. Quinn GC, Kidd JA, Lane JG. Modified frontonasal sinus flap surgery in standing horses: surgical findings and outcomes of 60 cases. UK Equine Vet J 2005;37(2): 138–42.
55. Woodford NS, Lane JG. Long-term retrospective study of 52 horses with sinunasal cysts. Equine Vet J 2006;38(3):198–202.
56. Freeman DE. Sinus disease (respiratory disease). Vet Clin North Am Equine Pract 2003;19(1):209–43.
57. Tremaine WH, Dixon PM. A long-term study of 277 cases of equine sinonasal disease. Part 2: treatments and results of treatments. UK Equine Vet J 2001;33(3):283–9.
58. Bell B, Baker GJ, Foreman JH. Progressive ethmoid hematoma: characteristics, cause, and treatment. Compend Contin Educ Pract Vet 1993;15(10):1391–8.

59. Specht TE, Colahan PT, Nixon AJ, et al. Ethmoidal hematoma in nine horses. J Am Vet Med Assoc 1990;197(5):613–6.

60. Rothaug PG, Tulleners EP. Neodymium:yttrium-aluminum-garnet laser-assisted excision of progressive ethmoid hematomas in horses: 20 cases (1986–1996). J Am Vet Med Assoc 1999;214(7):1037–41.

61. Frees KE, Gaughan EM, Lillich JD, et al. Severe complication after administration of formalin for treatment of progressive ethmoidal hematoma in a horse. J Am Vet Med Assoc 2001;219(7):950–2.

62. Anderson JD, Tulleners EP, Johnston JK, et al. Sternothyrohyoideus myectomy or staphylectomy for treatment of intermittent dorsal displacement of the soft palate in racehorses: 209 cases (1986–1991). J Am Vet Med Assoc 1995;206:1909–12.

63. Hogan PM, Palmer SE, Congelosi M. Transendoscopic laser cauterization of the soft palate as an adjunctive treatment for dorsal displacement in the racehorse. Proc Am Assoc Equine Pract 2002;48:228–30.

64. Woodie JB, Ducharme NG, Kanter P, et al. Surgical advancement of the larynx (laryngeal tie-forward) as a treatment for dorsal displacement of the soft palate in horses: a prospective study 2001–2004. UK Equine Vet J 2005;37(5):418–23.

65. Smith JJ, Embertson RM. Sternothyroideus myotomy, staphylectomy, and oral caudal soft palate photothermoplasty for treatment of dorsal displacement of the soft palate in 102 Thoroughbred racehorses. Vet Surg 2005;34(1):5–10.

66. Barakzai SZ, Johnson VS, Baird DH, et al. The efficacy of composite surgery for treatment of dorsal displacement of the soft palate in 53 racing Thoroughbreds. Equine Vet J 2003;36:175–9.

67. Reardon R, Fraser B, Heller J, et al. The use of race winnings, ratings and a performance index to assess the effect of thermocautery of the soft palate for treatment of horses with suspected intermittent dorsal displacement. A case-control study in 110 racing Thoroughbreds. UK Equine Vet J 2008;40(5):508–13.

68. Cheetham J, Pigott JH, Thorson LM, et al. Racing performance following the laryngeal tie-forward procedure: a case-controlled study. UK Equine Vet J 2008; 40(5):501–7.

69. Tate Jr. LP, Koch DB, Sembrat RF, et-al. Tracheal reconstruction by resection and end-to-end anastomoses in the horse. J Am Vet Med Assoc 1981;178:253–8.

70. Chesen AB, Rakestraw PC. Indications for and short- and long-term outcome of permanent tracheostomy performed in standing horses: 82 cases (1995–2005). J Am Vet Med Assoc 2008;232(9):1352–6.

71. Wong DM, Sponseller BA, Riedesel EA, et al. The use of intraluminal stents for tracheal collapse in two horses: case management and long-term treatment. Equine Vet Ed 2008;20(2):80–90.

Complications of Surgery for Diseases of the Guttural Pouch

David E. Freeman, MVB, PhD

KEYWORDS

• Guttural pouch • Horse • Mycosis • Tympany
• Empyema • Complications • Surgery

Guttural pouch diseases pose serious challenges in diagnosis and treatment. Complications from treatment are common and often life-threatening, largely because the unique anatomy of the guttural pouches brings them into intimate contact with the nervous, respiratory, and cardiovascular systems. There is little forgiveness for surgical errors, and so the surgeon should focus on ways to anticipate and prevent them. As with any disease, errors in diagnosis can set the stage for many surgical errors and must be recognized. Failure to produce a successful outcome after surgical treatment is as common with many guttural pouch diseases as with any other equine diseases, if not more so. The clinical signs, diagnostic procedures, and treatments for diseases of the guttural pouch have been covered elsewhere[1] and are beyond the scope of this article. This article deals with errors that can be expected after the most common surgical treatments for guttural pouch diseases.

GUTTURAL POUCH EMPYEMA

Response to medical treatment of empyema is usually satisfactory, but if it fails or if the purulent material becomes inspissated or forms chondroids, surgical drainage of the guttural pouch should be considered. In a study of 91 horses with guttural pouch empyema, 21% had chondroids, and horses with chondroids were more likely to have retropharyngeal and pharyngeal swelling than horses without this complication.[2] To avoid surgery, chondroids can be removed by maceration, repeated section of each mass by diathermic snare (Olympus Optical Co, Irving, Texas) or a wire loop, extraction by endoscopically guided grabbing forceps, a basket snare (Gomco Equipment, Chemetron Medical Products, Buffalo, New York), or a polyp retrieval basket (Cook Ltd, Bloomington, Indiana), followed by saline lavage.[1,3] Although these methods can yield a 44% success rate,[2] they can be time consuming. Special care must be taken to avoid overly aggressive lavage for removal of chondroids and inspissated

Department of Large Animal Clinical Sciences, College of Veterinary Medicine, University of Florida, Box 100136, Gainesville, FL 32610-0136, USA
E-mail address: freemand@vetmed.ufl.edu

Vet Clin Equine 24 (2009) 485–497
doi:10.1016/j.cveq.2008.10.003
0749-0739/08/$ – see front matter © 2009 Elsevier Inc. All rights reserved.
vetequine.theclinics.com

pus, because the pressure generated can rupture the guttural pouch at a point of weakness from inflammation and force septic contents into caudal tissue planes.[4] A standing surgical procedure through a modified Whitehouse approach also has been used successfully to remove chondroids and could be an alternative if the costs or risks of anesthesia are not acceptable.[5] If empyema is the result of occlusion of guttural pouch openings by adhesions, it can be treated by blunt division through a surgical approach to the guttural pouch[6] or by using a laser to establish a permanent pharyngeal fistula into the guttural pouch.[7]

Complications

Surgical approaches to the guttural pouches include hyovertebrotomy, Viborg's triangle, Whitehouse, and modified Whitehouse, all of which are fraught with the risk of nerve damage.[1] To avoid nerve damage during dissection, the guttural pouch lining is exposed beneath a covering of areolar tissue and punctured with the closed tips of scissors or a hemostat. This opening is enlarged by spreading its edges with a hemostat or fingers. With the Viborg's triangle approach, care must be taken to avoid the parotid duct superficially and branches of the vagus nerve along the floor of the guttural pouch. The guttural pouch is opened medial to the stylohyoid bone through the standard and modified Whitehouse approaches, and care must be taken to avoid the pharyngeal branch of the vagus nerve and the cranial laryngeal nerve, which are close to the incision.

Surgery of the guttural pouch through any approach should be a last resort because of risks of permanent dysphagia and other neurologic signs. These signs usually arise from damage to the vagus, particularly the pharyngeal branch, and the glossopharyngeal nerves. Identification of the guttural pouch lining and underlying nerves is difficult, especially in cases in which there is no distention, but it can be facilitated by a lighted endoscope inserted into the medial compartment. Mucosal inflammation complicates identification of normal anatomy, however. A fixed structure, such as the stylohyoid bone, should be used as a guide for deep dissection. The mucosa should not be incised with sharp instruments, and retractors should be applied with care to avoid nerve damage. Because all approaches enter the pouch cavity in the same approximate area, confined between rigid structures, none offers a clear-cut method of avoiding risk of nerve damage (**Figs. 1** and **2**).

GUTTURAL POUCH TYMPANY

Temporary alleviation of guttural pouch tympany can be achieved by needle decompression or an indwelling catheter, but surgery is required for definitive treatment. Temporary measures could delay surgery and predispose to empyema, bronchopneumonia,[8] and scarring in the cartilage of the pharyngeal ostium.[9] The affected guttural pouch is usually entered through Viborg's triangle or through a modified Whitehouse approach, and the median septum is fenestrated to allow egress of trapped air from the tympanitic pouch through the normal side. Alternatively, transendoscopic electrocautery can be used to create a fenestration in the septum or make a fistula into the guttural pouch through the pharyngeal recess or in the wall of the pharynx, caudal to the guttural pouch opening.[10,11] When bilateral involvement is suspected, the fenestration procedure can be combined with removal of a small segment (1.5 × 2.5 cm) of the medial lamina of the eustachian tube and associated mucosal fold of the plica salpingopharyngea. Bilateral partial resection of the caudal extent of the plica salpingopharyngea and fenestration of the median septum can be performed with laparoscopic instruments to reduce the risk of nerve damage.[8]

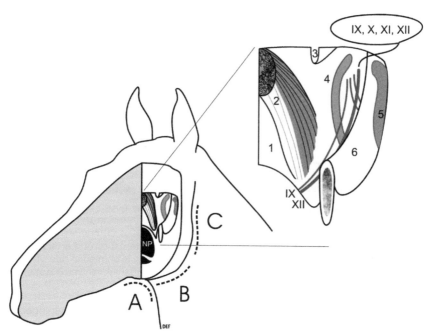

Fig.1. Anatomy of the interior of the left guttural pouch to demonstrate that the three standard approaches—Whitehouse, modified and regular (*A*), Viborg's triangle (*B*), and hyovertebrotomy (*C*)—approach from different sites but eventually must enter a confined part of the floor of the medial compartment between the stylohyoid bone (6) and the ventral straight muscles (2). The ICA and sympathetic trunk (4) and cranial nerves IX to XII and their branches are located in that confined area. 1, median septum; 3, cartilaginous part of the eustachian tube; 5, external carotid artery and maxillary artery; NP = nasopharynx.

Complications

The prognosis for full recovery after surgery for tympany is good,[12] even in foals with secondary empyema and pneumonia; however, nerve damage secondary to surgery can cause dysphagia, aspiration pneumonia, and death.[13] Although any surgical approach to the guttural pouch involves difficult and deep dissection between crucial nerves and vessels, the tympanitic pouch is easier to enter because the distended pouch lining is usually in a subcutaneous position and the nerves are more obvious than normal or have been displaced from the line of access. Chronic inflammation of the mucosa can prevent nerve identification, however, even if the interior is well illuminated with the endoscope.

Surgery for guttural pouch tympany needs to be repeated in some cases because of failure of the first procedure, and owners should be forewarned. In a report on standing laser surgery with sedation in 50 foals, 35 foals (70%) required only one surgery. A second operation was required in 7 foals during the initial hospitalization, and a second operation was performed during a second hospitalization in 8 foals.[12] Six of 7 foals that needed a second surgery were treated initially by combined fenestration of the median septum and resection of parts of the plica salpingopharyngea.[12] A repeat of the first surgery was successful in most of the foals that needed a second surgery.

The fenestration procedure can fail if the disease is bilateral, if the fenestration seals, or if the mucosal membrane was inadvertently removed from one side and the other

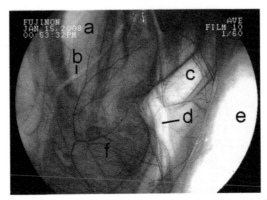

Fig. 2. Endoscopic anatomy of the interior of the left guttural pouch demonstrates structures on the floor of the guttural pouch that can be encountered in the approaches described in **Fig. 1**. Structures between the ventral straight muscles (a) and stylohyoid bone (not visible) are pharyngeal branch of the vagus nerve (b), external carotid artery (c), glossopharyngeal and hypoglossal nerves (d), stylopharyngeus muscle on medial side of the stylohyoid bone (e), and floor of the guttural pouch with retropharyngeal lymph nodes (f).

was left intact.[1,13,14] Resection of the mucosal fold of the plica salpingopharyngea can fail to relieve tympany if swelling and inflammation occur along the mucosal incision close to the pharyngeal orifice.[15] The salpingopharyngeal fistula can seal if the Foley catheter does not stay in place for the period required for the fistula to mature, if the fistula is created within the defective part of the pharyngeal ostium, or if the fistula is occluded by inflammation.[8,11,14]

Inaccurate distinction between unilateral and bilateral involvement is one possible cause of surgical failure. Radiographs are often misleading, and temporary decompression of the "apparently most distended pouch" is unlikely to cause the complete collapse that would be expected in unilateral cases. Based on most reports,[8,12,13,15] recurrence or complications can be expected in horses in which the initial surgery involved enlarging the pharyngeal ostium on the affected side. The effects of a salpingopharyngeal fistula on airway dynamics in racehorses are unknown or not established. Fenestration of the median septum should be the first and only surgery attempted in foals that lack strong clinical evidence of bilateral involvement. Although this approach fails if the condition is bilateral, it can be justified by its simplicity and the finding that even more aggressive approaches can require a second surgery.[8,12,13]

GUTTURAL POUCH MYCOSIS

Approximately 50% of horses with hemorrhage from guttural pouch mycosis die from this complication,[16] so vascular occlusion procedures become critical for management of this disease.[1] These procedures must be performed as soon as possible after the first bout of hemorrhage to prevent subsequent bouts that could render the horse a poor candidate for anesthesia and surgery. Delays in diagnosis or treatment can have fatal consequences, and affected horses should be treated as emergency cases. Although endoscopy is critical to making the diagnosis, a presumptive diagnosis can be made on the basis of the severity of spontaneous hemorrhage, especially if accompanied by neurologic signs referable to the cranial nerves and vagosympathetic trunk within the guttural pouch.[1]

Surgical treatment of guttural pouch mycosis should be directed at occlusion of the affected artery, as determined by endoscopy or arteriography. Accurate identification is not always possible, unless the lesion is discrete and situated on one artery only. If the lesion is extensive and overlies the internal and the external carotid arteries and branches of the latter, then both vessels are occluded. The artery most frequently eroded in guttural pouch mycosis is the internal carotid artery (ICA).

Complications: Ligation Procedures

A single ligature close to the origin of the ICA is sufficient to prevent fatal hemorrhage in most cases,[17] apparently because of gradual thrombosis of the stagnant column of blood distal to the ligature. Fatal or severe hemorrhage after proximal ligation of the ICA has been reported and can be attributed to retrograde flow from the cerebral arterial circle (circle of Willis) or ligation of the wrong vessel or an aberrant branch. Ligation of the ICA reduces flow to 19% of control values[18] but does not drop blood pressure distal to a ligature, so the ligature may not immediately prevent fatal hemorrhage.[19] Ligation distal to the site of arterial erosion is difficult and likely to damage the sympathetic nerve trunk.[20] Ligation of the ipsilateral common carotid artery in a horse bleeding from the ICA would increase flow in the affected artery and would be contraindicated; however, the same procedure might be of benefit in horses bleeding from the external carotid artery and its branches.[18] Although ligation of the major palatine artery could prevent retrograde flow, a combination of this procedure with occlusion of the external carotid artery and ICA can cause ischemic optic neuropathy and permanent blindness.[21]

Complications: Balloon-Tipped Catheters

The purpose of the balloon catheter technique is to allow immediate intravascular occlusion of the affected artery in the guttural pouch and prevent retrograde flow through the vascular defect. The ICA and the external carotid artery and branches are prone to persistent postoperative hemorrhage through retrograde flow. Complications of these methods have been reported and related to different aspects of the surgery and postoperative period, however.

Approach
The approach to the ICA involves dissection through fascia attaching the wing of the fascia to the parotid salivary gland, where it is possible to damage lobes of the parotid gland and cause some postoperative leakage of saliva. Large veins within the parotid gland are difficult to see and can be cut. The approach to the major palatine artery (for occlusion of retrograde flow to the external carotid artery and its branches) approximately 1 to 2 cm medial to the edge of the interalveolar space is difficult, and hemorrhage from the plexus of vessels in the palatine mucosa can prevent accurate identification of the artery. This artery is also small, and spasm induced by handling tends to reduce its size further. Careful and patient dissection close to the bony surface of the palate should be fruitful, and hemorrhage is rarely more than a constant oozing that can be controlled by pressure, clamping with hemostats, and electrocautery.

Errors in identification
It may be difficult to distinguish between the occipital and ICAs in some horses, especially horses with a thick throatlatch and horses in which both arteries arise as a single trunk and bifurcate at a variable distance from the common carotid artery. If both arteries arise in the normal fashion, the recommended method for identification is to dissect them both free and then elevate each one gently with umbilical tape or

a Penrose drain. It should be possible to demonstrate that the ICA lies deep to the occipital artery and that it courses more rostrally.

Aberrant branches

Aberrant branches of the ICA can complicate this surgery by causing brainstem lesions[22] or fatal hemorrhage by allowing retrograde flow to the eroded segment.[23] As much ICA as possible should be exposed by careful dissection toward the roof of the guttural pouch (approximately 6 cm), in the hope that any aberrant branch can be found and ligated.[23] Ligation of an accessible aberrant branch should prevent the catheter from entering it. The most troublesome aberration is an ICA that leads to the caudal cerebellar artery without following its usual pathway and places the inflated balloon in a position that causes brainstem neuronal necrosis.[22] If a catheter cannot be inserted to the required distance or passes beyond the 13-cm mark before it becomes arrested, then it is probably in an aberrant branch.

Catheterization of the affected artery should be monitored endoscopically to ensure that it is in the correct artery, although this can be difficult if landmarks are obscured by blood or the lesion. The catheter tip should be visible as it passes up the artery, and the balloon can be inflated at intervals to demonstrate its position. It does not distend the artery as dramatically as one would like, however, which can make it difficult to locate. Fluoroscopy is the method of choice to define aberrant branches and confirm occlusion of affected branches, but it is not always readily available in many hospitals.

Arterial penetration

On occasion, as the catheter is being inserted in the ICA, it penetrates the defect in the artery and enters the guttural pouch. Resistance to passage is lost as this happens, and a long segment of catheter can be advanced with ease. Fortunately, this mishap is rare, and when it occurs, it rarely triggers bleeding. Endoscopy of the pouch should help diagnose this complication. A 6-Fr venous thrombectomy catheter (Fogarty-Edwards Laboratories, Edwards Lifesciences, Irvine, California) is recommended to prevent this complication because it has a soft flexible tip that facilitates difficult negotiation through the bend on the roof of the guttural pouch and through the first bend in the sigmoid of the ICA. It also reduces the risk of arterial perforation at the defect eroded in the wall. On the other hand, the 6-Fr arterial embolectomy catheter, with its shorter and more rigid tip, is more likely to penetrate the arterial defect than the venous thrombectomy catheter.

A catheter that has penetrated the arterial defect can be redirected in several ways. One is to withdraw the catheter and re-advance it as often as needed while rotating the catheter to take advantage of any curvature in its shaft that would direct it away from the hole. If this approach fails, the balloon is inflated with saline, the catheter is withdrawn to snug the inflated balloon against the hole in the artery, and another catheter is passed alongside the first. With the hole blocked in this way, the second catheter should advance easily beyond this level. The first catheter can be removed and the second one advanced fully. If a second catheter is not available, the first one is left in but with the balloon inflated and snugged securely against the edges of the arterial defect to occlude and collapse the artery at this level. Another approach, which is more invasive, is to open the guttural pouch through a hyovertebrotomy and digitally block the hole in the artery as the catheter is passed to and beyond it. Regardless of the method of correction, any catheter placed after arterial penetration should be regarded as contaminated and be removed at or after 7 days.

Incisional infection

The most common complication of balloon catheter surgery is incisional infection that requires catheter removal and incisional drainage. With a catheter in the ICA, the shaft spans the mycotic plaque and bacteria can track from this to the incision. Infection is most likely if the distal arterial pressure displaces the balloon into the infected segment of artery, and such displacement should be prevented by using a fairly rigid catheter and inflating the balloon to its maximum diameter. With a catheter in the major palatine artery, the arteriotomy is performed through the oral mucosa, which could be a source of contamination. Because of this possibility and because the catheter cannot be protected by burying it at this site, it should be removed after approximately 7 days.

Catheter dislodgement
Blood pressure in the distal segment of ICA can force the inflated balloon to back into the infected segment. Such displacement and even delayed prolapse through the hole in the artery into the guttural pouch could favor development of incisional infection (see previous discussion). Hemorrhage is possible but rare after displacement. Catheters in the major palatine artery and transverse facial artery cannot be buried and are sufficiently exposed to get hooked on fixed objects and become prematurely extracted.

Balloon complications
Premature balloon deflation can be caused by inflating it with too much air, because air diffuses out of the balloon over time. Before the catheter is inserted, it should be primed beforehand with saline and filled and aspirated repeatedly with saline while the catheter tip is held below the syringe plunger. The needle should be left attached to the catheter until insertion is completed to prevent air ingress. Because the catheter is inserted into the ICA through a small arteriotomy in a confined space in the incision, a thumb forceps can be used to feed the tip of the catheter into the artery. This should be applied to the catheter body if possible and not to the balloon so the latter is not traumatized in any way or it will weaken and rupture. Despite the previously mentioned concerns about premature balloon deflation, a balloon of the size used should fill the artery sufficiently to induce thrombosis around it and rapid luminal occlusion. Despite the temptation to fill the balloon with a radiopaque compound so that it can be demonstrated radiographically in the artery, this is not recommended. Contrast materials tend to become inspissated within the balloon so that subsequent balloon deflation and catheter removal can be difficult or impossible.

Blindness
Blindness has not been reported after balloon catheter occlusion of the ICA only, although severe hemorrhage alone can cause blindness. Blindness has been reported after ligation of the external carotid artery and ICA,[24] although this might not be a consistent complication when these ligations are combined.[24] Balloon catheter occlusion of the maxillary artery does not cause blindness, even when combined with occlusion of the ICA.[25] By contrast, combined ligation of the external carotid and major palatine arteries can cause blindness when combined with ICA occlusion.[21] Blindness under these conditions can be attributed to the "steal phenomenon" (**Fig. 3**). The conditions for the steal phenomenon are met when a major artery is occluded and blood is diverted by backflow from collateral channels into the segment distal to the occlusion.[26] Owners should be warned of the possibility of unilateral blindness after any ligation technique for occlusion of the external carotid artery and its branches that pass within the guttural pouch.

Failure of surgery
The balloon-tipped catheter techniques should prevent hemorrhage in all horses in which they are used, provided that the balloon is placed in the desired location in

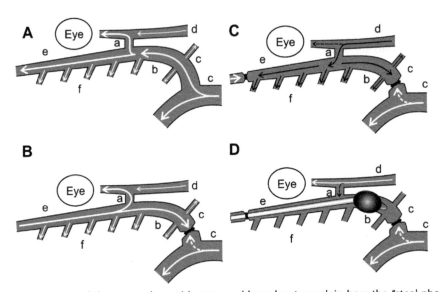

Fig. 3. Anatomy of the external carotid artery and branches to explain how the "steal phenomenon" can cause blindness after certain ligation procedures. (*A*) The major blood supply to the horse's eye is through the external ophthalmic artery (a), which originates from the maxillary artery (b), the direct continuation of the external carotid artery (c). The external ophthalmic artery anastomoses inconsistently with the internal ophthalmic artery (d), which is a branch from the ICA. The maxillary artery is continued as the major palatine artery (e), which is its largest terminal branch and joins with the same artery from the other side to form an arterial loop around the upper jaw. Branches (f) from the major palatine artery supply parts of the upper jaw. (*B*) When the external carotid artery is ligated, presumably the internal ophthalmic artery (from the arterial circle), other vessels, and retrograde flow through the external ophthalmic artery provide blood to the eye. Regardless of source, however, collateral flow to the eye might not be sufficient to prevent blindness under these conditions.[24] (*C*) If the major palatine artery and external carotid artery are ligated simultaneously, the potential for retrograde flow from the major palatine artery to the external ophthalmic artery is interrupted. Of greater importance, blood flowing into the external ophthalmic artery from remaining collateral sources can then drain into the maxillary and major palatine arteries (*black arrows*), if the reduced flow drops pressure sufficiently in these vessels to allow such backflow. These are substantial vessels, with large subsidiary arterial systems, and could drain off or "steal" a considerable amount of collateral flow from the external ophthalmic artery (*short black arrows*). (*D*) Ischemia and blindness follow. With a balloon catheter in the major palatine artery, the maxillary artery is fully occluded by the catheter shaft at the origin of the external ophthalmic artery so that a steal phenomenon is prevented (*broken black arrow*). As a result, all or most of blood flow from collateral channels that enter the external ophthalmic artery flows to the eye. Presumably subsidiary branches from the maxillary and major palatine arteries (f) receive blood flow from other sources after this procedure. Simultaneous occlusion of the ICA does not seem to increase the risk of blindness with this procedure, presumably because collateral channels through the contralateral ICA and other routes to the eye are sufficient.

the diseased artery. Without fluoroscopic guidance, such placement is achieved blindly, so that fatal hemorrhage can arise from failure to occlude the affected segment of ICA because the catheter was misdirected into an aberrant branch.[23] Many horses continue to have mild epistaxis after surgery, which is caused by continuous drainage of pooled blood from the guttural pouch, not from continued bleeding. Included as a measure of success with this procedure is resolution of the mycotic lesion caused by the arrest of blood flow through the affected segment;[27] however, this is questionable based on the author's experience.[28]

Newer Embolization Techniques

A detachable, self-sealing, latex balloon can effectively occlude the ICA[29] without the need for catheter removal, as sometimes is required with the nondetachable balloons. Combined with angiography, the detachable system also can be used to occlude aberrant vessels that originate at a distance from the origin of the ICA.[30] This procedure eliminates the need to protect redundant ends of catheters, which is necessary when nondetachable balloons are used.

A transarterial coil embolization technique can selectively occlude the arterial segments involved in a mycotic lesion in horses with guttural pouch mycosis.[31] The coil embolization technique combines angiographic studies to image and selectively embolize the affected vessels while identifying any aberrant branches or unusual vessels and sites of bleeding.[31] It is also less invasive than the original balloon catheter procedures and requires shorter anesthesia and shorter hospitalization. The surgical approach for coil embolization of all arteries in the guttural pouch is the common carotid artery exposed through a single incision (**Fig. 4**).

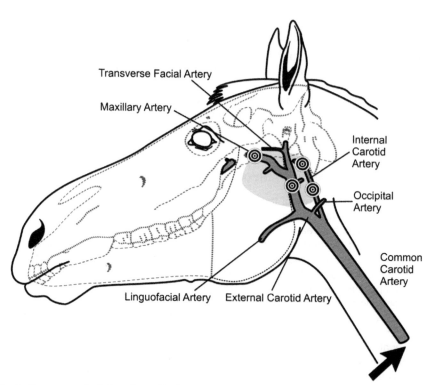

Fig. 4. Recommended sites for coil placement in the ICA and external carotid artery and branches. The arteriotomy is made in the common carotid artery for catheterization and delivery of all coils (*arrow*).

Approach

Exposure of the surgeon's hands to radiation during fluoroscopy is avoided by using the recommended distal location of the catheterization site on the common carotid artery.[31] Misdirection of the angiography catheter into the cranial thyroid artery during insertion is avoidable and can be corrected by withdrawing the catheter slightly and repositioning it into the common carotid artery under fluoroscopic guidance.[31] To prevent hematoma formation in the carotid sheath after catheter removal, the carotid arteriotomy should be closed with 5-0 silk or similar material.[31]

Air or clot embolization

Injection of air must be avoided by carefully expelling air from all syringes and performing injections with the plunger of the syringe upward. To avoid embolization of thrombi that may have formed within the catheter, heparinized saline is flushed and aspirated before injection of contrast agent.[1,31] Trauma to the vessel also should be avoided to prevent vasoconstriction, thrombosis, and difficulty in vascular filling.[1,31] The distal (cerebral) side of the lesion in the ICA is embolized first to protect the cerebral circulation from any intraoperative errors, such as air or clot embolization.[1,31]

Migration of embolization coils

Size of the coil is important because if it is too large, it does not coil fully within the artery and the tip might extend into and induce thrombosis at an undesirable site (such as in the arterial circle). Too small a coil might become dislodged and move away from the desired site. A coil slightly larger than the artery is placed first, and additional smaller imbricating embolization coils follow until complete occlusion is obtained.[31] For the distal ICA coil, diameters of 5 to 8 mm are usually necessary, although 3 mm may be needed in smaller horses or ponies.

The coil embolization technique was successful in 20 of 23 horses affected with guttural pouch mycosis.[32] The ability to selectively occlude affected vessels with a minimally invasive approach makes transarterial coil embolization the preferred treatment. Angiography is mandatory for anatomic identification and location of the vessels, exclusion of vascular anomalies, abnormal vascular connections between the ICA and the occipital artery, and correct positioning of the embolization coils.[31] If a connection is present between two embolization sites, continued bleeding could still occur, and such small branches must be occluded separately.

TEMPOROHYOID OSTEOARTHROPATHY (MIDDLE EAR DISEASE)

Unilateral partial ostectomy of the stylohyoid bone has merit as a prophylactic measure in horses with temporohyoid osteoarthropathy (middle ear disease) by creating a pseudoarthrosis between the cut ends of the bone, which decreases the forces on the ankylosed temporohyoid joint and prevents skull fractures.[33] This procedure can cause transient dysphagia or injury to the hypoglossal nerve.[33] When performed as a bilateral procedure, it causes permanent problems with prehension.[33] An additional complication associated with partial ostectomy is regrowth of the stylohyoid bone approximately 6 months after surgical resection and recurrence of clinical signs.[34] Because of this complication, a ceratohyoidectomy has been proposed to be a safer, easier, and more permanent surgical alternative.[34] The hypoglossal nerve and lingual branches of the mandibular and glossopharyngeal nerves are identified and gently retracted to protect them during surgery.

A potential complication of this procedure is iatrogenic skull fracture after surgical traction or manipulation of the ceratohyoid bone, so that the forces generated by these intraoperative maneuvers are transmitted through the ankylosed temporohyoid joint. Hypoglossal nerve paresis has been described after ceratohyoidectomy (**Fig. 5**), which

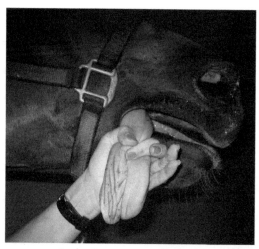

Fig. 5. Atrophy of tongue muscles on side of a ceratohyoidectomy (*left*), possibly caused by scarring in the surgery site.

appeared at necropsy to have resulted from fibrosis in the surgical incision and not from direct trauma to the nerve.[28] This paresis did not cause clinical signs and could go undetected unless the tongue was closely inspected after surgery for evidence of muscle atrophy.[28]

REFERENCES

1. Freeman DE, Hardy J. Diseases of the guttural pouch. In: Auer JA, Stick JA, editors. Equine surgery. 3rd edition. Philadelphia: WB Saunders Co.; 2005. p. 591–608.
2. Judy CE, Chaffin MK, Cohen ND. Empyema of the guttural pouch (auditory tube diverticulum) in horses: 91 cases (1977–1997). J Am Vet Med Assoc 1999;215: 1666–70.
3. Seahorn TL, Schumacher J. Nonsurgical removal of chondroid masses from the guttural pouches of two horses. J Am Vet Med Assoc 1991;199:368–9.
4. Fogle CA, Gerard MP, Johansson M, et al. Spontaneous rupture of the guttural pouch as a complication of treatment for guttural pouch empyema. Equine Vet Educ 2007;19:351–5.
5. Perkins JD, Schumacher J, Kelly G, et al. Standing surgical removal of inspissated guttural pouch exudate (chondroids) in ten horses. Vet Surg 2006;35: 658–62.
6. Verheyen K, Newton JR, Talbot NC, et al. Elimination of guttural pouch infection and inflammation in asymptomatic carriers of *Streptococcus equi*. Equine Vet J 2000;32:527–32.
7. Hawkins JF, Frank N, Sojka JE, et al. Fistulation of the auditory tube diverticulum (guttural pouch) with a neodymium:yttrium-aluminum-garnet laser for treatment of chronic empyema in two horses. J Am Vet Med Assoc 2001;218:405–7.
8. Schambourg MA, Marcoux M, Céleste C. Salpingoscopy for the treatment of recurrent guttural pouch tympany in a filly. Equine Vet Educ 2006;8:299–302.
9. Freeman DE. Clinical commentary: Guttural pouch tympany: a rare and difficult disease. Equine Vet Educ 2006;8:302–5.

10. Sullins KE. Endoscopic application of cutting current for upper respiratory surgery in the standing horse. Proc Am Assoc Equine Pract 1990;36:439–44.
11. Tate LP, Blikslager AT, Little EDE. Transendoscopic laser treatment of guttural pouch tympanites in eight foals. Vet Surg 1995;24:367–72.
12. Blazyczek I, Hamann H, Deegen E, et al. Retrospective analysis of 50 cases of guttural pouch tympany in foals. Vet Rec 2004;154:261–4.
13. McCue PM, Freeman DE, Donawick WJ. Guttural pouch tympany: 15 cases (1977–1986). J Am Vet Med Assoc 1989;194:1761–3.
14. Tetens J, Tulleners EP, Ross MW, et al. Transendoscopic contact neodymium: yttrium aluminum garnet laser treatment of tympany of the auditory tube diverticulum in two foals. J Am Vet Med Assoc 1994;204:1927–9.
15. Milne DW, Fessler JR. Tympanitis of the guttural pouch in a foal. J Am Vet Med Assoc 1972;161:61–4.
16. Cook WR. The clinical features of guttural pouch mycosis in the horse. Vet Rec 1968;83:336–45.
17. Greet TRC. Outcome of treatment in 35 cases of guttural pouch mycosis. Equine Vet J 1987;19:483–7.
18. Woodie JB, Ducharme NG, Gleed RD, et al. In horses with guttural pouch mycosis or after stylohyoid bone resection, what arterial ligation(s) could be effective in emergency treatment of a hemorrhagic crisis? Vet Surg 2003;31:498.
19. Freeman DE, Donawick WJ, Klein L. Effect of ligation on internal carotid artery blood pressure in horses. Vet Surg 1994;23:250–6.
20. Owen R. Epistaxis prevented by ligation of the internal carotid artery in the guttural pouch. Equine Vet J 1974;6:143–9.
21. Hardy J, Robertson JT, Wilkie DA. Ischemic optic neuropathy and blindness after arterial occlusion for treatment of guttural pouch mycosis in two horses. J Am Vet Med Assoc 1990;196:1631–4.
22. Bacon Miller C, Wilson DA, Martin DD, et al. Complications of balloon catheterization associated with aberrant cerebral arterial anatomy in a horse with guttural pouch mycosis. Vet Surg 1998;27:450–3.
23. Freeman DE, Staller GS, Maxson AD, et al. Unusual carotid artery branching that prevented arterial occlusion with a balloon-tipped catheter in a horse. Vet Surg 1993;22:531–4.
24. Smith KM, Barber SM. Guttural pouch hemorrhage associated with lesions of the maxillary artery in two horses. Can Vet J 1984;25:239–42.
25. Freeman DE, Ross MW, Donawick WJ, et al. Occlusion of the external carotid and maxillary arteries in the horse to prevent hemorrhage from guttural pouch mycosis. Vet Surg 1989;18:39–47.
26. Freeman DE, Ross MW, Donawick WJ. "Steal phenomenon" proposed as the cause of blindness after arterial occlusion for treatment of guttural pouch mycosis in horses. J Am Vet Med Assoc 1990;197:811–2.
27. Speirs VC, Harrison IW, van Veenendaal JC, et al. Is specific antifungal therapy necessary for the treatment of guttural pouch mycosis? Equine Vet J 1995;27:151–2.
28. Ernst NS, Freeman DE, MacKay RJ. Progression of mycosis of the auditory tube diverticulum (guttural pouch) after arterial occlusion in a horse with contralateral temporohyoid osteoarthropathy. J Am Vet Med Assoc 2006;229:1945–8.
29. Cheramie HS, Pleasant RS, Robertson JL, et al. Evaluation of a technique to occlude the internal carotid artery of horses. Vet Surg 1999;28:83–90.
30. Cheramie HS, Pleasant RS, Dabareiner RM, et al. Detachable latex balloon occlusion of an internal carotid artery with an aberrant branch in a horse with guttural

pouch (auditory tube diverticulum) mycosis: evaluation of a technique to occlude the internal carotid artery of horses. J Am Vet Med Assoc 2000;216:888–91.

31. Léveillé R, Hardy J, Robertson JT, et al. Transarterial coil embolization of the internal and external carotid and maxillary arteries for prevention of hemorrhage from guttural pouch mycosis in horses. Vet Surg 2000;29:389–97.

32. Lepage OM, Piccot-Crézollet C. Transarterial coil embolization in 31 horses (1999–2002) with guttural pouch mycosis: a 2-year follow-up. Equine Vet J 2005;37:430–4.

33. Blythe LL, Watrous BJ, Shires GMH, et al. Prophylactic partial stylohyoidostectomy for horses with osteoarthropathy of the temporohyoid joint. J Equine Vet Sci 1994;14:32–7.

34. Pease AP, Van Biervliet J, Dykes NL, et al. Complication of partial stylohyoidectomy for treatment of temporohyoid osteoarthropathy and an alternative surgical technique in three cases. Equine Vet J 2004;36:546–50.

Complications of Equine Oral Surgery

Padraic M. Dixon, MVB, PhD, MRCVS[a,b,*], Claire Hawkes, BVSc, MRCVS[a],
Neil Townsend, BSc, BVSc, MRCVS[a]

KEYWORDS

• Equine • Oral surgery • Dentistry • Oral surgery complications

The vast majority of equine oral procedures are dental-related and, unless great care is taken, almost all such procedures have the potential to cause marked short- or long-term damage to other oral structures. This review of the more common complications of oral surgery begins at the rostral oral cavity with procedures of the incisors, and then moves caudally to deal with complications related to procedures of wolf teeth and cheek teeth, including salivary duct disruption and dental sinusitis. Finally, complications associated with and maxillary and mandibular fractures are discussed.

COMPLICATIONS OF ORTHODONTIC TREATMENT OF OVERJET AND OVERBITE

The orthodontic treatment of overjet and overbite can be beneficial to many foals. However, such treatment in foals also has the potential to cause immediate and longer-term problems.[1–3]

Trauma to the Dorsal Buccal Nerve

The stab incision in the skin and cheeks, opposite the upper 06-07 or 07-08 interproximal spaces, should be made parallel with the facial crest and as dorsal as possible to help avoid damaging branches of the dorsal buccal nerve. Additionally, after one end of the wire has been introduced into the oral cavity (through a hypodermic needle inserted through the stab incision), some operators then withdraw the hypodermic needle and push the other end of the wire into the oral cavity parallel to the original strand. It is imperative that no soft tissues, which potentially could contain nerves, are trapped between the two wire strands. As soon as the foals recover from anesthesia, dysfunction of branches of the dorsal buccal nerve becomes apparent with ipsilateral flaccidity of the nostril and possibly partial flaccidity of the upper lip (**Fig. 1**).

[a] Division of Veterinary Clinical Studies, Easter Bush Veterinary Centre, Midlothian, Scotland, EH25 9RG, UK
[b] Department of Clinical Science, University of Edinburgh, Royal (Dick) School of Veterinary Studies, Midlothian, Scotland, UK
* Corresponding author. Division of Veterinary Clinical Studies, Easter Bush Veterinary Centre, Midlothian, Scotland, EH25 9RG, UK.
E-mail address: p.m.dixon@ed.ac.uk (P.M. Dixon).

Vet Clin Equine 24 (2009) 499–514
doi:10.1016/j.cveq.2008.10.001
0749-0739/08/$ – see front matter © 2009 Elsevier Inc. All rights reserved.

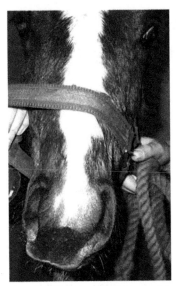

Fig. 1. This foal has partial left-sided facial paralysis caused by a hematoma at the buccal stab incision site while fitting an orthodontic brace for overjet. This neuropraxia resolved within 3 days.

Fortunately, such dysfunction (neuropraxia) is usually temporary. The cause is usually surgical bruising of one or more branches of the buccal nerve or local pressure from an adjacent hematoma. Many affected foals regain full tone in affected muscles within a week or so.[1,2] Nonsteroidal anti-inflammatory drug (NSAID) therapy (combined with anti–gastric ulcer therapy, such as omeprazole) may help speed up resolution of the neuropraxia. Even when severe structural damage to these nerves occurs, foals can often regain excellent or full function over the following 4 to 6 months through nerve regrowth.

Damage to the Greater Palatine Artery

When the Steinmann pin is inserted through the cheeks and interproximal spaces between the upper 06-07 (or 07-08), the pin should be directed dorsally to exit close to the gingival margin at the lateral edge of the hard palate. However, if the pin is inadvertently directed too dorsally, it may injure the greater palatine artery, causing an immediate and often severe oral hemorrhage. The hemorrhage should be controlled by applying local pressure with, for example, a surgical swab held in place with large curved artery forceps against the site of hemorrhage for 5 to 10 minutes. Ligation of this important artery (which is not an end artery) should be avoided. In any case, gaining access to this artery, situated in a groove of the palatine bone, is technically difficult.

Postoperative Pain and Nursing Problems

Some foals may have trouble suckling immediately following surgery, especially if an acrylic biteplate is fitted in addition to a wire brace (ie, fitted in cases that also have overbite). If the brace appears to be causing discomfort, the foal should be given low doses of NSAIDs and anti–gastric ulcer medication. An alternative plan in older cases is to wean the foal before this surgery. Orthodontic biteplates may also hurt the mare's udder (especially primiparous mares with small teats) and the mare may resent the foal suckling. Such mares should be milked for a few days and the foal bottle-fed with this milk before being gradually reintroduced to suckling the mare.[1–3]

Damage to Orthodontic Prostheses

Orthodontic wires may break unilaterally or bilaterally, causing the biteplate to loosen. Therefore, the foal's mouth should be inspected daily and broken wires should be immediately replaced, a procedure that usually requires general anesthesia.

Incisor and Gingival Damage

The orthodontic device invariably causes gingival injury, which may be hidden if an acrylic biteplate is also fitted. Incisors, especially the 01s (centrals), can become displaced, deformed, or even loosened by the prosthesis (**Fig. 2**). As these are deciduous incisors, such injuries are mainly of cosmetic concern.

COMPLICATIONS OF WOLF TOOTH EXTRACTION
Fracture of Wolf Tooth During Extraction

If the roots or adjacent apical aspects of wolf teeth fracture below the alveolar level during extraction, these (noninfected) dental fragments can be left behind and the alveoli will usually heal over fully. If however, wolf teeth fracture above the alveolar level, sharp protrusions of these teeth may cause marked gingival inflammation and pain when contacted by tack. Such horses may have more bitting-related problems postoperatively than they had before the (partial) extraction. Such dental remnants should be extracted under sedation and local analgesia. This procedure may require sharp rostrocaudal incision of adjacent gingiva to expose the fractured tooth and use of an osteotome or bone gouge and mallet to remove deeply embedded fragments.

Laceration of the Greater Palatine Artery in Adult Horses

If the dental elevator slips in a medial (palatal) direction during wolf tooth extraction, the greater palatine artery can be lacerated.[2,4] Initially, pressure should be applied to the bleeding site digitally, and then by placing a group of swabs or a large piece of cotton wool over the bleeding artery and taping these tightly around the upper jaw. Alternatively, a small folded towel can be placed in the mouth beneath the lacerated artery. The jaws should then be tied firmly together to put pressure on the artery. In any case, once pressure has been placed on the artery, such horses are best

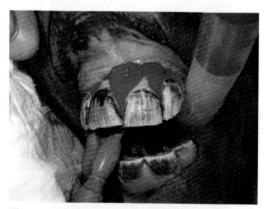

Fig. 2. These premaxillary central incisors (Triadan 701 and 801) have been slightly displaced by orthodontic bracing. Marked gingival inflammation and ulceration have also occurred because of jaw growth putting increased pressure on the orthodontic wires.

maintained with their head up (ie, on a headstand if they have been sedated) (**Fig. 3**). They are also best kept in a dark, deeply bedded stall until the hemorrhage stops.

WIDENING OF CHEEK TEETH DIASTEMATA
Pulpar Thermal Damage or Pulp Exposure

Widening of cheek teeth diastemata with high-speed carbide or diamond-coated burrs is increasingly used to prevent food impaction and painful periodontal disease, but this technique risks injuring the pulps of the (two) adjacent cheek teeth.[5,6] During cheek teeth diastemata widening, the burr should only be in contact with the adjacent teeth for approximately 5 seconds at a time and water should be intermittently sprayed over the cheek teeth being burred to prevent thermal pulpar damage. Excess dental tissue should not be removed from a tooth on one side of the diastema. Not all interproximal (interdental) spaces are at right angles to the cheek teeth row and, therefore, when widening such diagonally directed or curved interproximal spaces with a right-angled burr, great care must be taken to follow the actual interproximal space by constant use of an intraoral mirror or camera to prevent inadvertently exposing a pulp cavity.[5,6]

REDUCING OVERGROWTHS ON CHEEK TEETH
Pulpar Exposure or Thermal Injury During Cheek Teeth Reductions

The layer of occlusal secondary dentine overlying the pulp chambers of some cheek teeth can be as thin as 3 mm, even in adult horses. Consequently, there is great risk of causing pulpar exposure or thermal damage to such pulps when overgrowths on such teeth are reduced (rasped, floated), especially when using mechanical instruments. The risk of pulpar overheating is increased if dental instruments without water cooling or blunt mechanical burrs are used, if burrs are allowed to become clogged with dental

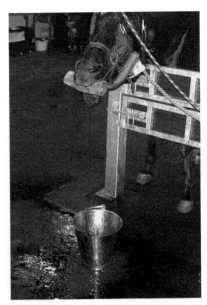

Fig. 3. This horse has profuse oral hemorrhage caused by iatrogenic laceration of the greater palatine artery during a dental extraction.

debris, or if burrs are kept in contact with the teeth for prolonged (ie, >10 seconds) periods while reducing overgrowths.[4] A thermally injured pulp suffers necrosis of a varying amount of the pulp horn tip and thus cannot lay down any further secondary dentine beneath the occlusal surface. When the existing occlusal dentine is worn away, pulpar exposure then occurs on the occlusal surface and food becomes impacted down the pulp chamber, which may cause subsequent periapical infection.[7,8]

In contrast to what was until recently common practice, very tall (ie, >1 cm) dental overgrowths should not be fully reduced at a single session, but should be reduced in stages at least 3 months apart (ie, maximum 5 mm at a time) to stimulate secondary dentine deposition of the underlying pulp horn tips and so help avoid pulpar exposure (**Fig. 4**).[4,8] Similarly, rounding-off of the rostral aspects of the 06s (ie, creating "bit seats") should not be performed aggressively, as unfortunately is common practice with some operators. When creating "bit-seats," the rostral aspect of the occlusal surface of the 06s should be reduced by just a few millimeters, as thermal pulpar damage or direct pulpar exposure (especially of the additional rostrally positioned [6th] pulp chamber in these Triadan 06 teeth) can easily be caused by this clinically unproven procedure. Signs of pulpar and later dental death may not be manifested until the tooth shows a sign of apical infection some years after this damage has been caused.

Fracture and Pulpar Exposure of the Mandibular Triadan 11 Cheek Teeth

Suspected "overgrowths" of the 311 and 411 should be carefully examined to ensure that they are in fact true overgrowths and not teeth of normal height lying in a very dorsally curved caudal mandible, which can be present in horses with a pronounced "curve of Spee" (especially Arabian horses and Welsh ponies).[4,8] If true overgrowths of the lower 11s are in fact present, they should, as noted above, be reduced in stages, preferably by using a mechanical instrument with a rotating disc. Manual shears ("molar cutters") or percussion guillotines (circular blades that encircle this caudal overgrowth) can fracture these teeth or remove too much of the overgrowth in one application and so cause pulpar exposure. Such dental fractures and pulpar exposure may lead to life-threatening cellulitis of the mandibular and pharyngeal areas (**Fig. 5**), airway obstruction, mandibular osteomyelitis, and at the very least will necessitate

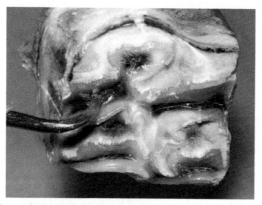

Fig. 4. One of the five pulps on this maxillary cheek tooth is exposed on the occlusal surface as demonstrated by the probe entering the secondary dentine above it. Food impaction and bacterial infection of pulp subsequent to such pulpar exposure make apical infection and loss of the tooth almost inevitable in a young cheek tooth such as this.

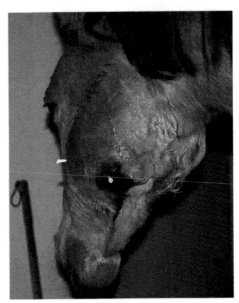

Fig. 5. Following iatrogenic trauma to the 311, this horse developed extensive cellulitis of the left mandibular area and now has widespread abscess formation in the masseter muscles. Pus is draining from two 14-gauge needles inserted in these muscles.

extraction of the fractured teeth, which will usually require a technically difficult cheek tooth repulsion through the likely infected masseter muscles and mandible.

COMPLICATIONS OF CHEEK TOOTH REPULSION

Repulsion under general anesthesia was the standard method for extracting equine cheek teeth for most of the 20th century. However, because of the necessity for general anesthesia and due to the high level of postoperative complications associated with cheek tooth repulsion, alternative techniques of cheek tooth extraction have been recently sought. Complications are common following cheek tooth repulsion because this procedure causes much traumatic damage to the alveoli and the supporting mandibular or maxillary bones. From 32% to 70% of horses undergoing cheek tooth repulsion require further surgical and nonsurgical treatments, and particularly so after maxillary cheek tooth repulsions.[9–12]

Trauma to the Infraorbital Nerve

When repulsing a caudal maxillary cheek tooth through a trephine opening, the punch may readily damage the infraorbital canal and nerve that directly overlay the apices of these cheek teeth. This damage is less likely to occur if the repulsion is performed through a larger maxillary osteotomy flap window that permits direct visualization of the affected apex and the overlying infraorbital canal, thus allowing more accurate placement of the punch. Repulsion of the upper 06s and 07s (occasionally of the 08s) that lie outside the maxillary sinuses also risks damaging the infraorbital nerve after it has exited the infraorbital foramen. If the infraorbital nerve is damaged, clinical signs often occur within hours and can include violent headshaking, distress, and rubbing (even excoriation) of the ipsilateral nostril on adjacent objects. Such cases often do not respond to NSAIDs or even opiate therapy, but some respond reasonably well to acetylpromazine, which has prolonged anxiolytic activity. Fortunately, many horses with infraorbital nerve damage show good resolution of clinical signs within 1 to 2 weeks following nerve injury. Concurrent antibiotic and NSAID therapy should also be given for approximately a week following injury to prevent infection of the exposed nerve due to inevitable bacterial contamination present at dental repulsion sites.

Repulsion Damage to Adjacent Teeth and Supporting Bones

Because of the varying angles of the cheek teeth's reserve crowns and apices in relation to their occlusal surface, the site of apical repulsion is often not directly above or below the clinical crown.[2,9,13] Therefore, unless the punch is accurately positioned under radiographic guidance, it can damage adjacent teeth at some stage during repulsion. Even punches that are initially positioned accurately can move during the repulsion procedure. Movement of the punch in a rostral or caudal direction during repulsion may cause damage to an adjacent cheek teeth. Fortunately, damage to an adjacent dental reserve crown or apex does not always devitalize the damaged tooth. A 2- to 3-week course of broad-spectrum antibiotic therapy should be administered (and lavage of the sinuses performed if a caudal maxillary cheek tooth is involved). The horse should be clinically reexamined (including detailed intraoral examination) and the damaged tooth re-radiographed 1 to 2 months later. If definitive clinical and radiographic evidence of apical infection is present at that time, the damaged tooth should be extracted, preferably by oral extraction.

Movement of the punch in a medial or a lateral direction during repulsion may damage supporting bones. For example, when repulsing a mandibular cheek tooth, the punch may penetrate or fracture the mandible medial or lateral to the tooth; or, when repulsing a maxillary cheek tooth, the punch may penetrate or fracture the hard palate or the lateral aspect of the maxillary bone. Such trauma to the surrounding supporting bones is usually well tolerated and even extensive fractures usually heal exceptionally well. Antibiotic therapy for 7 to 10 days following the repulsion may be beneficial to horses with iatrogenic fractures of the supporting bones. A limited number of these cases develop localized osteomyelitis (which requires prolonged antibiotic therapy) or develop sequestration of damaged bones, which requires curettage.

Delayed or Nonhealing of Alveolus

Following cheek tooth repulsion, post-extraction radiographs should be obtained, unless examination of the repulsed cheek tooth (which may be fragmented) indicates that the complete tooth has been repulsed. Digital examination of alveoli to assess for alveolar bone damage and in particular for the presence of intra-alveolar calcified tissue fragments is also essential after dental repulsion. Polymethylmethacrylate (PMMA) alveolar packing is often used to seal the communicating tract between the oral cavity and sinuses following repulsion of caudal maxillary cheek tooth because PMMA has increased retention as compared with other alveolar packing materials. The consequence of loss of alveolar packing at this site (ie, oromaxillary fistula formation) is very significant. Skin wounds associated with cheek tooth repulsion are usually highly contaminated and often discharge purulent material for a week or so postsurgery. The presence of very profuse, malodorous, or chronic discharge from repulsion wounds indicates delayed-healing or even nonhealing of an infected alveolus. The presence of food in this discharge suggests that loss of alveolar packing is the cause of the continuing alveolar infection and repulsion wound discharge.

Nonhealing alveoli should be examined per os to ensure that the alveolar packing is not loose or missing. Loose alveolar packing should be removed and the alveolus examined digitally and visually with a dental mirror (or endoscope). A few days follow-ing extraction, a normally healing alveolus will be fully covered by dark red, smooth granulation tissue, while the presence of exposed calcified tissue (white to pale brown in color) indicates the presence of sequestered alveolar bone or one or more residual dental fragments. Radiography of the affected alveolus should also be performed to further assess for the presence of more apically situated alveolar bone or dental frag-ments (**Fig. 6**).

Intra-alveolar dental fragments are usually radiographically identifiable, but larger, shell-like, alveolar sequestrae can be difficult to detect radiographically. However, such larger alveolar sequestrae may be detected by digital examination of alveoli per os (within a few weeks of extraction while there is room to allow this procedure) or by the use of an intraoral mirror or endoscope. Loose intra-alveolar sequestrae, which include most bony sequestrae, may be removed per os by digital manipulation, high-pressure lavage, or by using various right-angled dental picks and curettes. Right-angled, equine dental picks, with blades up to 10 cm long can be inserted into the periodontal space to separate residual dental fragments from the alveolar wall, or placed beneath sequestered alveolar bone fragments to dislodge them.

If dental fragments are firmly attached (especially following fracture of a tooth during repulsion), their removal can be aided in the sedated horse by first appropriately directing the tip of the dental pick blade between the wall of the alveolus and the dental fragment, while the distal aspect of the blade rests on the occlusal surface of the opposite tooth. The speculum is then slowly closed to allow the horse's powerful masticatory actions to loosen the fragments.[14] If dental fragments cannot be removed with dental picks because, for example, they are lying too deep in an alveolus or are hidden by granulation tissue, a Steinman pin may be used under radiographic guid-ance to repulse the fragments into the oral cavity (see **Fig. 6**). Rounded, dense, pearl-like areas of reactive cementum seldom cause postoperative intra-alveolar problems in the authors' opinions and need not necessarily be removed. If oral examination and postoperative radiographs show all the intra-alveolar fragments to be removed, the

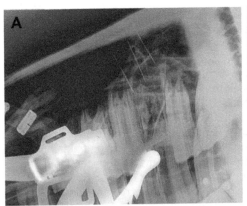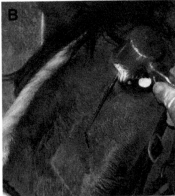

Fig. 6. (A) Latero-oblique radiograph of nonhealing alveolus that has some dental fragments remaining within it. A row of hypodermic needles has been placed in the overlying skin to facilitate repulsion of the dental fragments. (B) This horse is having an alveolar dental frag-ment repulsed under standing sedation. Note the row of skin staples above the Steinman pin that are used to radiographically guide the position of the Steinman pin (which appears excessively medially positioned). A full-mouth speculum is fitted, and the surgeon's left hand is in the horse's mouth and under the affected alveolus to detect movement of the re-sidual dental fragment and possible misplacement of the punch.

blood clot formed during the curettage procedure should be left in place to provide a substrate for granulation tissue formation and so facilitate alveolar healing.

Orosinus (Oromaxillary) Fistula

If loss of alveolar packing occurs following caudal maxillary cheek tooth (Triadan 08-11) repulsion, an orosinus fistula can develop.[2,11,13] Horses with an oromaxillary fistula should have the affected sinuses lavaged of food and exudate using an intrasinus catheter, and also by direct lavage through the repulsion site if it is still patent. Sinoscopy (direct sinus endoscopy) through the sinus portal can then be used to ensure the sinuses have been cleared of all food material and exudate. If the oromaxillary fistula is chronic, a sinus osteotomy is usually indicated to remove all food material and inspissated pus from the sinus. The affected alveolus should be digitally, visually, and radiographically examined to confirm the absence of dental or bony remnants that may be causing persistent alveolar infection and delayed healing. If the oromaxillary fistula is chronic, the alveolus should be curetted to remove oral and sinus epithelium lining the fistula. The alveolus should then be sealed with PMMA attached to the adjacent, dried, interproximal dental surfaces. Care should be taken not to insert the PMMA too deep into the alveolus because this also prevents alveolar healing. Excessive depth of insertion of PMMA is most likely to occur if the original repulsion site has healed or when retrograde pressure cannot be applied to the apical aspect of the PMMA packing in the alveolus.

Oronasal Fistula

If premature loss of alveolar packing occurs following repulsion of the rostral two or three maxillary cheek teeth (Triadan 06-08), an oronasal fistula can develop. The non-healing alveolus should be investigated and treated as described above (oromaxillary fistula). For problematic oronasal fistulas that do not respond to conventional treatment, a sliding mucoperiosteal flap procedure can be performed.[15] This involves making a full-thickness incision of the ipsilateral lips from the commisure to the level of the oronasal fistula to improve surgical access. Care should be taken to avoid branches of the dorsal buccal nerve at the caudal aspect of this incision. The fistula should be thoroughly curetted to remove epithelial tracts, food, exudate, and necrotic granulation tissue, and then lavaged clear of all debris. An incision is then made on the medial aspect of the fistula, down to the level of the hard palate. The palatal mucoperiosteum is then bluntly elevated over the width of the fistula with an appropriate periosteal elevator. This elevation is continued medially to just beyond the midline of the hard palate.

Transverse incisions are made in the palatal mucosa at the rostral and caudal aspects of the fistula to the midline of hard palate, taking care to place transfixing ligatures, both rostrally and caudally, around the greater palatine artery, unless the artery can be identified, dissected free, and left intact beneath the mucoperiosteal flap. The mobile mucoperiosteal flap can now be pulled laterally to close the defect. Buccal mucosal and submucosal flaps are created on the lateral aspect of the fistula, which is then firmly sutured to the free edge of the mucoperiosteal flap in two or three layers with absorbable sutures. The incisions on the rostral and caudal aspect of the fistula are similarly closed. The buccotomy incision is now closed in two or three layers. Semiliquid or mash feeds should be given for about 1 month to minimize stresses on the repairing tissues.

Postoperative Sinusitis Secondary to Cheek Tooth Extraction

Following cheek tooth extraction, persistent sinusitis in the absence of residual alveolar fragments or an orosinus fistula usually indicates the presence of inspissated pus or of necrotic dental or bone material remaining within the sinus, very often within the ventral conchal or rostral maxillary sinuses, even following extraction of more caudal cheek teeth, whose apices lie within the caudal maxillary sinus. Assessment of such cases requires radiography, including dorsoventral projections to detect empyema of the ventral conchal sinus and lateral-oblique views to examine for the presence of intra-alveolar sequestrae.

Sinoscopic examination is also of great use in such cases. Currently in our clinic, we use a frontal sinus approach with an endoscopically guided fenestration of the ventral conchal bulla (**Fig. 7**)[16] to allow examination of the lumen of the ventral conchal sinus. Direct trephination of either the rostral or caudal maxillary sinus may be performed. However, in horses 5 years old or younger, there is an increased risk of damaging a dental apex when trephining the rostral maxillary sinus directly.[17] If inspissated pus is detected in the sinuses, management of such cases involves complete removal of such exudate using either a maxillary sinus or a nasofrontal sinus osteotomy, which can readily be performed in the standing horse, as such concretions of pus will not readily be flushed out through the narrow nasomaxillary ostium.

Currently we favor a standing caudal maxillary sinus osteotomy in our clinic. Even in younger horses, the ventral conchal bulla can be safely accessed via a caudal maxillary osteotomy. The ventral conchal bulla can subsequently be opened and evacuated and the maxillary septum can also be broken and the rostral maxillary sinus safely examined and evacuated of any debris.

The sinuses should then be lavaged under high pressure with 10 to 15 L of lukewarm, dilute povidine iodine solution or saline to remove any smaller particles of inspissated pus or debris that may be hidden in one of the many and variable paranasal sinus recesses. Prior to closure, the surgical incision should be lavaged with 1 to 2 L of sterile saline. The bone flap is replaced and, if necessary, secured with one or two cerclage wires. The subcutaneous tissues are closed with absorbable sutures and the skin is stapled. The sinuses should be lavaged postoperatively (5–10 L twice a day) through a wide-bore catheter placed into the frontal sinus.

COMPLICATIONS OF ORAL EXTRACTION

Because oral extraction of cheek teeth is performed in the standing horse, the risks (and expense) of general anesthesia are removed. Unlike cheek tooth repulsion, the

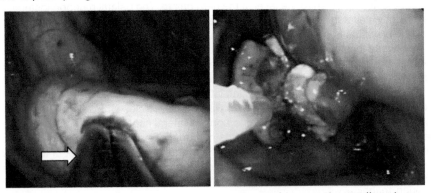

Fig. 7. (*Left*) Following creation of a small frontal sinus trephine opening to allow sinoscopy and access for a small rongeur. The rongeur (*arrow*) is inserted through the frontomaxillary opening and used to puncture and then break down the grossly normal ventral conchal bulla. Examination showed the lumen of the ventral conchal sinus to contain a small amount of inspissated pus (*right*), which was removed in this case with transendoscopic biopsy forceps and local lavage.

oral extraction technique does not require surgery of the supporting bones and, consequently, postoperative complications are uncommon and usually, when they do occur, are easy to treat.[18–20]

Fracture or Damage to Adjacent Teeth

When using dental separators to rostrocaudally loosen a cheek tooth that is being extracted, a narrow blade dental separator should be used initially, using slow sustained pressure on the instrument. The forceful use of dental separators, especially of wide-blade separators too early during the extraction process, can fracture or loosen adjacent cheek teeth, and can also fracture long roots on a cheek tooth being extracted. Additionally, before applying pressure that can fracture an adjacent cheek tooth, the operator must ensure that the separator blades are opposite the interproximal space between the affected cheek tooth and an adjacent cheek tooth and are not mistakenly placed in the normal vertical grooves present on the lateral and medial aspects of some cheek tooth.

When extracting an 07, separators should not be used between the 06 and 07 because their use will likely loosen the (healthy) 06 (because it has no rostral support) more than the diseased 07. Separators must also be used with great care when extracting caudal mandibular cheek teeth in horses with a marked curve of Spee, where the right-angled blades of the separator will not fit into the nonvertical interdental spaces of such cheek teeth, but might instead fracture them.[18,19] After a caudal (10 or 11) mandibular cheek tooth has been fully loosened during an oral extraction, a fulcrum must be used cautiously, in case the vertically directed elevating force fractures the caudally oriented reserve crowns of these teeth. It is preferable to loosen these cheek teeth digitally and then extract them in a rostrodorsally oblique direction with forceps.

Nonhealing Alveoli

Following oral extraction of infected cheek teeth that do not have an external sinus tract, the alveoli are usually packed with one or two surgical swabs or soft dental impression material. This packing should be removed a few weeks later if still present. Most alveoli will have healed significantly by this stage. If the alveoli have not healed by this time, they should be digitally palpated for the presence of roughened areas that are inevitably due to sequestration of areas of alveolar cortex.[18] Such sequestra should be removed digitally or by curettage. Intra-alveolar dental fragments are very rarely present following oral cheek tooth extraction. Specialized, long-handled, right-angled alveolar curettes (Kruuse Worldwide, Marslev, Denmark) are useful to curette the more caudal cheek teeth alveoli.

COMPLICATIONS OF MAXILLARY AND MANDIBULAR FRACTURE REPAIR

Except for complete fractures of the premaxilla (incisive bone) or the rostral mandible, the vast majority of other maxillary and mandibular fractures are relatively stable because of support from adjacent cheek teeth, undamaged maxillary bones, or the contralateral hemimandible. Consequently, external fixation of such fractures, although technically possible, is seldom necessary and in some cases may cause more harm than good. Due to the often contaminated nature of maxillary and mandibular fractures, which often communicate with the oral environment or are open externally, infection of, and drainage from, the site of fractures are common complications following repair. These infections usually respond slowly to a prolonged course of antibiotics.

Continuation of infection at the fracture site should prompt the clinician to investigate for the presence of sequestrum formation from avascular bone fragments or infection of adjacent (fractured or intact) teeth. Particularly with mandibular fractures in young horses, fractured and even obviously infected fractured cheek teeth should be left in place for at least 3 months, unless obviously loose (**Fig. 8**). Attempted removal of firmly attached infected or fractured cheek teeth before this time can result in catastrophic destabilization of the fracture site, which was effectively being splinted by the infected or fractured cheek teeth. Clinicians should just accept that there will be some discharge from external wounds or malodor of the breath during this time, until the primary fracture site has healed sufficiently to allow safe extraction of the damaged cheek tooth and curettage of the adjacent bones (see **Fig. 8**).

Bony sequestrae at the fracture site can sometimes be removed in the standing sedated patient via curettage, including curettage under radiographic guidance by inserting a row of hypodermic needles or skin staples in the adjacent skin. Excessive callus formation at the fracture site can be due to fracture instability during healing, as in the case of complete, rostral jaw fractures, or due to chronic infection of the fracture site, as outlined above. Depending upon the stage of healing, fracture stabilization can be performed (as described below). However, the majority of enlarged calluses will remodel significantly in the months following fracture repair, regardless of whether surgical or conservative methods were used.

Other complications encountered with maxillary and mandibular fractures can be specific to the technique employed for fracture stabilization. Tension band wires may loosen or break, resulting in fracture instability, local oral discomfort, or buccal ulceration. Even healthy cheek teeth that have had tension wires placed around them to stabilize a mandibular or maxillary fracture can become loose by the applied pressure, and may cause instability of the fracture. Such wires require tightening or replacement, depending on the stage of fracture healing. If adjacent cheek teeth are damaged by implants (Kirshner pins or screws), apical infection and eventual loss of cheek teeth can result. The use of a pinless external fixator reduces the risk of damage to dental structures. However, these fixators may cause bone sequestrum formation, problems caused by implant cycling and, as with other external fixators, risk getting caught on objects in the horse's stall and so become detached.[21] The potential for damage to soft tissue structures during external fixator placement (buccal nerve, salivary duct) has been discussed elsewhere in this article.

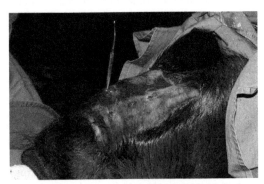

Fig. 8. Due to residual infection of a fractured cheek tooth at this site, this horse has a chronic sinus tract from a previously fractured left hemimandible. There is now good callus formation at the fracture site (note thickened hemimandible) and so the infected tooth can be carefully extracted.

Dynamic compression plates can be used to stabilize mandibular fractures, especially when placed more ventrally on the hemimandible in older horses with shorter reserve crowns. As noted earlier, in younger horses the screws can potentially damage multiple normal cheek teeth and cause infection. Plate/screw placement must be performed under radiographic guidance to avoid the cheek tooth apices. Plates can be more safely used to stabilize fractures of the rostral mandible ("bars of mouth" physiologic diastema). A disadvantage of this repair method is that the tension surface of the mandible is on its occlusal aspect. Therefore the ventrally placed plate is typically applied in a less than ideal position in terms of biomechanics, and the strong and prolonged forces of equine mastication can loosen such plates (**Fig. 9**).

Damage to Soft Tissues During Extraction

Oral extraction of caudal maxillary cheek teeth (10 or 11) and especially of a caudal supernumerary maxillary cheek tooth (12) risks damaging the soft palate (**Fig. 10**). This means that great care must be taken when placing the extraction forceps on the medial aspect of these cheek teeth. If the soft palate is deeply lacerated more than 2 cm from its lateral margin (where the horizontal part of the palatine bone ends), an oropharyngeal fistula may develop that may not be correctable because of poor surgical access.

Laceration of the Greater Palatine Artery

When extracting maxillary cheek teeth, especially with "claw type" dental extractors, it is sometimes necessary to mobilize and displace the gingiva on the medial aspect of the tooth to increase contact of the extractors on the (often very short) medial (palatal) aspect of the affected clinical crown. Care must be taken to avoid damage of the greater palatine artery during this procedure and adequate sedation of the patient is essential during the application or reapplication of extraction forceps on this tooth. Treatment of this sequel was described earlier.

COMPLICATIONS OF REMOVAL OF THE LATERAL ALVEOLAR PLATE (LATERAL BUCCOTOMY TECHNIQUE)
Buccal Nerve Damage

Removal of the lateral alveolar plate has mainly been used for extraction of the rostral upper three cheek teeth and the mandibular cheek tooth (via buccotomy or through

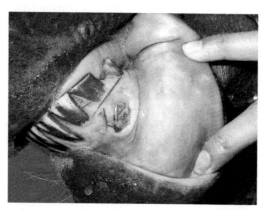

Fig. 9. A compression plate was used to stabilize the left hemimandible following removal of bone tumor. The rostrally fixed screws have loosened and allowed rostral migration of the plate, which is now protruding through the gingiva.

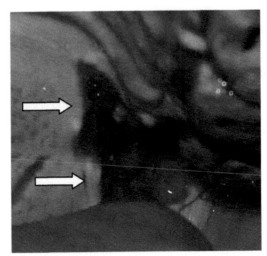

Fig. 10. This soft palate has been injured (*arrows*) during oral extraction of a 211 (empty alveolus is to the right of injury), but the injury was localized to the oral mucosa of the palate and it healed uneventfully. In any case, the horizontal plate of the palatine bone lies beneath the soft palate at this site.

the masseter muscle).[13,22,23] Incisions through the skin and underlying buccal muscle should be horizontal to reduce the risk of injuring the buccal nerves. Depending on which tooth is being extracted, the buccal nerve branch or branches and the parotid duct should be identified and surgically isolated if they cross the surgical field. This helps avoid accidental damage. Short- and long-term damage to the dorsal buccal nerve causes ipsilateral nostril and possibly lip paresis as previously discussed (see foal orthodontic procedures). Similar nerve injuries caused by a buccal stab incision may also occur during mandibular fracture fixation when wire is placed between the rostral cheek teeth.

Parotid Duct Damage

Damage to the parotid duct causes leakage of saliva from the surgical site, with this salivary flow increasing when the horse eats.[24–27] If the parotid duct damage is identified at the time of injury, the duct can be carefully repaired with fine absorbable sutures. Most lacerations of the parotid duct (or its branches) are not identified until after surgery when the horses eat. Fortunately, most of these lacerations spontaneously heal within 1 to 2 weeks and further investigations and surgical treatment can be deferred to beyond this period. Damage to the parotid duct can be confirmed by catheterizing the duct from its oral papilla (usually opposite the maxillary 08) under general anesthesia. Some more chronic fistulas may need surgical repair by suturing with or without the use of an indwelling catheter that acts like a stent as described elsewhere.[2,27] Alternatively, or following failure to repair the duct, chemical ablation of the parotid gland, including by using Lugol's iodine or 10% formalin solution, can be performed, but such chemical ablation of the parotid gland carries its own significant risks.

REFERENCES

1. Easley KJ. Basic equine orthodontics. In: Baker GJ, Easley KJ, editors. Equine dentistry. 2nd edition. London: WB Saunders; 2005. p. 249–66.

2. Dixon PM, Gerard MP. Oral cavity and salivary glands. In: Auer JA, Stick JA, editors. Equine surgery. 3rd edition. St Louis (MO): WB Saunders; 2006. p. 321–50.
3. Easley JK. Equine orthodontics. In: Focus on dentistry. American Association of Equine Practitioners, Indianapolis (IN) 2006, p 39–46.
4. Easley KJ. Corrective dental procedures. In: Baker GJ, Easley KJ, editors. Equine dentistry. 2nd edition. London: WB Saunders; 2005. p. 221–48.
5. Dixon PM, Barakzai SZ, Collins N, et al. Treatment of equine cheek teeth diastema by mechanical widening of diastemata in 60 horses. Equine Vet J 2006;39:22–8.
6. Collins N, Dixon PM. Diagnosis and management of equine diastemata. Clin Tech Equine Prac 2005;4:148–54.
7. Dacre IT. Equine dental pathology. In: Baker GJ, Easley KJ, editors. Equine dentistry. 2nd edition. London: WB Saunders; 2005. p. 91–109.
8. Dixon PM, Dacre IT. A review of equine dental disorders. Vet J 2005;169:165–87.
9. Dixon PM, Tremaine WH, McCann J, et al. Equine dental disease part 4: a long term study of 400 cases. Apical infections of cheek teeth. Equine Vet J 2000; 32:182–94.
10. Prichard MA, Hackett RP, Erb HN. Long-term outcome of tooth repulsion in horses a retrospective study of 61 cases. Vet Surg 1992;21:145–9.
11. Orsini PG, Ross MW, Hamir AN. Levator nasolabialis muscle transposition to prevent an orosinus fistula after tooth extraction in horses. Vet Surg 1992;21:150–6.
12. Tremaine WH, Dixon PM. Equine sinonasal disorders: a long-term study of 277 cases. Part II—treatment and long-term response to treatment. Equine Vet J 2001;33:283–9.
13. Tremaine HT, Lane JG. Exodontia. In: Baker GJ, Easley KJ, editors. Equine dentistry. 2nd edition. London: WB Saunders; 2005. p. 267–94.
14. Zaluski P, Davis MH. The use of dental picks for difficult extractions. In: Proceeding of American Association of Equine Practitioners, Focus on Dentistry. Indianapolis (IN): 2006. p. 322–4.
15. Barakzai SZ, Dixon PM. Sliding muco-periosteal hard palate flap for treatment of a persistent oro-nasal fistula. Equine Vet Educ 2005;17:287–91.
16. Smith MRW, Barakzai SZ, Lloyd D, et al. Diagnostic paranasal sinoscopy via a frontal sinus portal and ventral conchal bulla fenestration: clinical application in 13 horses with sinusitis. Proceedings, 44th Congress of the British Equine Veterinary Association, Harrogate, UK: 2005. p. 249.
17. Barakzai SZ, Kane-Smyth J, Lowles J, et al. Trephination of the equine rostral maxillary sinus: efficacy and safety of two trephine sites. Vet Surg 2008;37: 278–82.
18. Dixon PM, Dacre I, Dacre K, et al. Standing oral extraction of cheek teeth in 100 younger horses (1998–2003). Equine Vet J 2005;37:105–12.
19. Tremaine W.H. Oral extraction of equine cheek teeth, Equine Vet Educ 2004; 16:151–8.
20. Dixon PM. Dental extraction and endodontic techniques in horses. Comp Cont Educ Prac Vet 1997;19:628–39.
21. Auer JA. Management of cranio-maxillofacial fractures in the horse. Proceedings ECVS Annual Scientific Meeting, Basel: 2008. p. 57–61.
22. Evans LH, Tate LP, LaDow CS. Extraction of the equine 4th upper premolar and 1st and 2nd molars through a lateral buccotomy. Proc Am Assoc Equine Pract 1981;27:299–302.
23. Boussauw B. Indications and techniques for buccotomy. Proceedings of 42nd British Equine Veterinary Association Congress, Birmingham: 2003. p. 264.

24. Olivier A, Steenkamp G, Petrick SW, et al. Parotid duct laceration repair in two horses. Sth Afr Vet J 1998;69:108–11.
25. Schumacher J, Schumacher J. Diseases of the salivary glands and ducts of the horse. Equine Vet Educ 1995;7:313–9.
26. Newton SA, Knottenbelt DC, Daniel EA. Surgical repair of the parotid gland in a gelding. Vet Rec 1997;140:280–2.
27. Kannegieter NJ, Ecke P. Reconstruction of the parotid duct in a horse using an interposition polytetrafluoroethylene tube graft. Aust Vet J 1992;69:62–3.

Surgical Complications of Colic Surgery

Sarah Dukti, DVM*, Nathaniel White, DVM

KEYWORDS

• Horse • Colic • Laparotomy • Complications • Surgery

Colic is one of the most common and challenging problems that equine practitioners encounter. Although the majority of horses with colic can be treated with medical management, up to 10% of horses with colic require surgical intervention.[1] The decision for surgery is often straightforward based on historical and diagnostic information. However, some horses require further diagnostics and observation to determine if surgery is needed. Surgical intervention can be life saving. However, complications may arise during surgery, in the immediate postoperative period, or during long-term management, and often require further surgical intervention or medical management. This article addresses some of the more common surgical complications of abdominal surgery for colic to help prevent, recognize, and treat these complications.

INTRAOPERATIVE COMPLICATIONS

Complications that can occur during colic surgery include those related to anesthetics, abdominal distention, mesenteric or organ hemorrhage, mesenteric tearing, and intestinal rupture. Equine elective surgeries have an anesthetic-related death rate of 1 per 1250.[2] The risk of death attributed to equine general anesthesia has been reported to be 9.86 times greater in an emergency than for an elective surgical procedure. However, this number may be misleading because the study included horses euthanized during surgery because of a poor prognosis or financial concerns.[3] Nonetheless, general anesthesia carries an increased risk for emergency colic cases compared with that for elective surgeries.

Hypoxemia is the most common cause of cardiac arrest associated with anesthesia.[4] Abdominal distention may cause ventilatory problems leading to hypoxemia and should be addressed by aseptic needle decompression of distended portions of the gastrointestinal tract immediately upon opening the abdominal cavity. Care should be taken to minimize contamination by tunneling the needle through the serosa and submucosa and using gauzes soaked with a balanced electrolyte solution to

Department of Emergency Medicine and Surgery, Marion duPont Scott Equine Medical Center, Virginia-Maryland Regional College of Veterinary Medicine, P.O. Box 1938, Leesburg, VA 20177, USA
* Corresponding author.
E-mail address: sdukti@vt.edu (S. Dukti).

Vet Clin Equine 24 (2009) 515–534
doi:10.1016/j.cveq.2008.09.002
0749-0739/08/$ – see front matter © 2009 Elsevier Inc. All rights reserved.

vetequine.theclinics.com

prevent leakage from the puncture site (**Fig. 1**). Alternatively, a suture can be placed as the needle is withdrawn from the lumen of the bowel.

Anesthesia can also be complicated during reduction of intestinal strangulation when the blood trapped in the infarcted bowel is released into the general circulation. Acute decreases in blood pressure can occur. Treatment with heparin for experimental large colon strangulation was found to prevent the sudden drop in blood pressure and should be considered when large segments of intestine are released from a strangulation.[5]

Hemorrhage can occur during abdominal surgery as a result of either erosion of a strangulated vessel or of vessel rupture during the exploration of the abdomen or intestinal manipulation. Hemorrhage can occur at the epiploic foramen, an opening into the omental bursa from the peritoneal cavity. The epiploic foramen is bordered dorsally and dorsocranially by the caudate lobe of the liver, cranioventrally by the portal vein, and ventrally by the gastropancreatic fold.[6] Entrapment of the epiploic foramen has been reported for both the small intestine and large colon.[7–11] Fatal hemorrhage from the portal vein or, less commonly, the caudal vena cava has been reported during reduction of small-intestinal entrapment in the epiploic foramen.[7–9] The epiploic foramen is surgically inaccessible. Therefore repair cannot be attempted.[9] Other areas of hemorrhage that can occur during surgical exploration include mesenteric vessels (**Fig. 2**), enterotomy sites, and such organs as the liver or spleen.

Attempts should be made to locate any potential sources of hemorrhage. Primary repair of torn vessels may be attempted in select cases. However, ligation is often required. Mesenteric vessels that are incompletely ligated during intestinal resection can bleed immediately and often create a hematoma in the mesentery. Before abdominal closure, the mesentery and intestine at the site of anastomosis should be inspected for bleeding that may not have been apparent during the initial ligature placement. Vessels in the mesentery of the large colon are particularly susceptible to hemorrhage during or after ligation (**Fig. 3**). Careful dissection and double ligation of the vasculature in the colon is needed to prevent secondary hemorrhage. Hemorrhage from mesentery deep to the incision may be stopped temporarily by using intestinal staples to prevent further blood loss during the manipulation to expose the affected intestinal segment. Ligation of mesenteric vessels, if completed by staples, should also have a suture ligation to prevent hemorrhage if the staple should slip or release.

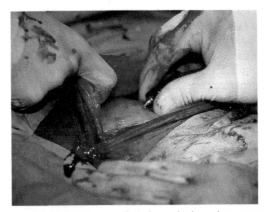

Fig. 1. Decompression using a needle tunneled through the submucosa while the cecum is still within the abdomen. Decompression relieves pressure on the diaphragm and helps to exteriorize the cecum and colon.

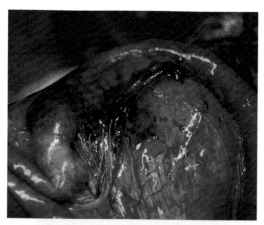

Fig. 2. Ruptured mesenteric vessel caused by incarceration of this small intestine within the epiploic foramen.

Generalized bleeding from the incision or intestine during surgery can indicate severe shock with disseminated intravascular coagulation. Oozing of the tissues at the abdominal incision, though rare, cannot be stopped by ligation of vessels and is generalized as a result of the coagulopathy. Immediate assessment of the horse's condition is needed because the prognosis for survival with this coagulopathy is poor.

Gastrointestinal rupture can be discovered or caused by the surgeon during colic surgery. In one retrospective study of 67 horses with peritonitis, none of the horses with gastrointestinal tract rupture survived (12 horses were euthanized and 2 died). Rupture sites included stomach (8 horses), large colon (3 horses), cecum (2 horses), and small colon (1 horse).[12] Gastrointestinal tract rupture may occur during correction of surgical lesion. If the rupture occurs outside of the abdominal cavity, care must be taken to prevent contamination of the abdominal cavity or incision (**Fig. 4**). The

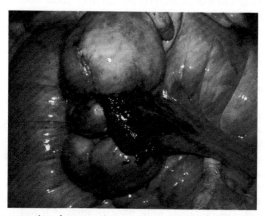

Fig. 3. After a colon resection, hemoperitoneum was evident and due to hemorrhage from the colonic vessels, which were ligated during surgery. Because of the numerous branching of the vasculature, bleeding may be possible even after multiple ligations of both veins and arteries. Care and inspection are required after releasing tension on the colon and mesentery to make sure bleeding does not occur.

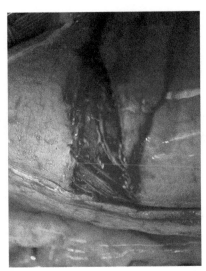

Fig. 4. A seromuscular tear caused by lifting the large colon distended with ingesta and fluid. The wall may also be friable because of the distension or ischemia. Suturing the defect is best accomplished after the colon is emptied to avoid more tearing by the suture.

ruptured segment of bowel should be isolated with drapes and the incision covered to prevent any leakage into the abdomen. Often the primary tear can be repaired. However, when tearing occurs in the large colon, enterotomy to empty the colon contents is often required to decrease the tension on the intestinal wall. Depending on the amount of contamination that occurs within the abdomen, lavage may be used at surgery to remove debris and bacteria. Because gross contamination may be spread throughout the abdomen with lavage at surgery, drain placement with lavage after surgery may be the best way to decrease the risk of generalized peritonitis. Alternatively, if the intestine is compromised, a resection should be completed to remove the damaged segment. If the amount of tension on the colon or cecal wall increases, the risk of rupture of the bowel during manipulation also increases. An enterotomy should be performed before removal of the entire colon or cecum from the abdomen. Enlargement of the incision may also be necessary to prevent increases in intraluminal pressure of bowel within the abdomen as the bowel is being removed from the abdomen.

POSTOPERATIVE COMPLICATIONS

Possible complications during the immediate postoperative period include incisional infection, evisceration, intra-abdominal hemorrhage, peritonitis, those associated with specific surgical procedures, obstruction from adhesions, and infarct/devitalization of tissue. Monitoring in the postoperative period is essential for early identification of these problems.

Incisional complications include peri-incisional edema, drainage, infection, suture sinus, and acute dehiscence.[13] Repeat laparotomy has been reported to increase the rate of incisional complications from 26% to 88%.[14] It has also been reported that the rate of incisional complication from abdominal exploration increases in acute abdominal disease when compared with that for horses undergoing primarily elective procedures. This study also found that incisions made in the muscular body wall had an increased rate of complication when compared with ventral midline celiotomies.[13]

Honnas and Cohen[15] found an increased risk of incisional complications associated with an enterotomy/resection. However, this has not been found in other studies.[14,16] Phillips and Walmsley[16] found an increased risk of incisional complications in horses with lesions involving the cecum or large colon and hypothesized that the weight of the colon at the surgical wound caused trauma. However, this has not been described in other reports.

Incisional Infection

Incisional infections present special problems, including increased risk of abdominal hernia. The incidence of incisional infection after ventral midline celiotomy for colic has been reported to range from 7.4% to 37%.[13–21] The relationship between development of incisional infections and the suture type and pattern used has been evaluated. Kobluk and colleagues[14] found an increased rate of incisional infection to be associated with a near-far-far-near suture versus a simple interrupted pattern. Honnas and Cohen[15] found an increased rate of incisional infection when polyglactin 910 was used for closure of the linea alba. Gibson and colleagues[22] found an increased rate of incisional hernia with chromic gut suture material. Bacterial culture at the time of incisional closure has not been beneficial in identifying incisional contaminates.[23] Mair and Smith[20] found a decreased rate of incisional infection when antibiotics were applied topically to the surgical wound at the time of closure, a finding that may warrant further investigation.

Many clinicians attempt to minimize contamination during the immediate postoperative period. Two studies have identified a decreased risk of incisional infection when an incise drape is applied to the surgical wound for recovery, though these drapes are easily dislodged during recovery.[14,23] Application of a stent bandage to the surgical wound for 3 days was found to increase the risk of incisional infection.[20] More recently, a study reported that application of an abdominal bandage post–exploratory laparotomy may help reduce the prevalence of incisional infection.[24] Currently, recommendations to decrease the risk of incisional infection include minimizing surgical time; ensuring that the surgical site is properly prepared, including adequate draping when an enterotomy is performed; and minimizing trauma to the surgical wound.[25] Although no one has clearly established a link between infection and suture material and pattern, closure should be performed with a minimally reactive suture material and overly large bites should be avoided to reduce the likelihood of excessive tension, which can lead to ischemia of the abdominal wall at the incision.[25] The optimal tissue bite size for adult horses has been reported to be 15 mm from the edge of the linea alba.[26]

If an incisional infection does occur, culture and sensitivity should be performed and drainage should be established. This may necessitate removal of skin and subcutaneous sutures. The use of local or systemic antimicrobials, while controversial, is often recommended if the horse is febrile after drainage has been established or if excessive edema or cellulitis is present at the surgical site.[25]

Incision Dehiscence

Acute dehiscence of an abdominal incision, though rare, is a potentially devastating complication after abdominal surgery. The reported rate of acute dehiscence following exploratory celiotomy has been reported to be less than 1% to 3%.[13,14,27] Stone and colleagues[27] found that an increased risk of dehiscence was associated with both an increased hematocrit in the first 12 hours postoperatively and an increased duration of surgery. The report suggested that interrupted appositional suture patterns were less likely than continuous patterns to dehisce.[27] However, continuous suture patterns in the linea alba have been shown to be stronger than interrupted sutures. Factors that may lead to incisional breakdown include abdominal distention, incisional trauma during surgery, recovery from general anesthesia or rolling postoperatively, and severe postoperative debility.[28] Disruption of the incision usually occurs in the first 3 to 8 days postoperatively and may be preceded by a brown serosanguinous discharge from the wound.[27] Bandaging or an abdominal girdle cannot prevent evisceration. Abdominal bandages applied to reduce risk of evisceration need to be checked frequently for opening of the incision and failure of the abdominal wall, which can progress rapidly.[27]

If dehiscence occurs, an abdominal bandage should be applied and the horse anesthetized to examine, decontaminate, and possibly repair the incision. If detected early with minimal bowel ischemia, superficial contamination can be removed with lavage and the intestine can be replaced in the abdomen. Surgical debridement of the incision should be completed to remove any necrotic or infected tissue. Closure requires full-thickness interrupted vertical mattress sutures using stainless steel wire (22 gauge) with stents approximately 2 to 3 cm apart and 5 cm from the wound edge for closure (**Fig. 5**).[27,29,30] The incision is brought into apposition and the skin left open for drainage and debridement during healing. If contamination has occurred, abdominal lavage should be completed at surgery and an abdominal catheter placed for subsequent lavage with the horse standing (see section on treatment of peritonitis).

Hemoperitoneum

Hemoperitoneum after surgery may be due to mesenteric bleeding from ligature failure or from the intestine at the enterotomy site. General anesthesia may decrease cardiac output and blood pressure, delaying onset of severe hemorrhage until recovery from anesthesia. In one report, life-threatening hemorrhage occurred in seven horses after enterotomy and anastomosis. These horses had incisions in the large colon (four had incisions at more than one site), suggesting that the large intestine may be more prone to incisional hemorrhage.[31] All seven horses had signs of acute hemorrhage, including tachycardia, pale mucous membranes, depression, muscle fasciculations, colic, and a severe decrease in packed cell volume. Medical therapy included 10% buffered formalin, intravenous fluid therapy, and whole blood transfusion. Two horses had repeat celiotomy. One horse at surgery had a bleeding artery that was identified and ligated at the site of the pelvic flexure enterotomy, while a second horse had a 25-cm blood clot

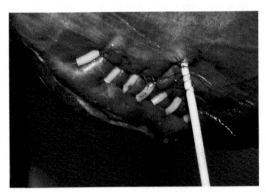

Fig. 5. Stainless steel wire tension sutures placed through the abdominal wall were used to close an abdominal incision that was dehiscing and necrotic. The wires can be adjusted to remove tension as the tissue swells and prevent the wires from cutting into the skin.

obstructing the lumen of the pelvic flexure. The clot was removed by a second enterotomy.[30]

Suture technique can play an important role in preventing hemorrhage at the enterotomy site. In a study comparing three techniques for closure of a pelvic flexure enterotomy, the full-thickness simple continuous pattern oversewn technique with a Cushing pattern was superior to other techniques because it apposed all layers and provided hemostasis.[32] Closure of the mucosa as a separate layer can result in hematoma formation between the mucosa and the submucosa.[32] In a retrospective study of horses with severe abdominal hemorrhage, all enterotomies were closed with a double inverting pattern, which theoretically might not have effectively occluded submucosal vessels.[31] If hemorrhage is suspected, aggressive medical therapy should be attempted, but surgical intervention may be required if the horse cannot be stabilized or a blood clot is occluding the lumen.

Transfusion, including intraoperative transfusion, may be necessary to keep up with blood loss. Autotransfusion can be completed by collecting blood from the abdomen and using the collected blood for transfusion. Because blood from the abdomen may be contaminated, such a transfusion should only be attempted if no other alternative is available.

Peritonitis

Peritonitis is a potential life-threatening complication of colic surgery [33] with a potential fatality rate of 30% to 67%.[12,34,35] Clinical signs of peritonitis include pyrexia, colic, weight loss, diarrhea, tachycardia, clinical evidence of dehydration, decreased borborygmi, and ileus.[12,35] Horses may have increased hyperechoic fluid identified with abdominal ultrasonography.[35] Diagnosis is made by abdominocentesis. Normal equine peritoneal fluid has a nucleated cell count of less than 5000 cells per microliter and a total protein of less than 2.5 g/dL. However, exploratory celiotomy in normal horses increases the nucleated cell count, total protein, percentage of neutrophils, and fibrinogen. Nucleated cell counts peak around day 4 at 200,000 cells per microliter and remain elevated at approximately 40,000 cells per microliter by day 6. The total protein reaches a peak around day 6 of approximately 6 g/dL.[36,37] This may complicate the diagnosis of peritonitis in the postoperative period.

Rodgers[38] reported that when evaluating peritoneal fluid, a serum/peritoneal glucose difference greater than 50 mg/dL or a pH less than 7.2 with glucose of less than 30 mg/dL is often found with septic peritonitis. Cytology should be performed to identify toxic or degenerative neutrophils or the presence of intracellular or extracellular bacteria to confirm septic peritonitis.[25] In 21 horses with septic peritonitis, Mair and colleagues[35] reported a case fatality rate of 57%. There was no association found between survival and hematologic values, serum chemistries, or cytology of peritoneal fluid. Hawkins and colleagues[12] reported a 60% case fatality in 67 horses with peritonitis. In this group, peritonitis after abdominal surgery resulted in higher mortality (56%) than peritonitis not associated with gastrointestinal rupture or surgery (43%). The other postoperative complications in nonsurvivors with peritonitis included incisional infection (10 horses), gastric reflux (9 horses), ileus (8 horses), diarrhea (7 horses), oral ulceration (5 horses), jugular thrombosis (3 horses), loose feces (2 horses), and laminitis (1 horse). Necropsy revealed fibrous adhesions in 8 of the 14 (57%) horses that did not survive. Hawkins and colleagues[12] found nonsurvivors had higher heart rates, red blood cell counts, creatinine levels, packed cell volumes, anion gaps, lower pH, and a greater number of bacterial species cultured from the peritoneal fluid. These horses were also more likely to exhibit signs of abdominal pain and circulatory shock, and to have a positive culture from the peritoneal sample.

Treatment for peritonitis must include stabilization of the patient and correction of the inciting cause if known. If a surgical complication, such as bowel necrosis or leakage from an anastomotic site, is suspected, exploratory celiotomy should be performed. Lavage at the time of surgery may be possible and an abdominal lavage system should be placed to allow for repeat peritoneal lavage after surgery to remove bacteria, foreign material, endotoxin, lysosomal enzymes, cellular debris, inflammatory mediators, fibrin, free fluid, and hemoglobin.[39] A 32F thoracic catheter or a Foley catheter is placed at the time of surgery distant (normally cranial to) the incision.[40] The drain is sutured and then wrapped in an abdominal bandage for recovery. Lavage consists of 10 to 20 L (20–40 mL/kg) of a balanced sterile electrolyte solution, such as lactated Ringer's solution, infused into the abdomen by gravity flow. The fluid is then immediately drained and the amount evacuated recorded. This is done once or twice daily. Normally, lavage is continued for no more than 3 days. The catheter can be left open for continual drainage but should be protected with a Heimlich valve or closed and kept as clean as possible between treatments. Abdominal drainage has also been shown to decrease abdominal adhesions.[40] It is theorized that lavage decreases adhesions by removing fibrin, inflammatory cells, and mediators from the abdomen and provides mechanical separation of the bowel loops.[40] Heparin may be added to the lavage solution or administered systemically (20–40 IU/kg) in an attempt to decrease peritoneal fibrin formation.[41] Open peritoneal drainage has also been suggested to treat horses with peritonitis as it has been used successfully in dogs and humans.[39,42,43] This may be possible as suggested by one study in horses that used temporary implantation of a permeable mesh within the abdominal wall permitting drainage of peritoneal fluid. However, the risk of mesh contamination and intestinal damage must be considered with this technique.[43] Horses should also receive broad-spectrum antimicrobial therapy effective against gram-positive, gram-negative, aerobic, and anaerobic bacteria and supportive therapy for dehydration, pain, and the potential for laminitis.[12]

Anastomosis Complications

Few reports have established the frequency or risk factors for intestinal anastomosis complications. In a study evaluating relaparatomy in 27 horses, problems involving an anastomosis were present in 9 cases (33%). These cases involved impaction at the anastomosis site (4 horses, 15%), intestinal kinking at the anastomosis (2 horses, 7.4%), and ischemia adjacent to the anastomosis site (3 horses, 11%).[44] Impaction at the anastomosis site may be due to the involution of excessive tissues during suturing, hematoma, ileus, stricture, or adhesion formation.[45] Further ischemia/necrosis may be due to inaccurate assessment of bowel viability at previous celiotomy, occlusion/kinking of vessels, or thrombus formation,[46] and can lead to anastomotic leakage or dehiscense (**Fig. 6**). Jejunojejunal intussusception has been reported at the site of functional end-to-end stapled anastomoses in 2 ponies, at a small intestinal transverse enterotomy site in ponies, and at the site of an end-to-end anastomosis in both a research horse and a clinical case.[47–50] Ileocecocolic intussusception has been reported as a complication of ileojejunocecostomy.[51] In general, repeat celiotomy is more often indicated in small-intestinal than in large-intestinal lesions.[45] Also, complications associated with the anastomosis are more often encountered in jejunocecostomies than jejunocecostomy.[17,19,52–54] More recently, it has been reported that an end-to-end jejunoileal anastomosis carries no greater risk than an end-to-end jejunojejunal anastomosis.[55] Horses treated for impaction of the small colon are at an increased risk of reimpaction of the small colon. Therefore, a pelvic flexure enterotomy should be performed at the first surgery to decrease this risk. However,

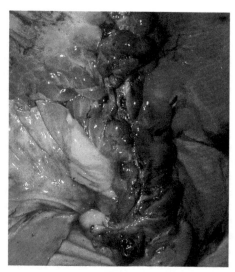

Fig. 6. Anastomosis leakage at the site of a large-colon resection. The colon appeared compromised and there was minimal sealing of the intestinal wall after surgery. The leakage caused fatal septic peritonitis and shock.

repeat celiotomy may be required if the impaction recurs.[56] Care in placing sutures to decrease tissue inversion and use of one suture line in the small intestine and two in the cecum or large colon is recommended to decrease anastomosis complications. When stricture due to unequal size of two bowel segments is anticipated, increasing the functional diameter of the smaller lumen can be accomplished by making an angled incision across the lumen to create equal length of tissue circumference (fish-mouth) for suturing. Increasing the size of a side-to-side stapled anastomosis can be completed by discharging the stapler in opposite directions along the bowel. While using this technique, care must be taken to ensure that both sides of the opening for introducing the gastrointestinal anastomosis stapler are properly closed as the staples may not always overlap.

Internal Hernia

Care should also be taken to close potential spaces within the abdomen that could cause internal herniation. For example, closing the mesenteric rent created during a jejunojejunostomy, the ileocecal fold during a jejunocecostomy, and any potential rents created during bypass surgery is recommended.[17,25] Defects in a recently closed mesentery are the most common causes of internal herniation. Usually, the small intestine becomes incarcerated and strangulated during herniation. Immediate relaparotomy is indicated if signs of pain or intestinal obstruction occur and persist after surgery as a mesenteric defect is a potential problem.

Intestinal Viability

Horses may also need a repeat celiotomy to reassess the viability of compromised bowel.[57,58] Most often this assessment is made by clinical observation. However, many techniques have been tried in the search for greater accuracy of assessment. Techniques that have been reported include clinical assessment, fluorescein dye, surface oximetry, Doppler ultrasonography, luminal pressure, and histopathology.[59–68]

Clinical assessment is based upon the color of the intestinal serosa and mucosa (if an enterotomy is performed or a resection completed), motility, and inability to rehydrate the surface with lavage solution.[59,62,63] Errors in clinical assessment occur. In one study, a population of research ponies was subjected to venous strangulation of the small intestine. Intestinal viability was assessed by clinical assessment, including color, wall thickness, motility, and pulse assessment. However, this study found that clinicians were only 54% accurate in predicting viability with a tendency of predicting nonviability when the intestine was able to recover. It was speculated that the clinicians were most often misled by edema and hemorrhage.[62]

One study compared clinical assessment to both fluorescein dye and Doppler ultrasonography in a small intestinal strangulation model. In this study, Doppler ultrasonography was the most accurate at 88% with clinical assessment and fluorescein dye found to both be 53% accurate. The fluorescein dye was found to be more accurate in determination of viability than nonviability.[62] Because edema and hemorrhage can prevent the fluorescence of bowel, this technique may predict nonviability even when the damage is not that severe.

Surface oximetry has also been explored as a technique to determine viability. A study was performed to determine normal surface oxygen partial pressure values for the pelvic flexure 55 ($\pm$ 13) mm Hg, jejunum 71 ($\pm$ 20) mm Hg, and ileum 61 ($\pm$ 8) mm Hg during general anesthesia for healthy horses.[64] These values have been used to assess colonic viability during large-colon volvulus in horses considered to have a nonviable large colon with values equal to or less the 20 mm Hg. Although this technique was found to be very accurate in predicting survival (88%), it was much less useful in predicting nonviability.[65]

Luminal pressure has also been used to evaluate intestinal viability in both small- and large-intestinal lesions. In one study evaluating the intraluminal pressure of horses with strangulating small-intestinal lesions, survivors were found to have a mean pressure of 6 cm H_2O and nonsurvivors had a mean pressure of 15 cm H_2O. Other studies have evaluated the intraluminal pressure of the large colon. One such study (set value 38 cm H_2O) was very accurate at predicting viability of the large colon (sensitivity 89%; specificity 91%).[66] A similar study evaluating horses with large-colon volvulus found intraluminal pressure (set point 38 cm H_2O) did not accurately predict survival. In horses that received correction of volvulus without resection, the sensitivity and specificity were 60% and 77%, respectively. In horses that had a resection, the sensitivity and specificity were 50% and 54%, respectively.[67]

Histology has been used to assess viability of the large colon by evaluating the percentage loss of surface epithelium, glandular epithelium, and the interstitium-to-crypt (I/C) ratio. Setting values for nonviability at 50% loss of glandular epithelium and I/C ratio greater than 3, clinicians were 94% accurate in predicting colonic viability.[68] These same researchers verified that colonic viability is relatively uniform across the entire region of strangulation.[69] During experimentally induced ischemia of the equine large colon, one study found the colon to be nonviable when the I/C was 3:1 with 95% loss of epithelium.[70]

Adhesions

Adhesions are a common complication of colic surgery, especially when horses have small-intestinal lesions. Ischemia-reperfusion and intraluminal distention cause serosal edema, leukocyte infiltration, and erythrocyte leakage leading to fibrin accumulation in the seromuscular layer of the small intestine, whereas the large-intestinal seromuscular layer does not develop the same severity of changes.[71,72] The rate of adhesion formation after small-intestinal surgery has been reported to be 6% to 26%, although these numbers may not reflect adhesions that do not become clinically relevant.[7,16,17,19,73,74] Adhesions are considered by some to be more common in foals and this has been supported in one research study. However, another study reporting on juvenile Thoroughbreds found the overall occurrence to be 8%, which is similar to reports in adult horses.[75,76] Foals between the ages of 15 days and 6 months were more likely than weanlings or yearlings to develop adhesions requiring surgical intervention.[75] Proper surgical technique, including gentle tissue handling, removal of damaged tissue, adequate hemostasis, and frequent lavage to keep the bowel moist, should be used to minimize adhesion formation.[25] The use of broad-spectrum antimicrobials, nonsteroidal anti-inflammatory drugs, and dimethyl sulfoxide has been shown to be effective in experimental studies to reduce adhesion formation.[77,78] After experimental ischemia-reperfusion of the small intestine in foals, gross adhesions were prevented by treatment with a combination of gentamicin and flunixin meglumine or by systemic administration of dimethyl sulfoxide. Gross adhesions were not prevented in foals treated with systemic heparin or intra-abdominal sodium carboxymethylcellulose (3%).[79] In contrast with these results, experimentally induced adhesions from intestinal ischemia were decreased in ponies by treatment with systemic heparin.[80] Furthermore, other experimental studies have reported that intraperitoneal 1% carboxymethylcellulose reduces the incidence of adhesions in adult horses by theoretically reducing trauma, acting as a lubricant, and acting as a mechanical barrier.[81–83] In another study, experimentally induced adhesions in ponies were decreased using a 0.4% sodium hyaluronate solution, whereas carboxymethylcellulose was not effective.[84] Other studies using an hyaluronate-carboxymethylcellulose membrane successfully decreased adhesions in both experimental trauma and at anastomosis sites.[85–87] This film applied to the anastomosis site has not been evaluated clinically but is recommended for use in the small intestine.

Carolina rinse, a tissue perfusate tested for organ transplant, has been shown to decrease reperfusion injury, migration of neutrophils into serosa, scarring, and fibroblast proliferation, which may decrease the incidence of adhesions. The authors recommend that it be applied topically and intraluminally rather than by direct injection as a perfusate into mesenteric arteries.[88–90] Currently this product is not manufactured but can be made from readily available compounds (**Box 1**).

Abdominal lavage is often used in an attempt to decrease adhesion formation. This may be done at surgery or through a passive or closed suction drain in the postoperative period. Although instillation of fluids may not be effective in reducing the formation of adhesions, the use of peritoneal lavage to remove fibrin and inflammatory mediators while mechanically separating bowel may be more effective.[91–93] Postoperative peritoneal lavage has been shown experimentally to decrease the frequency of adhesion formation.[92]

Omentectomy is another technique employed to reduce the frequency of adhesions. A retrospective study of 44 horses showed that omentectomy reduced the frequency of adhesion formation.[94] Despite proper surgical technique and use of many of the above therapeutics, adhesions are still a complication of colic surgery.

Horses that develop clinically apparent adhesions usually present with colic. Enterotomy and anastomosis sites are the most commonly involved with adhesions and mesenteric scarring. Adhesions and excessive scar formation cause strictures, intestinal kinks, and stricture of the blood vessels in affected mesentery. The result can be simple obstruction or local strangulation as the scar compresses the blood supply. These adhesions can cause chronic intermittent colic or acute obstruction. In some

---

Box 1
Carolina rinse solution G protocol

Glassware and equipment

    1-L graduated beaker

    1-L volumetric flask

    1-L autoclaved bottle

    0.2-μm bottle filter

    Stir bar

Components for 1-L solution

    1000-mL distilled deionized H_2O

    115-mM NaCl: 6.7 g/L

    5-mM KCl: 0.37 g

    1.30-mM $CaCl_2*2H_2O$: 0.19 g

    1-mM KH_2PO_4: 0.14 g

    1.2-mM $MgSO_4*7H_2O$: 0.30 g

    1-mM allopurinol: 0.14 g

    1-mM deferoxamine mesylate: 0.65 g

    3-mM glutathione: 0.92 g

    2-μM nicardipine: 1.02 mg

    200-μM adenosine: 0.065 g

    10-mM fructose: 1.8 g

    10-mM glucose: 1.8 g

    100-U/L insulin: 1 mL of 100 U/mL

    20-mM morpholinopanesulfonate: 4.2 g

    5-mM glycine: 0.37 g

Procedure

Put approximately 900 mL of distilled deionized H_2O in a 1-L beaker and stir. Then add each of the remaining components one at a time. Allopurinol can be dissolved in 1 mL of 1-N NaOH prior to addition. After all components are added, adjust the pH to 6.5 with 5-N NaOH. Transfer the solution to a 1-L volumetric flask and bring to a final volume of 1 L with distilled deionized H_2O.

Storage and glutathione addition

The solution can be stored at 4°C. However, in preparing solution for storage, glutathione should be omitted and then added just before use. This can be done by making 1 to 2 mL of a 3-M solution of reduced glutathione in distilled deionized H_2O. The solution can be sterile filtered through a 0.2-μm syringe filter. Using a sterile syringe, 1 mL of the sterile 3-M glutathione solution can be injected into the 1-L bottle of Carolina rinse solution yielding a final concentration of 3 mM.

To sterilize

The solution is sterile filtered through a 0.2-μm bottle filter into a sterile bottle.

cases, altering the diet to low bulk with pellets or soft forage can prevent colic, though the diet change may need to be permanent for the life of the horse.

The decision to explore the abdomen should be based on history and diagnostic findings. If surgery is called for, either bypass or removal of adhesions will be necessary. If the size of the adhesion mass is too large or cannot be removed because it cannot be elevated to the incision, bypass may be the least traumatic option with less adhesion formation postoperatively. Alternatively, removal of the adhesions is recommended if there is inflamed tissue, which will likely cause more adhesions in the future.

An alternative to celiotomy is a use of laparoscopy 7 to 10 days postoperatively to identify and possibly break down adhesions.[95,96] Diagnosis with laparoscopy has been shown to have a sensitivity of 82% and specificity of 66% in acute colic and 63% sensitivity and 33% specificity in chronic colic.[97] Use of laparoscopy is limited, depending on the position of adhesions or region of scarring as well as the position of the horse, standing or recumbent.

Recurrent Colic and Repeat Laparotomy

Numerous epidemiologic studies indicate that horses with colic are more likely to develop episodes of colic again and horses that have had colic surgery are more likely to have repeat episodes of colic.[18,98,99] Horses with displacement or volvulus of the large colon are at an increased risk of recurrence. Horses with large-colon volvulus have been reported to have a 5% to 8% chance of recurrence.[100,101] Reported recurrence rates of nephrosplenic entrapment are 7.5% to 8.5%.[102,103] The recurrence rate for either large-colon volvulus or displacement after one episode has been reported to be 15%.[104] Techniques recommended to prevent recurrence include large-colon resection, colopexy, or obliteration of the nephrosplenic space by either a flank lapartomy or laparoscopic approach.[104–120] These techniques are often best completed as an elective procedure if the intestine is compromised or anesthesia time is prolonged.

Survival rates after repeat celiotomy completed shortly after the initial surgery for a complication were reported to be from 36% to 56%. Long-term survival was reported as low as 20%.[6,7,17,33,44,45,57,58] In a recent study evaluating 300 horses undergoing surgical treatment of colic, relaparotomy was required in 10.6%. Short-term survival after relaparotomy was 50%. However, 40% of the horses requiring relaparotomy had episodes of colic necessitating additional surgery and long-term survival was found to be 22%.[44]

Incisional Hernia

The incidence of incisional hernia after ventral midline celiotomy in horses has been reported to range from 5.7% to 18%.[13–15,23,121] Studies have also reported that the risk of incisional hernia increases with relaparotomy. One study evaluating 142 horses reported an incisional hernia rate of 5.7% after one surgery and 12.5% after a second surgery.[14] Another study evaluating 300 horses undergoing colic surgery reported an incisional hernia rate of 8% with one surgery increasing to 25% after relapartomy.[44] Studies have found that incisional hernia is most often preceded by an incisional infection.[13,22,23] One study evaluating culture at the time of closure found the risk of incisional hernia to be 62.5 times greater when an incisional infection was present.[23] Another study found factors significantly associated with development of incisional hernias included incisional drainage, chromic gut (linea alba closure), previous ventral midline celiotomy, incisional edema, leukopenia postoperatively, and postoperative pain.[22] This study also reported that 20% of horses that develop incisional hernias have multiple smaller hernias along the incision.[22] Small hernias may not require surgical intervention and should be managed conservatively. However, if the hernia is large and pendulous or enlarges after turn out or exercise, repair is recommended.[29]

Ultrasound may be useful in the evaluation of the hernia. Adhesion of intestine to the hernial sac can complicate surgery and should be identified before surgery to avoid inadvertent incision into the bowel lumen. If surgical repair is required it should not be attempted until complete resolution of the incisional infection. Adequate time for maturation of the hernia ring and separated abdominal wall is required for adequate tissue strength for sutures. A minimum of 3 months is considered necessary after the initial surgery or when infection has been controlled.

Small hernias may be repaired primarily using a near-far-far-near or continuous suture pattern. Repair of large hernias requires diet modification to take tension off the abdominal wall at the time of the repair. If the abdominal wall can be apposed at surgery double-crossing continuous sutures placed by two surgeons helps to appose the abdominal wall and provides the strength needed for recovery (**Fig. 7**). If the abdominal wall cannot be apposed, the hernia should be repaired using a synthetic mesh and fascial overlay with a horizontal or vertical mattress suture.[25,29] Both polypropylene (Marlex, Davol, Cranston, Rhode Island) and plastic (Proxplast, Goshen Laboratories, Goshen, New York) mesh have been used for hernia repair.[25] Though the mesh can be successfully placed for hernia repair, problems with infection or rejection of the mesh can be serious and, therefore, use of mesh should avoided if possible.

Another option when the incision is still healing is the use of a postsurgical abdominal wrap (CM Heal, CM Equine Product, Norco, California), which has anecdotally been reported to allow healing of incisional hernias without surgery.[25] Abdominal support by bands or girdles should be fitted carefully to provide support while not causing sores on the back. These girdles often need to be used for 2 to 3 months for the full effect during healing of the incision.

This article has summarized some of the most common complications identified both during and after colic surgery that may require surgical intervention. Other medical complications may arise. However, for the most likely surgical complications that may be encountered, this article serves as a reference.

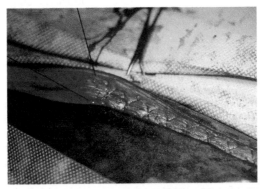

Fig. 7. Suturing of an incision using two strands of suture, each placed independently from opposite sides of the incision by two surgeons. The sutures cross as they are placed. The advantage of this pattern includes constant tension on the incision during the closure and the use of two sutures to ensure adequate holding in the tissue.

REFERENCES

1. Hillyer MH, Taylor FGR, French NP. A cross-sectional study of colic in horses on Thoroughbred training premises in the British Isles in 1997. Equine Vet J 2002; 33:380–5.
2. Mee AM, Cripps PJ, Jones RS. A retrospective study of mortality associated with general anaesthesia in horses: elective procedures. Vet Rec 1998;142:275.
3. Mee AM, Cripps PJ, Jones RS. A retrospective study of mortality associated with general anaesthesia in horse: emergency procedures. Vet Rec 1998;142:307.
4. Valverde A. Advances in inhalation anesthesia. In: Auer JA, Stick JA, editors. Equine surgery. 3rd edition. St Louis (MO): Saunders Elsevier; 2006. p. 219.
5. Provost MS, Stick JA, Patterson JS, et al. Effects of heparin treatment on colonic torsion-associated hemodynamic and plasma eicosanoid changes in anesthetized ponies. Am J Vet Res 1991;52(2):289–96.
6. Schmid A. Die Anatomie des Foramen epiploicum und seiner benachbarten Strukturen und diet Auswirkungen von Alter, Rasse und Geschlecht auf Darmstrangulation durch das Foramen epiploicum, Inguinalhernie, Lipoma pendulans und Invagination, Med Vet Thesis, Ludwig-Maximilians-Universitat, Munich; 1997.
7. Vachon AM, Fischer AT. Small-intestinal herniation through the epiploic foramen: 53 cases (1987–1993). Equine Vet J 1995;27(5):373.
8. Vasey JR. Incarceration of the small intestine by the epiploic foramen in fifteen horses. Can Vet J 1988;29:378.
9. Livesey MA, Little CB, Boyd C. Fatal hemorrhage associated with incarceration of small intestine by the epiploic foramen in three horses. Can Vet J 1991;32:434.
10. Freeman DE, Schaeffer DJ. Short-term survival after surgery for epiploic foramen entrapment compared with other strangulating diseases of the small intestine in horses. Equine Vet J 2005;37(4):292–5.
11. Forener JJ, Ringle MJ, Junkins DS, et al. Transection of the pelvic flexure to reduce incarceration of the large colon through the epiploic foramen in a horse. J Am Vet Med Assoc 1993;203:1312.
12. Hawkins JF, Bowman KF, Roberts MC, et al. Peritonitis in horses: 67 cases (1985–1990). J Am Vet Med Assoc 1993;203(2):284–8.
13. Wilson DA, Baker GJ, Boero MJ. Complications of celiotomy incisions in horses. Vet Surg 1995;24:506–14.
14. Kobluk CN, Ducharme NG, Lumsden JH, et al. Factors affecting incisional complication rates associated with colic surgery in horses: 78 cases (1983–1985). J Am Vet Med Assoc 1989;195:639.
15. Honnas CM, Cohen ND. Risk factors for wound infection following celiotomy in horses. J Am Vet Med Assoc 1997;210:78.
16. Phillips TJ, Walmsley JP. Retrospective analysis of the results of 151 exploratory laparotomies in horses with gastrointestinal disease. Equine Vet J 1993; 25(5):427.
17. Freeman DE, Hammock P, Baker GJ, et al. Short- and long-term survival and prevalence of post operative ileus after small intestinal surgery in the horse. Equine Vet J 2000;32(Suppl):42–51.
18. Proudman CJ, Smith JE, Edwards GB, et al. Long-term survival of equine surgical colic cases. Part 1: patterns of mortality and morbidity. Equine Vet J 2002;34: 432–7.
19. MacDonald MH, Pascoe JR, Stover SM, et al. Survival after small intestinal resection and anastomosis in horses. Vet Surg 1989;18:415–23.

20. Mair TS, Smith LF. Survival and complication rates in 300 horses undergoing surgical treatment of colic. Part 2: short-term complications. Equine Vet J 2005; 37(4):303–9.

21. Galuppo LD, Pascoe JR, Jang SS, et al. Evaluation of iodophor skin preparation techniques and factors influencing drainage from ventral midline incisions in horses. J Am Vet Med Assoc 1999;215:963–9.

22. Gibson KT, Curtis CR, Turner AS. Incisional hernias in the horse incidence and predisposing factors Vet Surgery 1989;18(5):360–6.

23. Ingle-Fehr JE, Baxter GM, Howard RD, et al. Bacterial culturing of ventral median celiotomies for prediction of postoperative incisional complications in horses. Vet Surg 1997;16:7–13.

24. Smith LJ, Mellor DJ, Marr CM, et al. Incisional complications following exploratory celiotomy: Does an abdominal bandage reduce the risk? Equine Vet J 2007;39(3):277–83.

25. Hardy J, Rakestraw PC. Postoperative care and complications associated with abdominal surgery. In: Auer JA, Stick JA, editors. Equine surgery. 3rd edition. St Louis (MO): Saunders Elsevier; 2006. p. 506–9.

26. Trostle SS, Wilson DG, Stone WC, et al. A study of the biomechanical properties of the adult equine linea alba: relationship of tissue bite size and suture material to breaking strength. Vet Surg 1994;23:435–41.

27. Stone WC, Lindsay WA, Mason ED, et al. Factors associated with acute wound dehiscence following equine abdominal surgery. Proceedings 4th Eq Colic Res Sym 1991. p. 52.

28. Tulleners EP. Incisional hernias with acute total dehiscence. In: Colahan PT, Merritt AM, Moore JN, et al, editors. Equine medicine and surgery. 5th edition. St Louis (MO): Mosby; 1999. p. 811.

29. Stick JA. Abdominal hernias. In: Auer JA, Stick JA, editors. Equine surgery. 3rd edition. St Louis (MO): Saunders Elsevier; 2006. p. 495.

30. Tulleners EP, Donawick WJ. Secondary closure of infected abdominal incisions in cattle and horses. J Am Vet Med Assoc 1983;182(12):1377–9.

31. Doyle AJ, Freeman DE, Rapp H, et al. Life-threatening hemorrhage from enterotomies and anastomoses in 7 horses. Vet Surg 2003;32:553–8.

32. Young RL, Snyder JR, Pascoe JR, et al. A comparison of three techniques for closure of pelvic flexure enterotomies in normal equine colon. Vet Surg 1991; 20:185–9.

33. Morton AJ, Blikslager AT. Surgical and postoperative factors influencing short-term survival of horses following small intestinal resection: 92 cases (1994–2001). Equine Vet J 2002;34(5):450–4.

34. Dyson S. Review of 30 cases of peritonitis in the horse. Equine Vet J 1983;15: 25–30.

35. Mair TS, Hillyer MH, Taylor FR. Peritonitis in adult horses: a review of 21 cases. Vet Rec 1990;126:567–70.

36. Dabareiner RM. Peritonitis in horses. In: Smith BP, editor. Large animal internal medicine. St Louis (MO): Mosby; 1996.

37. Santshi EM, Grindem CB, Tate LP. Peritoneal fluid analysis in ponies after abdominal surgery. Vet Surg 1988;17:6.

38. Rodgers L. Evaluation of peritoneal pH, glucose, and lactate dehydrogenase levels as an indicator of intra-abdominal sepsis. Proc Am Coll Vet Intern Med 1994;12:173.

39. Maetani S, Tobe T. Open peritoneal drainage as effective treatment for advanced peritonitis. Surgery 1981;90:804–9.

40. Hague BA, Honnas CM, Berridge BR, et al. Evaluation of postoperative peritoneal lavage in standing horses for prevention of experimentally induced abdominal adhesions. Vet Surg 1998;27:122–6.
41. Madaus M, Ahrenholz D, Simmons RL. The biology of peritonitis and implications for treatment. Surg Clin North Am 1988;68:431.
42. Woolfson JM, Dulisch ML. Open peritoneal drainage in the treatment of generalized peritonitis in 25 dogs and cats. Vet Surg 1986;15:27–32.
43. Chase JP, Beard WL, Bertone AL. Open peritoneal drainage in horses with experimentally induced peritonitis. Vet Surg 1996;25:189–94.
44. Mair TS, Smith LJ. Survival and complication rates in 300 horses undergoing surgical treatment of colic. Part 4: early (acute) relaparotomy. Equine Vet J 2005; 37(4):315–8.
45. Hainisch EK, Proudman CJ, Edwards GB. Indications, surgical intervention and outcome of relaparotomy in 27 cases. In: Proceedings of the European College of Veterinary Surgeons Annual Symposium, Glasgow, Scotland; 2003. p. 224.
46. Gerard MP, Bowman KF, Blikslager AT, et al. Jejunocolostomy or ileocolostomy for treatment of cecal impaction in horses: nine cases (1985–1995). J Am Vet Med Assoc 1996;209:1287.
47. Frankeny RL, Wilson DA, Messer NT, et al. Jejunal intussusception: a complication of functional end-end stapled anastomoses in two ponies. Vet Surg 1995;24: 515–7.
48. Lowe JE. Intussusception in three ponies following experimental enterotomy. Cornell Vet 1968;58:288.
49. Dean PW, Robertson JT, Jacobs RM. Comparison of suture materials and suture patterns for inverting intestinal anastomosis of the jejunum in the horse. Am J Vet Res 1985;46:2072–7.
50. Boswell JC, Schramme MC, Gains M. Jejunojejunal intussusception after an end-to end jejunojejunal anastamosis in a horse. Equine Vet Educ 2000;12(6): 303–6.
51. Schumacher J, Hanrahan L. Ileocecocolic intussusception as a sequel to jejunocecostomy in a mare. J Am Vet Med Assoc 1987;190(3):303–4.
52. Kersjes AW, Bras GE, Nemeth F, et al. Results of operative treatment of equine colic with special reference to surgery of the ileum. Vet Quart 1988;10:17–25.
53. Freeman DE. Surgery of the small intestine. Vet Clin N Am Equine Pract 1997; 13:261–301.
54. van den Boom R, van der Velden MA. Short- and long-term evaluation of surgical treatment of strangulating obstructions of the small intestine in horses: a review of 224 cases. Vet Quart 2001;23:109–15.
55. Rendle DI, Wood JL, Summerhays GES. End-to-end jejuno-ileal anastomosis following resection of strangulated small intestine in horses: a comparative study. Equine Vet J 2005;37(4):356–9.
56. Schumacher J, Mair T. Small colon obstruction in the mature horse. Equine Vet Educ 2002;68:27.
57. Huskamp B, Bonfig H. Relaparotomy as a therapeutic principle in postoperative complication of horses with colic. In: Proceedings of the 2nd Equine Colic Research Symposium, University of Georgia; 1985. p. 317–21.
58. Parker JE, Fubini SL, Todhunter RJ. Retrospective evaluation of repeat celiotomy in 53 horses with acute gastrointestinal disease. Vet Surg 1989;18:424–31.
59. Fischer AT. Colic: diagnosis, preoperative management, and surgical approaches. In: Auer JA, Stick JA, editors. Equine surgery. 3rd edition. St Louis (MO): Saunders Elsevier; 2006. p. 398–400.

60. Allen DJ, White NA, Tyler DE. Factors for prognostic use in equine obstructive small intestinal disease. J Am Vet Med Assoc 1986;189:777–80.

61. Snyder JR, Pascoe JR, Olander HF, et al. Vascular injury associated with naturally occurring strangulating obstructions of the equine large colon. Vet Surg 1990;19:446–55.

62. Freeman DE, Gentile DG, Richardon DW, et al. Comparison of clinical judgement, Doppler ultrasound, and fluorescein fluorescence as methods for predicting intestinal viability in the pony. Am J Vet Res 1988;49:895–900.

63. Sullins KE. Deterimination of intestinal viability and the decision to resect. In: White NA, Moore JN, editors. The equine acute abdomen. 1st edition. Philadelphia: WB Saunders; 1990.

64. Snyder JR, Pascoe JR Holland M, et al. Surface oximetry of healthy and ischemic equine intestine. Am J Vet Res 1986;47:2530–5.

65. Snyder JR, Pascoe JR, Meagher DM, et al. Surface oximetry for intraoperative assessment of colonic viability in horses. J Am Vet Med Assoc 1994;204:1786–9.

66. Moore RM, Hance SR, Hardy J, et al. Colonic luminal pressure in horses with strangulating and nonstrangulating obstruction of the large colon. Vet Surg 1996;25:134–41.

67. Mathis SC, Slone ED, Lynch TM, et al. Use of colonic luminal pressure to predict outcome after surgical treatment of strangulating large colon volvulus in horses. Vet Surg 2006;35(4):356–60.

68. Van Hoogmoed L, Snyder JR, Pascoe JR, et al. Use of pelvic flexure biopsies to predict survival after large colon torsion in horses. Vet Surg 2000;29:572–7.

69. Van Hoogmoed L, Snyder JR, Pascoe JR, et al. Evaluation of uniformity of morphological injury of the large colon following severe colonic torsion. Equine Vet J Suppl 2000;32:98–100.

70. Snyder JR, Olander HJ, Pascoe JR, et al. Morhphologic alterations observed during experimental ischemia of the equine large colon. Am J Vet Res 1988; 49(6):801–9.

71. Dabareiner RM, Sullins KE, White NA, et al. Serosal injury in the equine jejunum and ascending colon after ischemia-reperfusion or intraluminal distention and decompression. Vet Surg 2001;30:114.

72. Dabareiner RM, White NA, Donaldson LL. Effects of intraluminal distention and decompression on microvascular permeability and hemodynamics of the equine jejunum. Am J Vet Res 2001;62:225.

73. Freeman DE. Small intestine. In: Auer JA, Stick JA, editors. Equine surgery. 3rd edition. St Louis (MO): Saunders Elsevier; 2006. p. 428.

74. Baxter GM, Broome TE, Moore JN. Abdominal adhesions after small intestinal surgery in the horse. Vet Surg 1989;18:409.

75. Santschi EM, Slone DE, Embertson RM, et al. Colic surgery in 206 juvenile thoroughbreds: survival and racing results. Equine Vet J Suppl 2000;32:32.

76. Trevor PB, White NA, Sullins KE. Use of sodium hyaluronate to prevent adhesions in the horse and rabbit. Equine Colic Research Symposium 1991 [abstract].

77. Sullins KE, White NA, Lundin CS. Treatment of ischemia induced peritoneal adhesions in foals. Vet Surg 1991;20(5):348.

78. Freeman DE, Cimprich RE, Richardson DW, et al. Early mucosal healing and chronic changes in pony jejunum after various types of strangulation obstruction. Am J Vet Res 1988;49:810.

79. Sullins KE, White NA, Lundin CS, et al. Prevention of ischaemia-induced small intestinal adhesions in foals. Equine Vet J 2004;36:370.

80. Parker JE, Fubini SL, Car B. Prevention of intraabdominal adhesions in ponies by low-dose heparin therapy. Vet Surg 1987;16:459.
81. Moll HD, Shumacher J, Wright JC, et al. Evaluation of sodium carboxymethylcellulose for prevention of experimentally induced abdominal adhesions in ponies. Am J Vet Res 1991;42:88.
82. Murphy DJ, Peck LS, Detrisa CJ, et al. Use of a high-molecular-weight carboxymethylcellulose in a tissue protective solution for prevention of post operative abdominal adhesions in ponies. Am J Vet Res 2002;63:1448.
83. Hay WP, Mueller PO, Harmon B, et al. One percent sodium carboxymethylcellulose prevents experimentally induced abdominal adhesions in horses. Vet Surg 2001;30:223.
84. Eggleston RB, Mueller PO, Parviainen AK, et al. Effect of carboxymethylcellulose and hyaluronate solutions on jejunal healing in horses. Am J Vet Res 2004;65:637.
85. Mueller PO, Harmon BG, Hay WP, et al. Effect of carboxymethylcellulose and a hyaluronate-carboxymethylcellulose membrane on healing of intestinal anastomoses in horses. Am J Vet Res 2000;61:369.
86. Mueller PO, Hay WP, Harmon B, et al. Evaluation of a biosorbable hyaluronate-carboxymethylcellulose membrane for prevention of experimentally induced abdominal adhesions in horses. Vet Surg 2000;29:48.
87. Eggleston RB, Mueller E. Quandt JE, et al. Use of a hyaluronate membrane for jejunal anastomosis in horses. Am J Vet Res 2001;62:1314.
88. Dabareiner RM, White NA, Lemasters JJ. Effect of a reperfusion solution, "Carolina rinse," on intestinal vascular permeability and blood flow after jejunal ischemia and reperfusion in the horse. Vet Surg 1994;23(5):399.
89. Young BL, White NA, Donaldson LL, et al. Treatment of ischaemic jejunum with topical and intraluminal Carolina rinse. Equine Vet J 2002;34(5):469–74.
90. Dabareiner RM, White NA, Donaldson L. Evaluation of Carolina rinse solution as a treatment for ischaemia reperfusion of the equine jejunum. Equine Vet J 2003; 35(7):642–6.
91. Dunn DL, Barke RA, Ahrenholz DH. The adjuvant effect of peritoneal fluid in experimental peritonitis. Ann Surg 1984;199:37.
92. Hague BA, Honnas CM, Berridge BR, et al. Evaluation of standing postoperative peritoneal lavage for prevention of experimentally induced abdominal adhesions in horses. Vet Surg 1994;27:122–236.
93. Nieto JE, Snyder JR, Vatistas NJ, et al. Use of an active intra-abdominal drain in 67 horses. Vet Surg 2003;32:1.
94. Kuebelbec KL, Slone DE, May KA. Effect of omentectomy on adhesion formation in horses. Vet Surg 1998;27:132–7.
95. Boure LP, Pearce SG, Kerr CL, et al. Evaluation of laparoscopic adhesiolysis for the treatment of experimentally induced adhesions in pony foals. Am J Vet Res 2002;63(2):289–94.
96. Lansdowne JL, Boure LP, Pearce SG, et al. Comparison of two laparoscopic treatments for experimentally induced abdominal adhesions in pony foals. Am J Vet Res 2004;65(5):681–6.
97. Walmsley JP. Review of equine laparoscopy and an analysis of 148 laparoscopies in the horse. Equine Vet J 1999;31:456.
98. Tinker MK, White NA, Lessard P, et al. A prospective study of equine colic incidence, risk factors, and mortality rates. Equine Vet J 1997;29:448–53.
99. Cohen ND, Matejka PL, Honnas CM, et al. Case-control study of the association between various management factors and development of colic in horses. J Am Vet Med Assoc 1995;206:667–73.

100. Harrison IW. Equine large intestinal volvulus: a review of 124 cases. Vet Surg 1998;17:77–81.
101. Barclay WP, Foerner JJ, Phillips TN. Volvulus of the large colon in the horse. J Am Vet Med Assoc 1980;177:629–30.
102. Hardy J, Minton M, Robertson JT, et al. Nephrosplenic entrapment in the horse: a retrospective study of 174 cases. Equine Vet J Suppl 2000;32:95.
103. Baird AN, Cohen ND, Taylor TS, et al. Renosplenic entrapment of the large colon in horses: 57 cases (1983–1988). J Am Vet Med Assoc 1991;198:1423.
104. Hance SR, Embertson RM. Colopexy in broodmares: 44 cases(1986–1990). J Am Vet Med Assoc 1992;201(5):782–7.
105. Herthel DJ, Boles CL, Rick MC, et al. Partial large colon resection in the mare. Proc Am Assoc Equine Pract 1985;6(31):487–91.
106. Huskamp B, Kopf N. Die verlagerung des colon ascenden in den milznieren-raum beim pferd (2). Rierarztl Prax 1980;8:495–506.
107. Markel MD, Ford TS, Meagher DM. Colopexy of the left large colon to the right large colon in the horse. Vet Surg 1985;14:407–13.
108. Markel MD, Meagher DM, Richardson DW. Colopexy of the large colon in four horses. J Am Vet Med Assoc 1988;192:358–9.
109. Markel MD, Dreyfuss DJ, Meagher DM. Colopexy of the equine large colon: comparison of two techniques. J Am Vet Med Assoc 1988;192:354–7.
110. Markel MD, Richardson DW, Meagher DM, et al. Colopexy of the equine large colon: experimental and clinical results. Proc Am Assoc Equine Pract 1989; 34:45–52.
111. Markel MD. Prevention of large colon displacements and volvulus. Vet Clin N Am Equine Pract 1989;4:395–405.
112. Embertson RM, Hance SR. Effects of colopexy in the broodmare. Proc Am Assoc Equine Pract 1991;36:531–2.
113. Aright M, Ducharme NG, Horney FD, et al. Extensive large colon resection in 12 horses. Can Vet J 1987;28:245.
114. Bertone AL, Stashak TS, Sullins KE. Large colon resection and anastomosis in horses. J Am Vet Med Assoc 1986;188:612.
115. Boening K, von Saldern F. Resection of the left large colon in horses. In: Proceedings of the Second Colic Research Symposium; 1986. p. 337.
116. Ducharme NG, Burton JH, van Dreumel AA, et al. Extensive large colon resection in the pony. II. Digestibility studies and postmortem findings. Can J Vet Res 1987;51:76.
117. Ducharme NG, Horney FD, Baird JE, et al. Extensive large colon resection in the pony: I. surgical procedures and clinical results. Can J Vet Res 1987;51:66.
118. Marien T, Adriaenssen A, Hoeck FV, et al. Laparoscopic closure of the renosplenic space in standing horses. Vet Surg 2001;30:559.
119. Zekas LJ, Ramirez S, Brown MP. Ablation of the nephrosplenic space for treatment of recurring left dorsal displacement of the large colon in a racehorse. J Am Vet Med Assoc 1999;214:1361.
120. Epstein KL, Parente EJ. Laparoscopic obliteration of the nephrosplenic space using polypropylene mesh in five horses. Vet Surg 2006;35(5):431–7.
121. Mair TS, Smith LF. Survival and complication rates in 300 horses undergoing surgical treatment of colic. Part 3: long-term complications and survival. Equine Vet J 2005;37(4):310–4.

Colic: Nonsurgical Complications

Eileen Sullivan Hackett, DVM, MS*, Diana M. Hassel, DVM, PhD

KEYWORDS

- Colic • Horse • Postoperative complications • Ileus

Colic is a serious disease of horses and is the leading cause of death in horses in the United States aside from old age.[1] Colic surgery allows prolongation of life for many horses that would die without intervention. We are constantly in search of accurate survival statistics regarding the major types of colic lesions.[2–20] The development of nonsurgical complications may confound recovery from colic surgery. The authors attempt to outline the most common nonsurgical postoperative complications in this article. Early recognition and prompt appropriate treatment of common nonsurgical complications may improve survival of horses after surgery.

POSTOPERATIVE PAIN: RECOGNITION

The development of pain in a patient that has colic is the most prevalent postoperative complication[5,10] and requires early recognition of manifestations of pain, determination of the underlying cause, and effective management strategies to minimize perceived pain by the animal for its own sake and for that of the owner. The most obvious signs of pain in the equine patient after colic surgery may resemble those occurring in any patient with abdominal pain, such as pawing, rolling, stretching, turning the head toward the flank, kicking at the abdomen, repeated curling of the upper lip, trembling, posturing to urinate, straining to defecate, sweating, dog sitting, and repeatedly getting up and down. More subtle signs of pain may also occur that manifest as a depressed attitude and lack of interest in the surroundings, reduced appetite, lying down more than usual, tachycardia, and tachypnea. It is uncommon for adult horses undergoing ventral midline celiotomy to lie down in the postoperative period while hospitalized, particularly during daylight hours, unless they are painful. Lying down is of particular concern in the equine patient early after colic surgery because it may result in contamination of the surgical site and put the horse at an increased risk for incisional infection and other sequelae.

Foals may present an added challenge because the degree of abdominal pain does not always correlate with the severity of the disease. Although many of their signs of

Department of Clinical Sciences, Colorado State University, 300 West Drake Road, Fort Collins, Colorado 80523, USA
* Corresponding author.
E-mail address: Eileen.Hackett@colostate.edu (E.S. Hackett).

Vet Clin Equine 24 (2009) 535–555
doi:10.1016/j.cveq.2008.09.001
0749-0739/08/$ – see front matter

vetequine.theclinics.com

© 2009 Elsevier Inc. All rights reserved.

pain resemble those of adult horses, they may also exhibit tail flagging, persistent standing, and rolling up on their backs as indications that they are experiencing abdominal pain.[21]

POSTOPERATIVE PAIN: CAUSE

Classically, abdominal pain has been described as arising from bowel distention, spasm, mesenteric tension, ischemia, inflammation, peritonitis, or a combination of these factors.[22] Determination of the underlying cause of pain in the equine patient after colic surgery is of utmost concern because its presence may indicate the need for a second exploratory laparotomy. Timing from surgery may provide clues as to the nature of the painful episode. Horses experiencing pain while still in the recovery stall are more likely to be experiencing surgical and incisional pain rather than pain from a secondary lesion requiring surgical intervention. When this is the case, these horses generally respond to analgesic administration and become progressively more comfortable over the first 24 hours. Immediate postoperative pain may also be associated with more serious lesions, such as recurrence of bowel displacement, a strangulating lesion, or failure to identify all lesions eliciting pain at the time of surgery (eg, unidentified proximal small colon enterolith). Pain may also be observed in those horses exhibiting the systemic inflammatory response syndrome (SIRS) and endotoxemia secondary to surgical correction of a strangulating obstruction or inflammatory condition of the bowel.

Colic occurring after a period of hospitalization after surgery often requires a more extensive investigation. Determination of whether the cause of colic is medical or surgical in nature can be difficult. Because peritoneal fluid parameters may normally display marked abnormalities in the postoperative period,[23,24] interpretation of abdominal fluid parameters is not as clear-cut, unless septic peritonitis has developed.

Differentiating between small intestinal ileus and a postsurgical nonstrangulating obstructive lesion of the small intestine that requires a second laparotomy is a diagnostic challenge. In horses with surgical disease of the large intestine or cecum, recurrence of impaction or obstruction at the site of an enterotomy may occur and should be considered as a potential cause of postoperative colic. Results of abdominal ultrasound examination, response to gastric decompression, rectal palpation findings, and response to analgesics are common methods used to help identify the cause of pain in the postoperative period and to help identify whether a second exploratory celiotomy is indicated. A poor or short duration of response to analgesics can sometimes indicate a need for surgical exploration.[25]

In addition to determining and attempting to treat the underlying cause, the use of analgesic agents is an integral component of therapy. Pain management in the postoperative period can have a positive impact on the overall outcome and attenuate the proinflammatory cytokine response that occurs in response to tissue injury, anesthesia, pain, and stress.[26] Furthermore, because pain may lead to reflexive adrenergic activity, reduction of pain-induced sympathetic tone may enable a return of a more normal motility pattern in horses that have ileus or impaction colic.[27]

POSTOPERATIVE PAIN: MANAGEMENT STRATEGY

A multimodal approach should be used in treatment of postoperative colic pain. Using multiple analgesics concurrently allows a lower effective dosage and avoids the side effects seen with higher dosing. α_2-Adrenergic agonists are currently the most effective drugs for colic pain in horses and are considered the "gold standard" for visceral pain.[28,29] α_2-Adrenergic agonists can be given as single dose or continuously administered until desired analgesia is achieved. Side effects of these drugs include decreased gastrointestinal activity and delayed gastric emptying.[30] Detomidine has a greater effect on gastric emptying than xylazine and causes a dose-dependent decrease in gastric emptying.[31]

Butorphanol is an opioid analgesic with κ-receptor agonist and μ-receptor antagonist activity. Butorphanol is commonly administered to horses experiencing visceral pain and works synergistically with other analgesic drugs. Single doses of butorphanol alone increase gastric emptying time and also act synergistically with detomidine in this regard.[31] Butorphanol administered as a continuous rate intravenous infusion (CRI) results in fewer adverse behavioral and gastrointestinal effects.[32] In horses recovering from colic surgery, butorphanol administered as a CRI was shown to improve behavior scores and decrease plasma cortisol concentration.[33] Researchers believed butorphanol provided good analgesia that improved the immediate postoperative recovery characteristics.[33] Because butorphanol is a μ-receptor antagonist, many recommend against concurrent administration with μ-agonist opioid analgesics.[33]

Fentanyl, a synthetic μ-receptor agonist opioid drug, can be administered to horses as a CRI or transdermal patch. Pharmacokinetic data are available for fentanyl CRI in awake horses and horses undergoing general anesthesia.[34–36] Pharmacokinetic data are also available for horses receiving fentanyl administered as a transdermal patch, with several studies reporting variable absorption.[37–40] Fentanyl has not been shown to have a significant impact on the visceral pain threshold in horses and may have limited utility in horses with postoperative colic pain.[36] Fentanyl has been shown to act synergistically with nonsteroidal anti-inflammatory drugs (NSAIDS).[41] Rapid intravenous administration should be avoided because adverse behavioral effects may ensue.

Morphine is an opioid analgesic with μ- and κ-receptor activity. Use of morphine as an analgesic for visceral pain is usually avoided because the side effects of administration can include ileus, constipation, and central nervous system stimulation (**Fig. 1**). If morphine is used as an analgesic, there is evidence that the opioid antagonist N-methylnaltrexone can ameliorate negative effects on gastrointestinal function.[42]

NSAIDs are analgesics that exert their effect through blockage of the cyclooxygenase (COX) enzyme, decreasing production of eicosanoids from arachidonic acid. In the gastrointestinal tract, eicosanoids promote deleterious processes of pain,

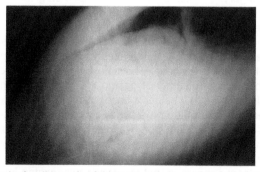

Fig. 1. Lateral abdominal radiograph of a miniature horse treated for colic by administration of morphine ad libitum for 5 consecutive days. Note the marked feed impaction of the large intestine secondary to delayed transit. This horse required surgical correction of the impaction and prolonged medical treatment.

inflammation, and vasoconstriction in addition to maintaining beneficial processes of motility and mucosal healing. For this reason, a potential side effect of NSAID administration is gastric and intestinal ulceration. Flunixin meglumine is the most commonly administered NSAID for visceral pain in horses. Flunixin meglumine inhibits COX-1 and COX-2 enzymes. Flunixin meglumine administration typically results in 6 to 8 hours of analgesia. At the authors' hospital, flunixin meglumine is commonly administered at a dose of 0.5 to 1.0 mg/kg and with a dose interval of 6 to 12 hours during the first 48 hours of the postoperative period.

ILEUS

Risk factors for gastrointestinal ileus are well outlined in the literature.[43–48] Recognized risk factors for small intestinal ileus include prolonged surgery and anesthetic time, small intestinal lesions (specifically strangulating lipoma lesions), and elevated packed cell volume.[43–45] Recognized risk factors for large intestinal ileus relevant to hospitalization include change of exercise routine; change in housing; recent transport; number of hours spent in a stable; lack of pasture access; feeding changes; previous colic episode; and recent anesthesia, including association with type of inhalant used.[46–48] Evaluation of each case for recognized risk factors may play a role in postoperative planning.

Recognition of the onset of gastrointestinal ileus is an important component of postoperative care. The most sensitive indicator is often heart rate. Other indicators include anorexia, abdominal pain, gross abdominal distention, and quiet behavior. On recognition, a nasogastric tube should be placed and siphoned without delay. If addressed promptly, severe gastric distention and resulting fatal perforation can be avoided. After nasogastric intubation, transcutaneous abdominal ultrasound and rectal examination may be performed, and information resulting from these three diagnostic procedures should be adequate to determine if the gastrointestinal ileus is primarily of large intestinal or small intestinal origin. Although abdominal ultrasound can be used to confirm gastric distention, therapeutic passage of a nasogastric tube should not be delayed by this diagnostic modality.[49] Small intestinal ileus is frequently associated with copious gastric reflux per nasogastric tube and small intestinal distention with or without sedimentation evident on ultrasonographic examination (**Figs. 2** and **3**). Large intestinal ileus is frequently associated with a feed-distended large colon palpable on rectal examination.

Small intestinal ileus is estimated to occur in roughly 1 in 5 to 1 in 10 horses undergoing colic surgery.[43,44] Horses that develop postsurgical small intestinal ileus have a greater likelihood of requiring a second celiotomy and a greater incidence of mortality.[44,45] Horses with gastric reflux have been shown to have an increased risk for developing renal insufficiency.[50] Treatment of small intestinal ileus is multimodal. Gastric decompression can be used therapeutically and to monitor response to therapy or clinical course of disease. The time interval of gastric decompression should be such that a large quantity of gastric fluid sequestration is avoided. It is the clinician's preference as to whether a nasogastric tube is placed periodically or left indwelling. Decisions are made on a "case by case" basis and may be related to the quantity of reflux or patient compliance. Serious consequences can result from repeated intubation or maintenance of a continuously indwelling nasogastric tube. These serious comorbidities include pharyngeal trauma and esophageal rupture.[51] An additional concern is that indwelling nasogastric intubation has been shown experimentally to delay gastric emptying time nearly 60%.[52]

Crystalloid fluid therapy should be adjusted according to measured gastric losses. Serum electrolytes should be monitored and corrected as needed. The adult horse

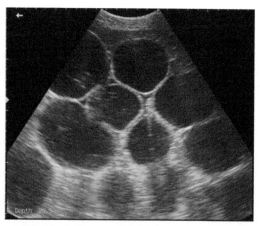

Fig. 2. Transcutaneous abdominal ultrasonographic image reveals multiple loops of small intestinal fluid distention.

maintenance fluid rate (2 mL/kg/h) plus the quantity of gastric reflux (L/h) equals the total hourly crystalloid fluid requirement. Serum electrolytes should be monitored and corrected by means of intravenous fluid additives as needed. Electrolyte abnormalities that can be anticipated are hypokalemia and hypocalcemia.[53] Hypocalcemia should be avoided because smooth muscle responsible for gastrointestinal motility and vascular tone relies on extracellular fluid free calcium for strength of contraction. Hydration status can be monitored objectively by frequent measurement of packed cell volume, serum total protein, and urine specific gravity. Circulating volume can also be objectively monitored through use of a dedicated catheter used to measure central venous pressure. Subjective assessment of hydration and circulating volume includes mucous membrane moisture, capillary refill time, heart rate, pulse quality, skin turgor, jugular refill time, frequency of urination, thirst, and peripheral

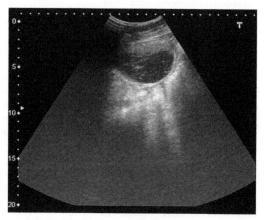

Fig. 3. Transcutaneous abdominal ultrasonographic image reveals sedimentation of intestinal contents within a loop of small intestine. Sedimentation implies long-standing adynamic ileus.

temperature. Partial or total parenteral nutrition should be considered in horses that have long-standing small intestinal ileus.

Prokinetic therapy is commonly pursued in horses that have refractory postoperative small intestinal ileus (**Table 1**). A survey of diplomates of the American College of Veterinary Surgeons published in 2004 revealed that 2% lidocaine was the most commonly prescribed prokinetic for postoperative ileus, followed by erythromycin and metoclopramide.[54] All three of these drugs have been shown to increase the contractile amplitude in vitro in different regions of the gastrointestinal tract.[55] Lidocaine affects contractile amplitude in the proximal duodenum; erythromycin in the pyloric antrum and middle jejunum; and metoclopramide in the pyloric antrum, proximal duodenum, and middle jejunum.[55] Literature demonstrating the positive prokinetic effects of these drugs in vivo is less definitive. Lidocaine is well tolerated in horses after colic surgery and has been shown to decrease jejunal distention and peritoneal fluid accumulation when used prophylactically in the postoperative period, although gastrointestinal activity and outcome were unaffected.[56] In another report, lidocaine administration significantly improved time to resolution and fecal passage and resulted in shorter hospitalization stays in horses when used after the development of postoperative reflux.[57] Lidocaine treatment in normal horses has not been shown to increase gastrointestinal motility.[58] In addition, continuous intravenous administration of lidocaine has not been shown to be effective in an experimental model of visceral pain in horses.[59] Gastrointestinal disease may alter the pharmacokinetic disposition of lidocaine in horses undergoing colic surgery when compared with normal horses.[60] Concurrent use of highly protein-bound drugs may displace lidocaine and increase unbound concentration, increasing the risk for toxicity.[61] Lidocaine toxicity is commonly manifested as tremors, muscle fasciculations, somnolence, or collapse. Treatment of lidocaine toxicity is interruption of the continuous intravenous infusion until signs resolve. Care should be taken to maintain the safety of personnel during toxic episodes. At the authors' hospital, horses undergoing colic surgery receive a 50-μg/kg/min infusion of lidocaine during the course of surgery, and

Table 1
Commonly administered prokinetic therapies in the horse

Drug	Indication	Dose	Mechanism
Erythromycin	Small intestinal ileus, improves gastric emptying	0.5–1.0 mg/kg IV; give over 60 minutes q 6–8 hours	Motilin receptor stimulation
Lidocaine	Small intestinal ileus	0.05 mg/kg/min by continuous IV infusion	Analgesia, sympathoadrenal inhibition, anti-inflammatory
Metoclopramide	Small intestinal ileus	0.01–0.05 mg/kg/h by continuous IV infusion 0.25–0.5 mg/kg IV; give over 30–60 minutes q 6–8 hours	Dopamine antagonist
Neostigmine	Large intestinal ileus	0.005–0.02 mg/kg IM or SQ	Cholinesterase inhibitor

Abbreviations: IM, intramuscular; IV, intravenous; q, every; SQ, subcutaneous.

most continue on a 50-μg/kg/min lidocaine infusion for the first 12 to 24 hours of the postoperative period.

Erythromycin is a macrolide antibiotic and prokinetic agent. Erythromycin is thought to exert its prokinetic effect through stimulation of motilin receptors. In the horse, motilin receptors are found within the duodenum, jejunum, cecum, and colonic pelvic flexure and are most concentrated in the duodenum and proximal gastrointestinal tract.[62] In an experimental model of postoperative ileus, erythromycin significantly increased ileal and colonic pelvic flexure activity.[63] Erythromycin has also been shown to increase gastric emptying in normal horses.[64] As a note of caution, erythromycin use has been associated with acute colitis in horses.[65] There are no published studies demonstrating the efficacy of erythromycin in naturally occurring adynamic postoperative ileus in horses.

Metoclopramide, a dopamine antagonist, can be administered as an intermittent or continuous infusion.[66] Metoclopramide has been shown to increase myomechanical activity in the jejunum and ileum of normal horses.[67] Other experimental studies have failed to show an effect on jejunal and colonic pelvic flexure activity.[68] Efficacy in preventing or treating postoperative ileus, in addition to decreasing mortality, is only empirically supported. Signs of toxicity include excitement and restlessness. Adverse behavioral effects are attributable to dopaminergic antagonism in the central nervous system as metoclopramide crosses the blood-brain barrier.[66] Caution should be used in its administration, and horses should be monitored for adverse behavioral effects.

Limitations in the treatment of small intestinal ileus stem from the direct physical injury sustained by the myogenic structure and myenteric neurologic control structures. Small intestinal distention alone, commonly seen oral to resection margins of small intestinal obstructive diseases or with clinically severe ileus, is known to cause injury as a result of ischemia.[69] Histologically, proximal jejunal resection borders in horses with naturally occurring small intestinal lesions demonstrate hemorrhage, edema, and neutrophilic infiltrate.[70] Strangulating small intestinal lesions can even result in cellular apoptosis within the distant intestinal tract, presumably attributable to SIRS.[71] Jejunal intraluminal distention and ischemia evaluated experimentally decreased motilin receptor expression in the intraluminal distention group.[72] Investigators suggest that a diminished prokinetic response in horses that have gastrointestinal disease may be attributable to receptor down-regulation secondary to inflammation. This is consistent with other researchers' findings that the contractile response to cisapride, erythromycin, and metoclopramide is decreased after jejunal distention.[73] An improved survival rate has not been shown with prokinetic use in horses that have postoperative ileus.[74]

Therapy for large intestinal ileus consists of intravenous and oral fluids, laxatives, oil as a marker of transit, hand-walking or turnout, analgesics with minimal motility effects, acupuncture, and prokinetic drugs. Oral fluid therapy has been a topic of recent study by Lopes and colleagues.[75] Experimental results revealed that a balanced electrolyte solution administered orally was the best method for hydrating colonic contents. This oral electrolyte solution can be conveniently mixed patient-side by combining table salt (3 tsp), lite salt (1 tsp), and baking soda (4 tsp) with fresh water (5 L). Nonselective NSAIDs should be used with caution because of documented deleterious effects on colonic motility.[76,77] COX-2–selective NSAIDS may be preferable if colonic motility is compromised.[77] Neostigmine given at 5 to 10 mg intramuscularly or subcutaneously was the most commonly administered prokinetic drug for large colon impaction by surgeons currently performing colic surgery.[54] Neostigmine, a cholinesterase inhibitor, is used almost exclusively for motility disorders of the large bowel because it has been shown experimentally to decrease gastric emptying and small intestinal motility.[78] Potassium penicillin G has been shown to have a direct positive effect on large bowel myoelectric activity.[79]

Limitations in treatment of large intestinal ileus stem from the direct physical injury sustained by the neural and contractile elements of the intestine in the course of disease. Interstitial cells of Cajal, responsible for gastrointestinal pacemaker activity, are significantly reduced in horses that have large intestinal disorders.[80] Circular muscle undergoes an increased incidence of cellular apoptosis after simple obstructive diseases of the large colon.[56] Gastrointestinal dysfunction may be refractory to treatment if sufficient injury occurs. Prevention of large intestinal ileus should be aimed at known risk factors. Feeding of concentrates to horses that have primary large colon disease should be limited.[48,81] Use of morphine should also be avoided.[82] Horses in high-risk categories should be monitored closely and treated appropriately if large colonic transit time is delayed.

COLITIS

The development of diarrhea in the equine patient after colic surgery occurs frequently, with a reported prevalence as high as 53.2%, with severe diarrhea (colitis) occurring in 27.5% of horses in one study.[83] The prevalence of colitis as a postoperative complication seems to vary by geographic region or surgical facility, because a more recent study described a much lower 3.2% occurrence of colitis in the researchers' colic population.[5] The differences may, in part, be reflective of criteria used to define colitis. The nature of the disease process also likely has an impact because those horses with sand and feed impactions of the large intestine[84] and large colon volvulus[85] seem to be at higher risk. Although primarily considered to be a complication with surgical diseases of the ascending and descending colon, diarrhea was reported as a complication in 21.4% of horses with incarceration of the small intestine through the gastrosplenic ligament.[86]

Equine patients with positive fecal cultures for Salmonella spp after colic surgery are at increased risk for development of diarrhea compared with those not shedding the organism,[84] and Clostridium spp are important causative agents of diarrhea in horses as well.[87] Changes in the intestinal flora of horses that have colic may allow for proliferation of enteric pathogens. The combination of perioperative broad-spectrum antimicrobial treatment; damage to the integrity of the gastrointestinal tract; surgical evacuation of normal gastrointestinal contents and associated flora; and the stress of surgery, anesthesia, and the disease process itself places these horses at increased risk for the development of colitis. In most cases of postoperative colitis, a specific pathogen is not identified. Pathogenic strains of other bacterial species, such as Escherichia coli,[88] need to be investigated as potential agents causing colitis in horses.

The key to treatment in the case of postoperative colitis is effective prevention or early recognition and treatment. Di-tri-octahedral (DTO)–smectite is a natural hydrated aluminomagnesium silicate that is commercially available for use in horses (Bio-Sponge, Platinum Performance, Buellton, California). DTO-smectite has been shown to adsorb substances, such as endotoxins and exotoxins, in the human gastrointestinal tract effectively and, more recently, to bind equine-origin Clostridium difficile toxins A and B in addition to Clostridium perfringens enterotoxin and α-, β-, and β_2-exotoxins in vitro without any effect on bacterial growth or the action of metronidazole.[89,90] An in vivo clinical trial on the prevention of diarrhea in equine patients after colic surgery revealed a marked reduction in the prevalence of postoperative diarrhea and improved clinical and hematologic parameters in horses receiving prophylactic treatment with DTO-smectite in the perioperative period compared with controls.[91]

The authors currently use DTO-smectite at an initial dosage of l to 2 lb every 12 to 24 hours in mature horses for the treatment and prevention of colitis when there is a perceived increased risk for the development of colitis and when diarrhea develops in the postoperative period. Examples of when it may be used routinely in equine patients after colic surgery include those horses that have colonic volvulus with vascular compromise to the colon, large colon impactions, and surgical diseases of the small colon. It is also routinely administered during the course of surgery by means of an intra-luminal route (0.5–1 lb in water [1 L]) in those patients undergoing enterotomy of the pelvic flexure as a component of their surgical therapy. Treatment with DTO-smectite seems to have few if any adverse effects in mature horses and foals, and anecdotal reports suggest that it is effective at reducing the volume and duration of acute diarrhea in horses.

Other therapies for the treatment and prevention of postoperative colitis include the use of various forms of probiotics, including commercially available products and fecal transfaunation. The theoretic benefit of probiotic use is to aid in restoration of a balanced nonpathogenic bacterial population, which is considered to be the primary defense mechanism against colonization of pathogenic bacteria.[92] Investigation of the efficacy of probiotic therapy in the treatment and prevention of colitis in horses is somewhat limited. A clinical trial performed on equine patients after colic surgery eval-uating two commercially available probiotic products demonstrated no effect of either product on *Salmonella* shedding, prevalence of diarrhea, or length of hospitalization.[84] A more recent study evaluating the efficacy of administration of *Saccharomyces boulardii* for the treatment of acute enterocolitis in horses did demonstrate a beneficial effect on reducing the severity and duration of clinical signs.[93] Conversely, *Lactoba-cillus pentosus* WE7 was evaluated in foals for the prevention of neonatal diarrhea in a randomized clinical trial and was found to have detrimental effects, resulting in an increased prevalence of diarrhea and requirement for veterinary intervention.[94] This raises the obvious concern for the need for safety and efficacy studies before the routine use of probiotics in horses. In addition, quality control of commercially available veterinary probiotic products is apparently low, with inaccurate label descriptions of most products,[95] again emphasizing the need for additional species-specific randomized clinical trials.

When prevention is ineffective in the development of postoperative colitis, efforts must be directed toward supportive care, including fluid volume replacement, electro-lyte balance, colloidal support, use of NSAIDs, endotoxin-binding strategies, systemic antimicrobials when appropriate, and adequate enteral nutrition when possible. Preventative strategies toward other common complications, such as laminitis, renal failure, and thrombophlebitis, are also indicated.

Systemic antimicrobial use in the perioperative period is well recognized and used by most surgeons performing equine colic surgery.[96] The use of systemic antimicro-bials as a component of management in postoperative colitis is controversial, however, because antimicrobial-induced colitis is a well-known and highly life-threatening entity. Factors used to dictate the necessity for continued or reinstituted intravenous antimicrobial therapy include the presence of a known surgical-related infection and profound leukopenia with neutropenia (<2000 neutrophils per microliter) in a clinically ill or febrile horse. Concurrent therapy with oral metronidazole in those horses with suspected anaerobic infection or clostridial colitis may be appropriate.

In horses developing colitis in the postoperative period, fecal cultures for *Salmonella* spp and *Clostridium* spp and their toxins are appropriate, along with isolation of the horse from other hospitalized patients and institution of proper biosecurity protocols.

Therapy for colitis has been thoroughly discussed elsewhere,[85,97] but a few recent equine-specific publications are worthy of discussion. Lidocaine used as a constant rate infusion has become a common first-line method of treatment for postoperative ileus by many surgeons.[54] More recent research suggests that its anti-inflammatory effects on the gastrointestinal tract may play a more important role than its direct prokinetic effects,[98] perhaps increasing its utility for treatment of a wider range of gastrointestinal disturbances, such as colitis. Lidocaine inhibits neutrophil adhesion, phagocytosis, and the production of free radicals.[99] Therapy with the NSAID flunixin meglumine remains a key component of therapy for endotoxemia and colitis, although the use of flunixin has been shown to impair recovery of intestinal barrier function in compromised equine jejunum,[100] potentially leading to increased absorption of endotoxin from the gastrointestinal tract. In a model of ischemic-injured jejunum, lidocaine administered as a constant rate infusion concurrently with flunixin ameliorated the inhibitory effects of flunixin meglumine on recovery of the mucosal barrier from ischemic injury.[101] Although models of ischemic injury within the equine jejunum do not closely mimic a clinical case of postoperative colitis, these preliminary findings merit further study of the potential benefits of lidocaine constant rate infusion therapy in the equine patient that has colitis and endotoxemia.

ENDOTOXEMIA AND SYSTEMIC INFLAMMATORY RESPONSE SYNDROME

Endotoxemia and the resulting SIRS are common in horses recovering from surgical gastrointestinal disease. Endotoxin is a well-conserved lipid moiety of gram-negative bacteria found in abundance in the gastrointestinal lumen. Horses are exquisitely sensitive to even small amounts of endotoxin. Under experimental conditions, when endotoxin is administered intravenously, signs include anxiety, sweating, tachycardia, and intestinal stasis.[102] In horses with naturally occurring disease, signs of endotoxemia are similar and include hyperemic mucous membranes, ileus, and hypotensive shock. These signs are attributable primarily to endotoxin's prostaglandin-mediated effects on tissues.[102]

Treatment of endotoxemia includes supportive intravenous crystalloid fluid therapy, enteral adsorbents to aid in prevention of systemic absorption, and administration of agents capable of binding endotoxin and clearing it from the plasma. Small-volume resuscitation with hypertonic saline solution and hetastarch has been shown to prevent endotoxin-associated hypocalcemia when compared with large-volume crystalloid administration under experimental conditions, although a drop in mean arterial pressure and changes in additional hemodynamic parameters were not ameliorated.[103,104] Polymyxin B, an antimicrobial, is capable of binding endotoxin and is effective at reducing negative effects if administered after the onset of endotoxemia.[105,106] Caution should be exercised when administering polymyxin B because of concern about nephrotoxicity, although this has not been reported in horses when they are given polymyxin the at low dosages required for antiendotoxin treatment.

COAGULOPATHY

Since coagulation dysfunction in association with equine gastrointestinal disease was first reported in 1983, a firm link has been established between these two disease processes.[107-110] The association of equine gastrointestinal disease and coagulation abnormalities is likely attributable to increased levels of circulating endotoxin and endothelial release of tissue factor creating a prothrombotic environment, although sympathetic activation may play a role.[111-113] Coagulation dysfunction is of particular concern because associated disease processes can lead to poor end-organ oxygenation and failure. Direct and indirect tests of coagulation function include platelet count, mucosal bleeding time, activated clotting time, activated partial thromboplastin time (aPTT), prothrombin time (PT), plasma fibrinogen concentration, fibrin degradation product concentration (FDP), D-dimer concentration, thrombin-antithrombin complex level, antithrombin activity (AT), and thromboelastography (TEG). The sheer number of coagulation tests may seem overwhelming. Recent reports have documented subclinical disseminated intravascular coagulation in horses by analyzing the following six tests: PT, aPTT, AT, FDP, platelet count, and plasma fibrinogen level. The prognosis for horses that develop coagulation dysfunction is markedly diminished, and mortality may be increased. A recent report identified coagulation abnormalities in 70% of horses treated surgically for large colon volvulus and found horses with a postoperative coagulation profile consisting of four of six abnormal coagulation test results had 47:1 odds of euthanasia.[114] Subclinical disseminated intravascular coagulation has also been associated with an eight times greater mortality rate in horses with naturally occurring colitis.[115] Of concern is using therapies in these cases that are known to exacerbate coagulation abnormalities. This has been the subject of recent study. Hetastarch colloid administration, at recommended doses of 10 mL/kg, has not been shown to exacerbate coagulation dysfunction attributable to endotoxemia.[103]

Although coagulation dysfunction in equine patients after colic surgery can be used as a prognostic indicator or signal of severity of disease, treatment of these disorders is difficult. In addition to supportive care and routine treatments for endotoxemia, heparin, an anticoagulant, has been used in horses that have colic to prevent disorders of coagulation. In a prospective study of horses that had naturally occurring colic disease, low-molecular-weight heparin was shown to have fewer side effects than unfractionated heparin.[116]

CATHETER-ASSOCIATED THROMBOPHLEBITIS

Thrombophlebitis is an unwelcome sequela to intravenous catheterization. In one study, when compared with controls, hospitalized horses with a jugular catheter were more likely to develop thrombophlebitis if they had large intestinal disease, hypoproteinemia, salmonellosis, or endotoxemia.[117] In another study evaluating equine patients after colic surgery specifically, 7 of 38 horses developed thrombophlebitis.[118] Factors associated with thrombophlebitis in this study were dwell time of catheter and related state of debilitation. These results are similar to those of another study that identified dwell time, presence of fever, and diarrhea as risk factors positively associated with vein thrombosis in horses treated with intravenous fluids.[119] Clinical signs of thrombophlebitis include firm swelling, heat, pain in the area overlying the catheter insertion site, and fever. The catheter insertion site and jugular vein should be frequently monitored in equine patients after colic surgery. Ultrasonographic examination can be used to confirm thrombophlebitis and monitor response to treatment.[120] Ultrasound can also be used to determine the best site of aspiration for bacterial culture and sensitivity testing.[120]

LAMINITIS

Multiple studies have identified an association between the development of laminitis and the presence of various diseases of the gastrointestinal tract.[121–124] Most recently, Parsons and colleagues[125] recognized clinical manifestations of endotoxemia, as defined by hyperemia of the mucous membranes, along with supportive laboratory findings of neutropenia with toxic changes, as a significant risk factor for the development of acute laminitis. Hospitalized horses were at a fivefold increased risk for developing laminitis if they had clinically evident endotoxemia, compared with horses without evidence of endotoxemia.[83] Interestingly, the experimental administration of endotoxin does not predictably cause laminitis in horses, although exposure to endotoxin does have well-documented effects on the equine digital vasculature.[126,127] Ideas on the pathophysiology of laminitis are numerous, with the two most popular theories relevant to postoperative colic consisting of the vascular or hemodynamic theory versus the metabolic or enzymatic theory.[128] Some suggest that it is products of the inflammatory activity at the level of the gastrointestinal tract rather than the direct effect of circulating endotoxin or vasoactive amines that may trigger the vascular events that result in laminitis secondary to gastrointestinal disease.[129] It has been proposed that laminitis triggers factors, hypothesized to reach the lamellar tissues by means of the circulation, that contribute to increased activity of matrix metalloproteinases and proinflammatory cytokines within the laminar tissues, in turn, leading to laminar separation and the clinically evident acute phase of laminitis.[130,131] Because evidence for vascular and metabolic theories exists, perhaps the two mechanisms occur simultaneously in naturally acquired laminitis.[128]

Regardless of the pathogenesis, the first consideration in the management of an equine patient after colic surgery at risk for laminitis is to provide maximum effort toward repairing the primary disease process that has or is likely to lead to the development of laminitis. This often entails aggressive antiendotoxic and anti-inflammatory therapy for those horses that have ischemic or inflammatory disease, placing them at increased risk for developing laminitis. This may consist of the use of NSAIDs, polymyxin-B, DTO-smectite administration, and J-5 plasma, in addition to intravenous fluid support.[89,106,132] Recent research by Cook and colleagues[101] suggests that a constant rate infusion of lidocaine used in combination with flunixin meglumine attenuates the flunixin-induced impairment in mucosal barrier recovery and subsequent endotoxin absorption in ischemic injured jejunum. Although primarily used by equine surgeons as a prokinetic agent, these new research findings support an alternative role in the battle against endotoxemia.[54] Further evaluation is necessary to determine whether these experimental results prove useful in the clinical arena.

Once the acute phase of laminitis has begun, much of the injury to the lamina has already occurred; thus, the key to successful treatment of laminitis is prevention. Identifying patients at risk during the developmental stage of laminitis, before the onset of clinical signs, is a key component to success in the application of preventive treatments. These may include, but are not limited to, equine patients after colic surgery demonstrating clinical and clinicopathologic manifestations of endotoxemia, horses with a history of prior episodes of laminitis, those with a known history or clinical signs of pituitary pars intermedia dysfunction or hyperinsulinemia and equine metabolic syndrome, and certain breeds (eg, Andalusian horses).[133–135] Alford and colleagues[136] suggest that thoroughbred horses may be at decreased risk. If it is a routine practice to pull shoes at the time of surgery, exercise caution during the postoperative period with regard to hand-walking exercise or even stall confinement on pavement or other hard surfaces, particularly in mature overweight horses not accustomed to being barefoot. Early reapplication of shoes, extra deep bedding, or application of Soft-Ride equine boots (Soft-Ride, Inc., Vermilion, Ohio) may be appropriate in these cases.

The most promising preventative treatment in high-risk equine patients after colic surgery consists of the application of continuous cryotherapy to the distal limbs. Cryotherapy induces digital vasoconstriction and induces a profound hypometabolic effect, which is considered to be the most important mechanism by which cold limits the severity of an injury.[137] Continuous distal limb cryotherapy during the developmental stage of laminitis has the potential to preserve the lamellar tissue until the systemic insult has abated. Data from experimental models of laminitis and limited clinical anecdotal evidence suggest that continuous distal limb cryotherapy is an effective method for prevention of laminitis.[137] The challenge lies in the application of the cooling method. Current recommendations suggest cooling of the limb through the upper third metacarpal region for 48 to 72 hours or until clinical signs of endotoxemia have abated, because cooling the feet alone is inadequate.[137] This generally requires the use of a large adapted tub and immobilization of the horse by means of stocks or cross-tying. This is a less than optimal scenario for the application of a preventive treatment for a disease that occurs relatively infrequently. The authors use a modified method in high-risk patients consisting of continuous application of ice in empty 5-L intravenous fluid bags taped in place to the upper pastern and fetlock region. Although perhaps suboptimal in terms of effectiveness, this method allows ambulation of the horses in their stalls. A potential future therapy that is currently under investigation includes trials of proteinase inhibitor therapy specifically targeted at hoof wall matrix metalloproteinases.[137]

Although laminitis is a relatively infrequent complication observed in the equine patient after colic surgery, many of our equine patients after colic surgery have endotoxemia, placing them at increased risk.[123,138] When laminitis occurs in its acute severe form in endotoxemic patients, it is often life threatening, and therefore remains a significant postoperative complication that requires diligent and effective preventive treatment methods.

POSTOPERATIVE FEVER

The development of fever in the postoperative period is common in equine patients that have colic. The cause of persistent postoperative fever should be thoroughly investigated because it may dictate changes in therapy and alter the morbidity and mortality of the patient. The most common causes of postoperative fever consist of endotoxemia or SIRS secondary to the primary gastrointestinal lesion, infection of the ventral midline incision, and septic thrombophlebitis. Ultrasound evaluation of the incision and jugular vein may provide useful insight into whether an infection is present or developing. Other less common causes to consider are bacterial pneumonia, pleuropneumonia, peritonitis, and viral respiratory disease. Auscultation of the thorax and trachea, including a rebreathing examination, and ultrasound evaluation of the lungs and pleural cavity should provide information pertaining to bacterial diseases of the lung. Nasal swabs for isolation of viral respiratory pathogens may also prove useful when other causes of fever have been ruled out. Septic peritonitis may be recognized by means of abdominal ultrasound and abdominal paracentesis. White blood cell counts must be interpreted with caution in equine patients after colic surgery because they may remain persistently elevated in the absence of peritoneal sepsis. Other means to substantiate the significance of peritonitis may include the presence of large quantities of free peritoneal fluid with or without fibrin tags visualized on ultrasound, fluid analysis indicating the presence of degenerate neutrophils or bacteria, low pH of peritoneal fluid (<7.3), and low glucose concentration in peritoneal fluid compared with systemic blood glucose concentration (>50-mg/dL difference).

REFERENCES

1. Traub-Dargatz JL, Kopral CA, Seitzinger AH, et al. Estimate of the national incidence of and operation-level risk factors for colic among horses in the United States, spring 1998 to spring 1999. J Am Vet Med Assoc 2001;219(1):67–71.

2. Hughes KJ, Dowling BA, Matthews SA, et al. Results of surgical treatment of colic in miniature breed horses: 11 cases. Aust Vet J 2003;81(5):260–4.

3. Mair TS, Smith LJ. Survival and complication rates in 300 horses undergoing surgical treatment of colic. Part 4: early (acute) relaparotomy. Equine Vet J 2005; 37(4):315–8.

4. Mair TS, Smith LJ. Survival and complication rates in 300 horses undergoing surgical treatment of colic. Part 3: long-term complications and survival. Equine Vet J 2005;37(4):310–4.

5. Mair TS, Smith LJ. Survival and complication rates in 300 horses undergoing surgical treatment of colic. Part 2: short-term complications. Equine Vet J 2005;37(4):303–9.

6. Mair TS, Smith LJ. Survival and complication rates in 300 horses undergoing surgical treatment of colic. Part 1: short-term survival following a single laparotomy. Equine Vet J 2005;37(4):296–302.

7. Santschi EM, Slone DE, Embertson RM, et al. Colic surgery in 206 juvenile thoroughbreds: survival and racing results. Equine Vet J Suppl 2000;(32):32–6.

8. Dugdale AH, Langford J, Senior JM, et al. The effect of inotropic and/or vasopressor support on postoperative survival following equine colic surgery. Vet Anaesth Analg 2007;34(2):82–8.

9. Proudman CJ, Smith JE, Edwards GB, et al. Long-term survival of equine surgical colic cases. Part 2: modelling postoperative survival. Equine Vet J 2002; 34(5):438–43.

10. Proudman CJ, Smith JE, Edwards GB, et al. Long-term survival of equine surgical colic cases. Part 1: patterns of mortality and morbidity. Equine Vet J 2002; 34(5):432–7.

11. Proudman CJ, Edwards GB, Barnes J, et al. Modelling long-term survival of horses following surgery for large intestinal disease. Equine Vet J 2005;37(4): 366–70.

12. Proudman CJ, Edwards GB, Barnes J, et al. Factors affecting long-term survival of horses recovering from surgery of the small intestine. Equine Vet J 2005;37(4): 360–5.

13. Proudman CJ, Edwards GB, Barnes J. Differential survival in horses requiring end-to-end jejunojejunal anastomosis compared to those requiring side-to-side jejunocaecal anastomosis. Equine Vet J 2007;39(2):181–5.

14. Blikslager AT, Roberts MC. Accuracy of clinicians in predicting site and type of lesion as well as outcome in horses with colic. J Am Vet Med Assoc 1995; 207(11):1444–7.

15. Freeman DE, Hammock P, Baker GJ, et al. Short- and long-term survival and prevalence of postoperative ileus after small intestinal surgery in the horse. Equine Vet J Suppl 2000;(32):42–51.

16. Freeman DE, Schaeffer DJ. Short-term survival after surgery for epiploic foramen entrapment compared with other strangulating diseases of the small intestine in horses. Equine Vet J 2005;37(4):292–5.

17. Johnston K, Holcombe SJ, Hauptman JG. Plasma lactate as a predictor of colonic viability and survival after 360 degrees volvulus of the ascending colon in horses. Vet Surg 2007;36(6):563–7.

18. Garcia-Seco E, Wilson DA, Kramer J, et al. Prevalence and risk factors associated with outcome of surgical removal of pedunculated lipomas in horses: 102 cases (1987–2002). J Am Vet Med Assoc 2005;226(9):1529–37.

19. Hassel DM, Langer DL, Snyder JR, et al. Evaluation of enterolithiasis in equids: 900 cases (1973–1996). J Am Vet Med Assoc 1999;214(2):233–7.

20. Mair TS, Smith LJ, Sherlock CE. Evidence-based gastrointestinal surgery in horses. Vet Clin North Am Equine Pract 2007;23(2):267–92.
21. Bryant JE, Gaughan EM. Abdominal surgery in neonatal foals. Vet Clin North Am Equine Pract 2005;21(2):511–35, viii.
22. Hay WP, Moore JN. Management of pain in horses with colic. Compend Contin Educ Pract Vet 1997;19:987–90.
23. Santschi EM, Grindem CB, Tate LP Jr, et al. Peritoneal fluid analysis in ponies after abdominal surgery. Vet Surg 1988;17(1):6–9.
24. Hanson RR, Nixon AJ, Gronwall R, et al. Evaluation of peritoneal fluid following intestinal resection and anastomosis in horses. Am J Vet Res 1992;53(2):216–21.
25. White NA, Elward A, Moga KS, et al. Use of web-based data collection to evaluate analgesic administration and the decision for surgery in horses with colic. Equine Vet J 2005;37(4):347–50.
26. Shavit Y, Fridel K, Beilin B. Postoperative pain management and proinflammatory cytokines: animal and human studies. J Neuroimmune Pharmacol 2006; 1(4):443–51.
27. White NA. Medical management of the colic patient. Proceedings of the 34th Annual Convention of the American Association of Equine Practitioners. Golden, CO, December 1998.
28. Jochle W, Moore JN, Brown J, et al. Comparison of detomidine, butorphanol, flunixin meglumine and xylazine in clinical cases of equine colic. Equine Vet J Suppl 1989;(7):111–6.
29. Muir WW, Robertson JT. Visceral analgesia: effects of xylazine, butorphanol, meperidine, and pentazocine in horses. Am J Vet Res 1985;46(10):2081–4.
30. Doherty TJ, Andrews FM, Provenza MK, et al. The effect of sedation on gastric emptying of a liquid marker in ponies. Vet Surg 1999;28(5):375–9.
31. Sutton DG, Preston T, Christley RM, et al. The effects of xylazine, detomidine, acepromazine and butorphanol on equine solid phase gastric emptying rate. Equine Vet J 2002;34(5):486–92.
32. Sellon DC, Monroe VL, Roberts MC, et al. Pharmacokinetics and adverse effects of butorphanol administered by single intravenous injection or continuous intravenous infusion in horses. Am J Vet Res 2001;62(2):183–9.
33. Sellon DC, Roberts MC, Blikslager AT, et al. Effects of continuous rate intravenous infusion of butorphanol on physiologic and outcome variables in horses after celiotomy. J Vet Intern Med 2004;18(4):555–63.
34. Thomasy SM, Mama KR, Whitley K, et al. Influence of general anaesthesia on the pharmacokinetics of intravenous fentanyl and its primary metabolite in horses. Equine Vet J 2007;39(1):54–8.
35. Thomasy SM, Steffey EP, Mama KR, et al. The effects of i.v. fentanyl administration on the minimum alveolar concentration of isoflurane in horses. Br J Anaesth 2006;97(2):232–7.
36. Sanchez LC, Robertson SA, Maxwell LK, et al. Effect of fentanyl on visceral and somatic nociception in conscious horses. J Vet Intern Med 2007;21(5):1067–75.
37. Maxwell LK, Thomasy SM, Slovis N, et al. Pharmacokinetics of fentanyl following intravenous and transdermal administration in horses. Equine Vet J 2003;35(5): 484–90.
38. Mills PC, Cross SE. Regional differences in transdermal penetration of fentanyl through equine skin. Res Vet Sci 2007;82(2):252–6.
39. Orsini JA, Moate PJ, Kuersten K, et al. Pharmacokinetics of fentanyl delivered transdermally in healthy adult horses—variability among horses and its clinical implications. J Vet Pharmacol Ther 2006;29(6):539–46.

40. Eberspacher E, Stanley S, Rezende M, et al. Pharmacokinetics and tolerance of transdermal fentanyl administration in foals. Vet Anaesth Analg 2008.

41. Thomasy SM, Slovis N, Maxwell LK, et al. Transdermal fentanyl combined with nonsteroidal anti-inflammatory drugs for analgesia in horses. J Vet Intern Med 2004;18(4):550–4.

42. Boscan P, Van Hoogmoed LM, Pypendop BH, et al. Pharmacokinetics of the opioid antagonist N-methylnaltrexone and evaluation of its effects on gastrointestinal tract function in horses treated or not treated with morphine. Am J Vet Res 2006;67(6):998–1004.

43. Cohen ND, Lester GD, Sanchez LC, et al. Evaluation of risk factors associated with development of postoperative ileus in horses. J Am Vet Med Assoc 2004; 225(7):1070–8.

44. Blikslager AT, Bowman KF, Levine JF, et al. Evaluation of factors associated with postoperative ileus in horses: 31 cases (1990–1992). J Am Vet Med Assoc 1994; 205(12):1748–52.

45. French NP, Smith J, Edwards GB, et al. Equine surgical colic: risk factors for postoperative complications. Equine Vet J 2002;34(5):444–9.

46. Durongphongtorn S, McDonell WN, Kerr CL, et al. Comparison of hemodynamic, clinicopathologic, and gastrointestinal motility effects and recovery characteristics of anesthesia with isoflurane and halothane in horses undergoing arthroscopic surgery. Am J Vet Res 2006;67(1):32–42.

47. Senior JM, Pinchbeck GL, Allister R, et al. Post anaesthetic colic in horses: a preventable complication? Equine Vet J 2006;38(5):479–84.

48. Hillyer MH, Taylor FG, Proudman CJ, et al. Case control study to identify risk factors for simple colonic obstruction and distension colic in horses. Equine Vet J 2002;34(5):455–63.

49. Lores M, Stryhn H, McDuffee L, et al. Transcutaneous ultrasonographic evaluation of gastric distension with fluid in horses. Am J Vet Res 2007;68(2):153–7.

50. Groover ES, Woolums AR, Cole DJ, et al. Risk factors associated with renal insufficiency in horses with primary gastrointestinal disease: 26 cases (2000–2003). J Am Vet Med Assoc 2006;228(4):572–7.

51. Hardy J, Stewart RH, Beard WL, et al. Complications of nasogastric intubation in horses: nine cases (1987, 1989). J Am Vet Med Assoc 1992;201(3):483–6.

52. Cruz AM, Li R, Kenney DG, et al. Effects of indwelling nasogastric intubation on gastric emptying of a liquid marker in horses. Am J Vet Res 2006;67(7):1100–4.

53. Garcia-Lopez JM, Provost PJ, Rush JE, et al. Prevalence and prognostic importance of hypomagnesemia and hypocalcemia in horses that have colic surgery. Am J Vet Res 2001;62(1):7–12.

54. Van Hoogmoed L, Nieto JE, Snyder JR, et al. Survey of prokinetic use in horses with gastrointestinal injury. Vet Surg 2004;33(3):279–85.

55. Nieto JE, Rakestraw PC, Snyder JR, et al. In vitro effects of erythromycin, lidocaine, and metoclopramide on smooth muscle from the pyloric antrum, proximal portion of the duodenum, and middle portion of the jejunum of horses. Am J Vet Res 2000;61(4):413–9.

56. Brianceau P, Chevalier H, Karas A, et al. Intravenous lidocaine and small-intestinal size, abdominal fluid, and outcome after colic surgery in horses. J Vet Intern Med 2002;16(6):736–41.

57. Malone E, Ensink J, Turner T, et al. Intravenous continuous infusion of lidocaine for treatment of equine ileus. Vet Surg 2006;35(1):60–6.

58. Milligan M, Beard W, Kukanich B, et al. The effect of lidocaine on postoperative jejunal motility in normal horses. Vet Surg 2007;36(3):214–20.

59. Robertson SA, Sanchez LC, Merritt AM, et al. Effect of systemic lidocaine on visceral and somatic nociception in conscious horses. Equine Vet J 2005; 37(2):122–7.

60. Feary DJ, Mama KR, Thomasy SM, et al. Influence of gastrointestinal tract disease on pharmacokinetics of lidocaine after intravenous infusion in anesthetized horses. Am J Vet Res 2006;67(2):317–22.

61. Milligan M, Kukanich B, Beard W, et al. The disposition of lidocaine during a 12-hour intravenous infusion to postoperative horses. J Vet Pharmacol Ther 2006;29(6):495–9.

62. Koenig JB, Cote N, LaMarre J, et al. Binding of radiolabeled porcine motilin and erythromycin lactobionate to smooth muscle membranes in various segments of the equine gastrointestinal tract. Am J Vet Res 2002;63(11):1545–50.

63. Roussel AJ, Hooper RN, Cohen ND, et al. Prokinetic effects of erythromycin on the ileum, cecum, and pelvic flexure of horses during the postoperative period. Am J Vet Res 2000;61(4):420–4.

64. Ringger NC, Lester GD, Neuwirth L, et al. Effect of bethanechol or erythromycin on gastric emptying in horses. Am J Vet Res 1996;57(12):1771–5.

65. Gustafsson A, Baverud V, Gunnarsson A, et al. The association of erythromycin ethylsuccinate with acute colitis in horses in Sweden. Equine Vet J 1997;29(4): 314–8.

66. Eades SC, Moore JN. Antagonism of a specific dopaminergic receptor agonist with metoclopramide in horses. Am J Vet Res 1993;54(1):122–5.

67. Hunt JM, Gerring EL. A preliminary study of the effects of metoclopramide on equine gut activity. J Vet Pharmacol Ther 1986;9(1):109–12.

68. Sojka JE, Adams SB, Lamar CH, et al. Effect of butorphanol, pentazocine, meperidine, or metoclopramide on intestinal motility in female ponies. Am J Vet Res 1988;49(4):527–9.

69. Dabareiner RM, White NA, Donaldson LL. Effects of intraluminal distention and decompression on microvascular permeability and hemodynamics of the equine jejunum. Am J Vet Res 2001;62(2):225–36.

70. Gerard MP, Blikslager AT, Roberts MC, et al. The characteristics of intestinal injury peripheral to strangulating obstruction lesions in the equine small intestine. Equine Vet J 1999;31(4):331–5.

71. Rowe EL, White NA, Buechner-Maxwell V, et al. Detection of apoptotic cells in intestines from horses with and without gastrointestinal tract disease. Am J Vet Res 2003;64(8):982–8.

72. Koenig JB, Sawhney S, Cote N, et al. Effect of intraluminal distension or ischemic strangulation obstruction of the equine jejunum on jejunal motilin receptors and binding of erythromycin lactobionate. Am J Vet Res 2006;67(5):815–20.

73. Nieto JE, Van Hoogmoed LM, Spier SJ, et al. Use of an extracorporeal circuit to evaluate effects of intraluminal distention and decompression on the equine jejunum. Am J Vet Res 2002;63(2):267–75.

74. Smith MA, Edwards GB, Dallap BL, et al. Evaluation of the clinical efficacy of prokinetic drugs in the management of post-operative ileus: can retrospective data help us? Vet J 2005;170(2):230–6.

75. Lopes MA, White NA 2nd, Donaldson L, et al. Effects of enteral and intravenous fluid therapy, magnesium sulfate, and sodium sulfate on colonic contents and feces in horses. Am J Vet Res 2004;65(5):695–704.

76. Van Hoogmoed LM, Snyder JR, Harmon FA. In vitro investigation of the effects of cyclooxygenase-2 inhibitors on contractile activity of the equine dorsal and ventral colon. Am J Vet Res 2002;63(11):1496–500.

77. Van Hoogmoed LM, Snyder JR, Harmon F. In vitro investigation of the effect of prostaglandins and nonsteroidal anti-inflammatory drugs on contractile activity of the equine smooth muscle of the dorsal colon, ventral colon, and pelvic flexure. Am J Vet Res 2000;61(10):1259–66.

78. Adams SB, Lamar CH, Masty J. Motility of the distal portion of the jejunum and pelvic flexure in ponies: effects of six drugs. Am J Vet Res 1984;45(4):795–9.

79. Roussel AJ, Hooper RN, Cohen ND, et al. Evaluation of the effects of penicillin G potassium and potassium chloride on the motility of the large intestine in horses. Am J Vet Res 2003;64(11):1360–3.

80. Fintl C, Hudson NP, Mayhew IG, et al. Interstitial cells of Cajal (ICC) in equine colic: an immunohistochemical study of horses with obstructive disorders of the small and large intestines. Equine Vet J 2004;36(6):474–9.

81. Lopes MA, White NA 2nd, Crisman MV, et al. Effects of feeding large amounts of grain on colonic contents and feces in horses. Am J Vet Res 2004;65(5):687–94.

82. Senior JM, Pinchbeck GL, Dugdale AH, et al. Retrospective study of the risk factors and prevalence of colic in horses after orthopaedic surgery. Vet Rec 2004; 155(11):321–5.

83. Cohen ND, Honnas CM. Risk factors associated with development of diarrhea in horses after celiotomy for colic: 190 cases (1990–1994). J Am Vet Med Assoc 1996;209(4):810–3.

84. Parraga ME, Spier SJ, Thurmond M, et al. A clinical trial of probiotic administration for prevention of Salmonella shedding in the postoperative period in horses with colic. J Vet Intern Med 1997;11(1):36–41.

85. Southwood LL. Postoperative management of the large colon volvulus patient. Vet Clin North Am Equine Pract 2004;20(1):167–97.

86. Jenei TM, Garcia-Lopez JM, Provost PJ, et al. Surgical management of small intestinal incarceration through the gastrosplenic ligament: 14 cases (1994–2006). J Am Vet Med Assoc 2007;231(8):1221–4.

87. Donaldson MT, Palmer JE. Prevalence of Clostridium perfringens enterotoxin and Clostridium difficile toxin A in feces of horses with diarrhea and colic. J Am Vet Med Assoc 1999;215(3):358–61.

88. DebRoy C, Maddox CW. Identification of virulence attributes of gastrointestinal Escherichia coli isolates of veterinary significance. Anim Health Res Rev 2001; 2(2):129–40.

89. Weese JS, Cote NM, deGannes RV. Evaluation of in vitro properties of di-tri-octahedral smectite on clostridial toxins and growth. Equine Vet J 2003;35(7): 638–41.

90. Lawler JB, Hassel DM, Magnuson RJ, et al. Adsorptive effects of di-tri-octahedral smectite on Clostridium perfringens alpha, beta, and beta-2 exotoxins and equine colostral antibodies. Am J Vet Res 2008;69(2):233–9.

91. Hassel DM, Smith PA, Nieto JE, et al. Di-tri-octahedral smectite for the prevention of post-operative diarrhea in equids with surgical disease of the large intestine: results of a randomized clinical trial [abstract]. Vet Surg 2004;33(5):E11.

92. Fuller R. Probiotics in human medicine. Gut 1991;32(4):439–42.

93. Desrochers AM, Dolente BA, Roy MF, et al. Efficacy of Saccharomyces boulardii for treatment of horses with acute enterocolitis. J Am Vet Med Assoc 2005; 227(6):954–9.

94. Weese JS, Rousseau J. Evaluation of Lactobacillus pentosus WE7 for prevention of diarrhea in neonatal foals. J Am Vet Med Assoc 2005;226(12):2031–4.

95. Weese JS. Microbiologic evaluation of commercial probiotics. J Am Vet Med Assoc 2002;220(6):794–7.

96. Traub-Dargatz JL, George JL, Dargatz DA, et al. Survey of complications and antimicrobial use in equine patients at veterinary teaching hospitals that underwent surgery because of colic. J Am Vet Med Assoc 2002;220(9):1359–65.
97. Feary DJ, Hassel DM. Enteritis and colitis in horses. Vet Clin North Am Equine Pract 2006;22(2):437–79, ix.
98. Cook VL, Blikslager AT. Use of systemically administered lidocaine in horses with gastrointestinal tract disease. J Am Vet Med Assoc 2008;232(8):1144–8.
99. Azuma Y, Shinohara M, Wang PL, et al. Comparison of inhibitory effects of local anesthetics on immune functions of neutrophils. Int J Immunopharmacol 2000; 22(10):789–96.
100. Tomlinson JE, Wilder BO, Young KM, et al. Effects of flunixin meglumine or etodolac treatment on mucosal recovery of equine jejunum after ischemia. Am J Vet Res 2004;65(6):761–9.
101. Cook VL, Jones Shults J, McDowell M, et al. Attenuation of ischaemic injury in the equine jejunum by administration of systemic lidocaine. Equine Vet J 2008;40(4):353–7.
102. King JN, Gerring EL. The action of low dose endotoxin on equine bowel motility. Equine Vet J 1991;23(1):11–7.
103. Pantaleon LG, Furr MO, McKenzie HC, et al. Effects of small- and large-volume resuscitation on coagulation and electrolytes during experimental endotoxemia in anesthetized horses. J Vet Intern Med 2007;21(6):1374–9.
104. Pantaleon LG, Furr MO, McKenzie HC 2nd, et al. Cardiovascular and pulmonary effects of hetastarch plus hypertonic saline solutions during experimental endotoxemia in anesthetized horses. J Vet Intern Med 2006;20(6):1422–8.
105. Durando MM, MacKay RJ, Linda S, et al. Effects of polymyxin B and Salmonella typhimurium antiserum on horses given endotoxin intravenously. Am J Vet Res 1994;55(7):921–7.
106. Barton MH, Parviainen A, Norton N. Polymyxin B protects horses against induced endotoxaemia in vivo. Equine Vet J 2004;36(5):397–401.
107. Morris DD, Beech J. Disseminated intravascular coagulation in six horses. J Am Vet Med Assoc 1983;183(10):1067–72.
108. Johnstone IB, McAndrew KH, Baird JD. Early detection and successful reversal of disseminated intravascular coagulation in a thoroughbred mare presented with a history of diarrhoea and colic. Equine Vet J 1986;18(4):337–40.
109. Welch RD, Watkins JP, Taylor TS, et al. Disseminated intravascular coagulation associated with colic in 23 horses (1984–1989). J Vet Intern Med 1992;6(1): 29–35.
110. Prasse KW, Topper MJ, Moore JN, et al. Analysis of hemostasis in horses with colic. J Am Vet Med Assoc 1993;203(5):685–93.
111. Roth RI. Hemoglobin enhances the production of tissue factor by endothelial cells in response to bacterial endotoxin. Blood 1994;83(10):2860–5.
112. Hinchcliff KW, Rush BR, Farris JW. Evaluation of plasma catecholamine and serum cortisol concentrations in horses with colic. J Am Vet Med Assoc 2005; 227(2):276–80.
113. Guyton HJA. The autonomic nervous system; the adrenal medulla. In: Textbook of medical physiology. Philadelphia: (W.B. Saunders Company); 2005.
114. Dallap BL, Dolente B, Boston R. Coagulation profiles in 27 horses with large colon volvulus. J Vet Emerg Crit Care 2003;13(4):215–25.
115. Dolente BA, Wilkins PA, Boston RC. Clinicopathologic evidence of disseminated intravascular coagulation in horses with acute colitis. J Am Vet Med Assoc 2002; 220(7):1034–8.

116. Feige K, Schwarzwald CC, Bombeli T. Comparison of unfractioned and low molecular weight heparin for prophylaxis of coagulopathies in 52 horses with colic: a randomised double-blind clinical trial. Equine Vet J 2003;35(5):506–13.
117. Dolente BA, Beech J, Lindborg S, et al. Evaluation of risk factors for development of catheter-associated jugular thrombophlebitis in horses: 50 cases (1993–1998). J Am Vet Med Assoc 2005;227(7):1134–41.
118. Lankveld DP, Ensink JM, van Dijk P, et al. Factors influencing the occurrence of thrombophlebitis after post-surgical long-term intravenous catheterization of colic horses: a study of 38 cases. J Vet Med A Physiol Pathol Clin Med 2001; 48(9):545–52.
119. Traub-Dargatz JL, Dargatz DA. A retrospective study of vein thrombosis in horses treated with intravenous fluids in a veterinary teaching hospital. J Vet Intern Med 1994;8(4):264–6.
120. Gardner SY, Reef VB, Spencer PA. Ultrasonographic evaluation of horses with thrombophlebitis of the jugular vein: 46 cases (1985–1988). J Am Vet Med Assoc 1991;199(3):370–3.
121. Cohen ND, Parson EM, Seahorn TL, et al. Prevalence and factors associated with development of laminitis in horses with duodenitis/proximal jejunitis: 33 cases (1985–1991). J Am Vet Med Assoc 1994;204(2):250–4.
122. Cohen ND, Woods AM. Characteristics and risk factors for failure of horses with acute diarrhea to survive: 122 cases (1990–1996). J Am Vet Med Assoc 1999; 214(3):382–90.
123. Hunt JM, Edwards GB, Clarke KW. Incidence, diagnosis and treatment of postoperative complications in colic cases. Equine Vet J 1986;18(4):264–70.
124. Slater MR, Hood DM, Carter GK. Descriptive epidemiological study of equine laminitis. Equine Vet J 1995;27(5):364–7.
125. Parsons CS, Orsini JA, Krafty R, et al. Risk factors for development of acute laminitis in horses during hospitalization: 73 cases (1997–2004). J Am Vet Med Assoc 2007;230(6):885–9.
126. Rodgerson DH, Belknap JK, Moore JN, et al. Investigation of mRNA expression of tumor necrosis factor-alpha, interleukin-1beta, and cyclooxygenase-2 in cultured equine digital artery smooth muscle cells after exposure to endotoxin. Am J Vet Res 2001;62(12):1957–63.
127. Zerpa H, Vega F, Vasquez J, et al. Effect of acute sublethal endotoxaemia on in vitro digital vascular reactivity in horses. J Vet Med A Physiol Pathol Clin Med 2005;52(2):67–73.
128. Moore RM, Eades SC, Stokes AM. Evidence for vascular and enzymatic events in the pathophysiology of acute laminitis: which pathway is responsible for initiation of this process in horses? Equine Vet J 2004;36(3):204–9.
129. Merritt A. Where does the subject of black walnut extract-induced laminitis fit into a colic symposium? Equine Vet J 2005;37(4):289–91.
130. Pollitt CC, Pass MA, Pollitt S. Batimastat (BB-94) inhibits matrix metalloproteinases of equine laminitis. Equine Vet J Suppl 1998;(26):119–24.
131. Belknap JK, Giguere S, Pettigrew A, et al. Lamellar pro-inflammatory cytokine expression patterns in laminitis at the developmental stage and at the onset of lameness: innate vs. adaptive immune response. Equine Vet J 2007;39(1):42–7.
132. Sykes BW, Furr MO. Equine endotoxaemia—a state-of-the-art review of therapy. Aust Vet J 2005;83(1–2):45–50.
133. Munoz E, Arguelles D, Areste L, et al. Retrospective analysis of exploratory laparotomies in 192 Andalusian horses and 276 horses of other breeds. Vet Rec 2008;162(10):303–6.

134. Treiber KH, Kronfeld DS, Geor RJ. Insulin resistance in equids: possible role in laminitis. J Nutr 2006;136(Suppl 7):2094S–8S.
135. Johnson PJ, Messer NT, Ganjam VK. Cushing's syndromes, insulin resistance and endocrinopathic laminitis. Equine Vet J 2004;36(3):194–8.
136. Alford P, Geller S, Richrdson B, et al. A multicenter, matched case-control study of risk factors for equine laminitis. Prev Vet Med 2001;49(3–4):209–22.
137. Pollitt CC. Laminitis: what treatment at what stage? Paper presented at: 10th Geneva Congress of Equine Medicine and Surgery. Geneva (CH), December 11–13, 2007.
138. Phillips TJ, Walmsley JP. Retrospective analysis of the results of 151 exploratory laparotomies in horses with gastrointestinal disease. Equine Vet J 1993;25(5): 427–31.

Complications of Laparoscopic Surgery

Dean A. Hendrickson, DVM, MS

KEYWORDS

- Laparoscopy • Complications
- Minimally invasive surgery • Bowel puncture • Hemorrhage

Laparoscopy is a minimally invasive surgical technique that has gained prominence in both the human and equine surgical arena in the past 20 years.[1] As with all surgical techniques, complications occur. The biggest question in surgery is not if there will be complications, but rather how will the surgeon respond to them? The purpose of this article is to describe surgical complications associated with laparoscopy, how to avoid them, how to recognize them if they do happen, and how to deal with them in the most expedient method possible. The article will be broken down into complications of sedation, anesthesia, positioning, the general surgical approach, and finally complications associated with specific surgical procedures.

One of the early papers on avoiding laparoscopic complications in human medicine was published in 1974.[2] In this summary, morbidity and side effects with respect to laparoscopy were estimated at 5%, with emergency situations requiring laparotomy estimated at 1%. The overall mortality was published at three deaths per 12,000 cases. The paper also described suggestions for preventing complications. The main sections of the report dealt with; training, case selection, equipment, anesthesia, pneumoperitoneum, insertion of the laparoscope, insertion of the operating cannula, and operative techniques. Nearly 30 years later, Philosophe,[3] reported on avoiding complications of laparoscopic surgery. He reiterated that vigilance in anesthesia, positioning, bladder decompression, trocar placement, electrosurgery, and postoperative care can prevent most injuries. Major areas of complications noted in the paper were: vascular injury during cannula placement, bowel injury (thermal and mechanical), and urological injury (thermal and mechanical). Wadlund[4] described the benefits of laparoscopic surgery to include; smaller incisions, decreased hospital stay, decreased recovery time, better surgical visualization, and magnification of anatomy and pathology. Important steps in limiting complications included strict compliance

Department of Clinical Sciences, James L. Voss Veterinary Teaching Hospital, College of Veterinary Medicine and Biomedical Sciences, 1620 Campus Delivery, Colorado State University, Fort Collins, CO 80523-1678, USA

E-mail address: Dean.hendrickson@colostate.edu

Vet Clin Equine 24 (2009) 557–571
doi:10.1016/j.cveq.2008.09.003
0749-0739/08/$ – see front matter © 2009 Elsevier Inc. All rights reserved.

vetequine.theclinics.com

with patient selection and care during the surgical procedure. Of particular concern in patient selection was limiting the acceptance of obese and pregnant patients while recognizing the potential for adhesions in patients with previous surgical histories. With regards to surgical procedure, one of the main concerns was the establishment of pneumoperitoneum and its effects on pulmonary, circulatory, and renal systems, along with coagulation disorders of lower extremities, peritoneal inflammation and intestinal ileus. The most common vessel involved was the right common iliac artery. Regardless of the complication, it is important to be able to diagnose the occurrence as soon as possible to limit the negative effects of the problem. Shettko[5] identified similar possible complications in the equine patient. In a large retrospective study of 158 laparoscopies,[6] fewer than 5% of the horses showed signs of postoperative discomfort and only two horses needed further therapy. Retroperitoneal insufflation occurred primarily in obese horses, and bowel puncture happened only one time. Splenic puncture occurred four times with unguarded obturators. A more common complication was puncture of the caudal epigastric artery and vein, and the circumflex iliac vessels.

TRAINING

As always, the best way to deal with a complication is to prevent it from happening. It has been stated that knowing how to manage complications is important, but knowing how to avoid them is prudent and intelligent, and will prevent heartache for both patient and surgeon.[3] Training is a critical step in all types of surgery. However, endoscopic surgery has an even greater requirement for training. The operative procedure is performed on a three-dimensional patient while viewing a two-dimensional monitor. The body wall provides a fulcrum in such a way that to move the tip of the instrument or telescope, the handle or camera must be moved in the opposite direction. The amount of movement required to change the position of the instrument or telescope tip is dependent on the amount of instrument on the inside and outside of the body wall. For instance, if the instrument is pushed into the abdomen as far as possible, it will require less movement of the handle to get the same amount of movement at the tip than it would if the instrument was mostly withdrawn from the abdomen. Depth perception is limited from working with a two-dimensional monitor, and the positioning of the portals can make hand movements very difficult. It is best to be able to have portals placed so that the telescope can be between the portals and there are approximately 30 degrees between the instruments and the telescope; or a total of 60 degrees between the instruments. Either a larger distance or smaller distance between instruments will make coordinated hand movements more difficult. Proper portal placement is generally easy to achieve in the dorsally recumbent horse, but is more difficult in the flank approach due to the limited access of the flank. Proper training will involve inanimate trainers and time spent with laparoscopic surgeons that are skilled in the techniques desired by the new surgeon.

Because not all complications will be eliminated by good training, it is important to be able to identify what has gone wrong as quickly as possible and to fix the problem to limit the consequences to the patient. The rest of this article will be devoted to recognizing and treating horses with complications associated with laparoscopy.

COMPLICATIONS WITH SEDATION

Standing laparoscopy is generally performed using sedation and local anesthetic. The author prefers to use either detomidine as an epidural (40 μg/kg brought to a total of 12–15 mL in the first or second coccygeal space) or given intravenously to effect

(20 mg detomidine in 1 L of polyionic fluids). The reported dose for epidural detomidine was 60 μg/kg.[7] In my experience, this dose is too high and it is not uncommon for horses to get very sedate and unstable, or even to fall down (**Fig. 1**).[8] If the horse becomes too sedate and unsteady, surgical stimuli may be enough to improve the horse's depth of sedation. However, it must be noted that if you have already placed instruments, and the horse collapses, it can be very detrimental to your instruments (**Fig. 2**). In general, it is better to give the horse some time to recover before placing portals and instruments.

COMPLICATIONS WITH ANESTHESIA

All of the traditional complications associated with general anesthesia can be present with laparoscopy. Only those complications that are unique to, or exacerbated by, laparoscopy will be discussed in this section. Carbon dioxide is the most commonly used gas for abdominal distension in laparoscopy. It is safe to use with electrosurgery and is soluble in blood which limits the development of gas emboli.[9] Studies in both people and horses show an increase in $PaCO_2$, acidosis, and end tidal CO_2.[9,10] These changes are thought to be easily reversible in healthy patients, but could cause problems in patients with pulmonary problems. It is recommended that particular care be taken to monitor the parameters most likely to change with insufflation and to adapt ventilation to best keep them in check.[9] Consequently, as described later in positioning problems, laparoscopy under general anesthesia should not be performed without adequate monitoring potential and positive pressure ventilation.

COMPLICATIONS WITH POSITIONING
Standing

Not every horse is compatible with standing surgery under sedation and local anesthesia. It is important when looking at patient selection to be sure that the horse will stand in the stocks for the procedure. In the author's experience, the most likely times for the horse to jump out of the stocks include; epidural placement, portal placement, and grasping the testis or ovary before local anesthetic blockade. It is worthwhile to ask the owner if the horse tolerates being tied, being placed in stocks, and being injected. If the horse is very difficult to inject, standing surgery is probably not the best option. In one study it was determined that the pneumoperitoneum associated with standing laparoscopy does not cause adverse alterations in cardiopulmonary, hematology, or

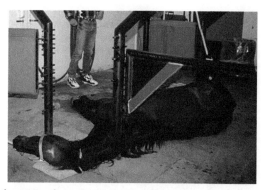

Fig. 1. A horse that has gone down in the stocks after a 60 μg/kg dose of detomidine hydrochloride in the caudal epidural space.

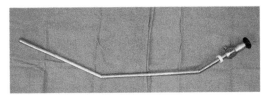

Fig. 2. A bent laparoscope after the horse went down in the stocks.

plasma chemistry variables, but does induce a mild peritoneal inflammatory response.[11]

Dorsal Recumbency

Ventral laparoscopy requires positioning the horse in dorsal recumbency. In most cases of surgery in the caudal abdomen, the horse will need to be placed into Trendelenberg position where the head is tilted down and the hind quarters up. This allows the viscera to be moved forward using the effects of gravity. This provides two potentials for complications: first, inappropriate pressure of the viscera on the diaphragm, and second, the possibility of the horse slipping off the table. To avoid the complication of the extra pressure on the diaphragm, the anesthesiologist must have the ability to perform positive pressure ventilation. To avoid the complication of slipping off the table the horse can be tied to the table (**Fig. 3**). In some surgeries, such as laparoscopic ovariectomy in dorsal recumbency, the table needs to be able to tilt at least 30 degrees. If the table will not tilt this far, it will be very difficult to perform the procedure. A study should be performed to determine if tilting the horse side to side as they do in small animal ovariectomies would be beneficial in gaining access to the ovarian pedicle without the need to tip into Trendelenberg position. Peripheral nerve injury has been reported in humans undergoing laparoscopic procedures.[3] To the author's knowledge this has not been a reported complication in equine laparoscopy.

Draping

Standard water impermeable drapes should be used for laparoscopy, regardless of the positioning of the patient. This is especially true for standing procedures where the dorsum is not clipped or aseptically prepared. The hair at the edges of the surgical

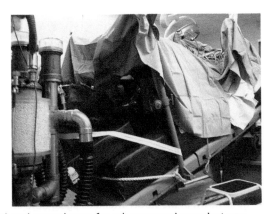

Fig. 3. A horse in dorsal recumbency for a laparoscopic ovariectomy.

region almost always remains damp and will wick through a water permeable drape. Fixing the drape to the patient for standing procedures can be challenging. During standing surgery, the patients are only sedated and will often move during the procedure. They also maintain skin sensation. It is possible to deposit local anesthetic where the towel clamps will go, but it is generally difficult to find the blebs under the drapes. The author chooses to not use local anesthetic, but to apply the towel clamps very slowly to limit response of the horse. Another option is to use a skin stapler to attach the drape to the horse (John Walmsley, personal communication, 2007). This is another opportunity for the horse to jump out of the stocks. While not proven, it is the author's opinion that using a caudal epidural with detomidine for sedation will reduce the responsiveness of horses to towel clamp placement when compared with sedation by intravenous techniques.

COMPLICATIONS WITH GENERAL LAPAROSCOPIC SURGICAL APPROACH
Standing

After the horses are sedated, blocked and draped, most surgeons will insufflate before cannula placement. Various insufflation cannulas have been described for laparoscopic surgery. In the author's experience, the spring-loaded Veress needle from human laparoscopy, is too short and too small in diameter for equine flank insufflation. The author has used a standard mare urinary catheter that has been straightened, a large diameter mare urinary catheter that has been straightened, an 11 mm diameter cannula with a blunt obturator, and a controlled access cannula (**Fig. 4**). The mare urinary catheters are effective as they have blunt ends and the larger diameter catheter is less likely to penetrate bowel. However, when compared with the 11 mm cannula with a blunt obturator, there is no obvious benefit to using a urinary catheter. In fact, using the cannula with the blunt obturator, makes it possible to assess placement within the peritoneal space before insufflation, reducing the possibility of retroperitoneal insufflation. The controlled access cannula is designed to screw into the body wall while monitoring with the laparoscope. It is better to have a zero degree laparoscope for placing the screw in cannulas; however, the camera can be canted at an angle with 30 degree laparoscopes when placing a screw in cannula. In a study of cannula insertion techniques in standing horses, problems with insufflation or cannula insertion occurred in 12 out of 40 horses.[12] Six horses had peritoneal detachment, four had splenic puncture, and two had descending colon puncture. The complications were primarily seen in the groups using a Veress needle or a 12-gauge catheter. Horses in the group that included an optical cannula had significantly fewer problems. As soon as the peritoneum is penetrated, insufflation can begin. Complications that occur

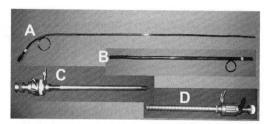

Fig. 4. Insufflation cannulas. (A) Standard mare urinary catheter. (B) Large-diameter mare urinary catheter. (C) 11 mm diameter cannula with a blunt obturator (Surgical Direct, Deland, Florida). (D) Controlled access cannula (Karl Storz Veterinary Endoscopy America, Goleta, California).

during insufflation include retroperitoneal insufflation, laceration of the circumflex iliac artery, bowel puncture, and splenic puncture.

Retroperitoneal insufflation, if significant, may be enough to stop the procedure and force the surgeon to come back in two to three weeks to redo the surgery. The insufflation cannula should be placed in a slow, but consistent, method to reduce the possibility of pushing the peritoneum away from the body wall. The best way to confirm entry into the peritoneal space is to directly visualize the bowel with a laparoscope. If using a mare urinary catheter or some other insufflation technique, entry into the peritoneal space is indicated when air is sucked into the peritoneal space after penetration of the peritoneum. The abdomen in a normal horse will have a slight negative pressure due to the weight of the viscera on the ventral body wall. In general the insufflator will have a reading of −3 to −5 mm Hg immediately upon entering the peritoneal space. This will not be the case in horses that have had recent abdominal surgery, or where a large amount of distended bowel is present. Consequently, when using anything other than an operative cannula, it is beneficial to have the room quiet to listen to the air entering the abdominal cavity. Another indication of retroperitoneal insufflation is where the intra-abdominal pressure increases rapidly when insufflation begins. In some cases where retroperitoneal insufflation has occurred, a cannula can be placed into the last intercostal space for insufflation. It is the author's opinion that the peritoneum is more rigidly attached in the caudal thoracic region than in the flank region, most likely because of less retroperitoneal fat.

The circumflex iliac artery is located at the dorsal aspect of the internal abdominal oblique muscle, often in the region of the middle portal. The incision for the middle portal should include the skin, subcutaneous region, and the fascia of the external abdominal oblique muscle. If the incision is carried further, it is possible to incise the artery. The use of pyramidal-shaped, sharp obturators is not recommended in the flank region as they are more likely to lacerate the artery. Sharp obturators should be used only for penetration of the peritoneum after using a blunt obturator for the muscle layers (**Fig. 5**). If the artery is encountered during placement of a cannula, sequellae include bleeding from the incision, hematoma in the body wall, or bleeding along the cannula and telescope. In some cases the blood drips off from the scope and onto the lens making visualization difficult. Fortunately, the scope is generally moved to the dorsal cannula for surgery which obviates the visibility problem. In some cases the bleeding is severe enough to require ligation of the vessel. In those instances, the skin incision is sharply enlarged and the external abdominal oblique bluntly enlarged to find the vessel and ligate it. This is not necessarily easy, and can make the situation stressful. The author likes to pack the enlarged incision with a laparotomy sponge then get ready to ligate the vessel. The light cord can be disconnected from the laparoscope to provide excellent light to help with visibility during vessel ligation. It is then possible to continue the surgical procedure.

One of the most serious complications associated with laparoscopic surgery is that of bowel puncture (**Fig. 6**). The use of sharp instruments such as sharp obturators, trocar catheters, or aggressive penetration techniques increase the possibility of bowel puncture. Other considerations include the volume of gas and ingesta within the bowel. One way to reduce the possibility of bowel puncture is to make sure there is limited gas and ingesta distension of the bowel. This is obviously more achievable in elective procedures when the patient can be held off feed. While there have not been any studies looking at ingesta loads with different feed withholding times, it is generally accepted that 18 to 24 hours off feed for standing procedures and 24 to 36 hours off feed for dorsally recumbent procedures is adequate to reduce the bulk of ingesta in the colon. The author has not experienced any problems with gas

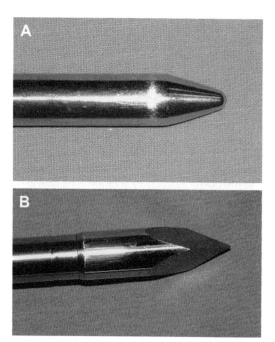

Fig. 5. Close-up view of the tips of a blunt (*A*) and a sharp (*B*) obturator.

distention in the horse with a prolonged feed withholding time. However, it is common in camelid species to have a problem with gas distention if the animals have feed withheld for an extended period of time. It is possible that providing a low-bulk diet would still allow working space in the abdomen without potential intestinal upset that can occur with limited food intake. Water should not be withheld at any point. It has been suggested that it is safer to approach the left hemi abdomen because the spleen is generally positioned next to the body wall, limiting the opportunity to puncture bowel.[1] It is however, possible to puncture the bowel from both sides of the abdomen and from the ventral aspect of the abdomen as well. Using blunt obturators and

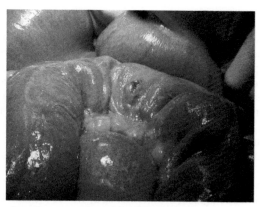

Fig. 6. Descending colon after puncture with a blunt obturator.

controlled entry force will limit the possibility of puncturing bowel. If the surgeon is concerned about bowel puncture, controlled access cannulas can be used (see **Fig. 4**). These cannulas are designed to place a zero degree laparoscope into the cannula: place the cannula through the skin incision, and screw the cannula through the body wall and into the peritoneal space. This technique provides a very safe way to enter the peritoneal space, but does not work well with a 30 degree telescope. If the surgeon punctures the bowel, the insufflator should be turned off and the tip of the telescope directed dorsally to keep the bowel on the telescope. If only penicillin has been used preoperatively, broad spectrum antibiotics with gram negative coverage should be given. The skin and body wall incision should be enlarged to exteriorize the affected bowel from the abdomen, the scope and cannula removed, and the bowel perforation closed and the bowel thoroughly lavaged. The bowel is then replaced into the peritoneal cavity; the body wall incision should be copiously lavaged and closed. The surgery should then be terminated and the clients alerted to the problem. Antibiotic coverage is generally continued for five days, and the horse discharged. The surgery can be reattempted in two to three weeks. While it may seem like a good idea to remove the scope and cannula as soon as a puncture is diagnosed, the increased intraluminal pressure secondary to insufflation will cause more contamination if the cannula is removed before isolation from the peritoneal space. It is also difficult to find the perforated portion of bowel after it drops into the abdomen with other bowel, making treatment difficult. In the cases where the puncture has been identified, the bowel isolated and closed, and supportive therapy pursued, the horses have all recovered without incident. However, in the one case where the puncture was not identified, the horse was eventually euthanized.

Splenic puncture can create a field contaminated by blood, but rarely is a problem postoperatively for the horse. Blunt obturators or controlled access cannulas will limit the possibility of puncturing the spleen. There have been no reported treatments necessary for splenic puncture. Fibrin glues have been used in other species, but have not been used in horses.[13]

It is possible to have subcutaneous emphysema postoperatively from the intra-abdominal carbon dioxide escaping from the incisions as the horse begins to move around after surgery. It has been theorized that removing the insufflation gas from the peritoneal space after surgery would reduce this problem, however there are no studies available to confirm this. The horses do not seem to be affected by the subcutaneous emphysema.

Dorsal Recumbency

Similar complications can be seen with dorsal recumbent laparoscopy as with standing laparoscopy. Retroperitoneal insufflation is less likely because an open approach can be used to determine proper placement of the cannula within the peritoneal space. When an open approach is performed, skin, subcutaneous tissue, linea alba, and peritoneum are all sharply incised and a blunt cannula introduced into the abdomen. Controlled access cannulas can also be used for dorsally recumbent procedures, but are actually more difficult to use because of the thin body wall in this location.

The caudal epigastric vessels are generally found at the abaxial portion of the rectus abdominus muscle. While it is difficult to see the vessels from the external aspect of the body wall, it is possible to see them with the telescope from the internal aspect of the abdomen. In young horses it is possible to determine the location of the vessels by directing the telescope against the internal body wall at the location of the vessels, thereby transilluminating them. Secondary portal placement can then be performed. If the vessels are inadvertently affected they can be ligated by placing a needle into the skin incision, passing it through the body wall while visualizing with the telescope, back out the body wall, and tied. The portal is then moved to a different position.

Bowel puncture is corrected as described in the section on standing surgery. It is important to leave the telescope and cannula in place until the bowel has been exteriorized through the enlarged incision. When the cannula is removed prematurely, the bowel contents can be pressurized and disseminated throughout the peritoneal cavity.

The author is aware of one case where a horse suffered a rupture of the diaphragm while in dorsal recumbency secondary to increased intra-abdominal pressure. An insufflator was not used and pressures were not constantly monitored. The procedure was converted to an open approach with laparoscopic assistance. A mesh was stapled to the diaphragm and the original procedure completed. It would therefore seem to be important to monitor the intra-abdominal pressure and limit the maximum pressure to 20 mm Hg.

The following sections will identify specific complications associated with selected surgical procedures.

CRYPTORCHID CASTRATION

The most common complication associated with cyrptorchid castration is hemorrhage at the castration stump. This most often occurs with improper techniques associated with ligation or cauterization of the mesorchium. When placing ligating loops, the tension should be let off from the mesorchium before final tightening of the loop (**Fig. 7**). If hemorrhage occurs, another ligating loop, vascular clip, or application of an electrosurgical modality should be performed. It is easier to identify bleeding in a standing horse after amputation of the testis than in a dorsally recumbent horse (**Fig. 8**).

Another complication associated with laparoscopic cryptorchidectomy is when the testis is dropped after amputation and before removal from the abdomen. There are no reports of these testes becoming revascularized after amputation, but since the possibility exists, every effort should be made to find the dropped testis and to remove it from the peritoneal space. Early reports suggesting that it would be

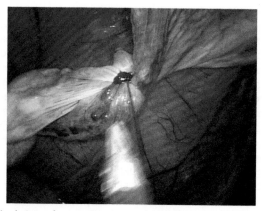

Fig. 7. Intra-abdominal view of a standing laparoscopic cryptorchidectomy while the ligating loop is being tightened.

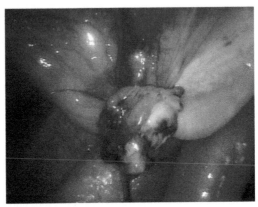

Fig. 8. Intra-abdominal view of a standing laparoscopic cryptorchidectomy after the mesorchium has been ligated and amputated.

safe to leave inguinal testes in situ after ligation of the mesorchium were promising.[14] However, two case reports described revascularization of the testicular parenchyma after successful ligation of the mesorchium.[15,16] In both reports it was suggested that the testicle was revascularized from an alternate blood supply than the spermatic cord. In a large study of laparoscopic castration, 5.6% of inguinally retained and 3.4% of normally descended testes were revascularized via the cremaster and or external pudendal artery.[17] Their conclusion was that laparoscopic castration without orchidectomy is not recommended in the case of inguinal cryptorchids or normal stallions. However, they had no problems with the ligated intra-abdominal testes. The author is not sure that it is good surgical technique to leave structures in the abdomen to undergo aseptic necrosis when it is relatively easy to minimally enlarge the incision to remove the testis. Therefore, if the dropped testis cannot be found laparoscopically, a portal should be enlarged and the surgeon should explore the abdomen to retrieve the testes rather than leave it in the abdomen.

Incomplete anesthesia of the testis or mesorchium can lead to excess movement.[18] If this is encountered, further local anesthesia should be used.

OVARIECTOMY

Similar hemorrhage concerns occur with laparoscopic ovariectomy. However as the vascular supply to the ovary is generally more substantial than that with the testis, hemorrhage may be more common. In a brief communication, the complication of ligature slippage and subsequent electrosurgery is described.[19] In one study using an ultrasonic cutting and coagulating device, most of the horses required further hemostasis in the form of vascular clips (**Fig. 9**).[20] It is important to reduce the size of the vascular pedicle before applying ligating loops (**Fig. 10**). This will reduce the amount of tissue in the ligature which will add security to the ligation. The author always places two ligating loops on the ovarian pedicle due to the larger vessel size. If hemorrhage occurs, techniques such as additional ligating loops, application of vascular clips, or application of electrosurgical devices should be performed.

Similar to cryptorchid castration, it is possible to drop the ovary after amputation and before removal from the abdomen. The ovary seems more prone to dropping as it is generally very dense and often larger than an intra-abdominal testis. Consequently it is important to make a large enough incision in the skin and body wall to

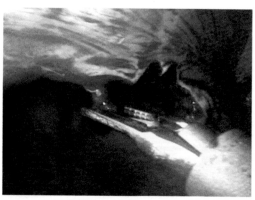

Fig. 9. Intra-abdominal view of a standing laparoscopic ovariectomy using an ultrasonic cutting and coagulating hand piece with a vascular clip.

easily remove the ovary from the abdomen. The author uses acute claw grasping forceps to remove both ovaries and testes from the abdomen (**Fig. 11**). As soon as the ovary is visible in the body wall incision, additional ochsner forceps are applied to the ovary to aid in removal. Only one report was found that described leaving transected ovaries in the abdomen after surgery.[21] In this report, surgery was performed on fillies, aged four to five months. The ovarian pedicles were transected using electrosurgery and left within the abdomen after amputation. Ten weeks following surgery, the fillies were euthanized and the abdomens explored. Four of the 20 ovaries were free floating in the abdomen and 16 were caught up in the omentum. It is unknown what would happen if the same thing were done in a mature mare. Similarly, the author is not aware of any studies on ligation of the ovarian pedicle while leaving the ovary to undergo avascular necrosis. Without appropriate information on the potential for revascularization in the mature mare, it cannot be recommended to leave transected or ligated ovaries, and every effort should be made to find ovaries that are dropped

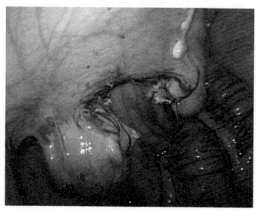

Fig. 10. Intra-abdominal view of a standing laparoscopic ovariectomy where the caudal pole of the ovary has been sharply transected.

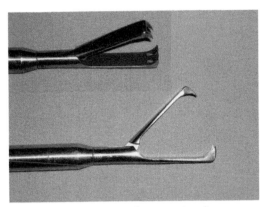

Fig. 11. Close-up view of the tips of an acute claw grasping forceps.

during removal. In one case, the author had to enlarge the incision and do a hand-assisted localization of the dropped ovary to remove it from the abdomen.

When performing standing ovariectomies, desensitization of the ovarian pedicle with local anesthetic will reduce movement of the horse, making the surgery easier to perform. Incomplete anesthesia is best remedied by adding more local anesthesia to the mesovarium.[22]

ABDOMINAL EXPLORATION

The biggest complication associated with abdominal exploration is not planning ahead in communications with the owner with respect to what is possible when performing laparoscopic exploration.[23] Abdominal exploration is best when performed on a horse where you have an expectation of finding something. Abdominal exploration in a horse where there are no reasonable expectations are generally unrewarding. Only the dorsal contents of the abdominal cavity can be evaluated in standing surgery, and the ventral contents during dorsally recumbent surgery.

NEPHROSPLENIC SPACE ABLATION

Hemorrhage is the most common complication noted when performing laparoscopic nephrosplenic space ablations. Hemorrhage is generally not of any significance, and is thought to be beneficial as it seems to encourage a better adhesion of the spleen to the peritoneum. Other complications include future displacement of the large colon. Ablation of the nephrosplenic space only removes one possible location for the large colon to become entrapped, it does not preclude continued movement of the large colon.[24]

URINARY SURGERY

Laparoscopy has been used for repair of ruptured bladders and the removal of uroliths. In a paper by Edwards and colleagues,[25] a ruptured bladder in a foal was repaired by staples and the foal subsequently formed bladder stones. It was suggested that nonabsorbable staples should not be used to repair bladder defects as they may be a source of further stone formation. When performing laparoscopic or laparoscopic urolith removal, the biggest potential complication is contamination of the peritoneal cavity. Presurgical lavage of the bladder through a urinary catheter, preoperative antibiotics, and adherence to aseptic technique are all valuable steps in reducing the possibility and consequence of peritoneal contamination.

POSTOPERATIVE PERIOD

There is little information in the equine literature regarding postoperative infections in horses undergoing laparoscopic surgery. In the human literature, a summary paper showed a reduced rate of postoperative infection in laparoscopic cholecystectomy (1.1%) when compared with an open cholecystectomy (4%); with similar results in urinary and pulmonary infections.[26] Their conclusion was that laparoscopic surgery was associated with better preservation of immune function and an reduction of the inflammatory response when compared with open surgery. In another paper, it was suggested that there was an increased rate of intra-abdominal abscessation after laparoscopic appendectomy when compared with an open appendectomy.[27] Comments were made that the increased abscess formation might be due to aggressive manipulation of the infected appendix during laparoscopic appendectomy and increased use of irrigation fluid possibly producing greater contamination. Adhesions of the omentum has been described in ponies undergoing laparoscopic surgery.[28] Eight foals had surgery to reduce experimental adhesions, and five of them formed adhesions of the omentum to the portal sites. The author has not seen any adhesions to portal sites in any cases where a second surgery was performed or where a post-mortem evaluation was performed after laparoscopic surgery had been performed.

THORACOSCOPY

There have not been a lot of reports of complications with equine thoracoscopy. The most common problems have been associated with and incomplete mediastinum where both sides of the thorax will fill with air. It is critical to have suction available when performing standing thoracoscopy in cases where the mediastinum is not complete. The author had one such case where it was obvious that the contralateral lung was collapsing at the same rate as the ipsilateral lung during a standing thoracoscopy. It is recommended that the pneumothorax should be created slowly to determine the ability of the horse to cope with the respiratory change. Portal incisions should only include the skin and subcutaneous tissues with blunt penetration of the muscle layers. This will reduce the likelihood of postoperative leakage.[29] Local anesthetic blockade of the intercostals nerves may improve the horse's response to portal manipulation.

SUMMARY

The best defense against surgical complications is a thorough training program designed to limit common problems associated with minimally invasive surgery. A thorough understanding of the anatomy will help the surgeon work in the three-dimensional environment while being limited to two dimensions on the monitor. It is critical to be able to convert the surgery to an open procedure if there are problems with the equipment or the patient.

REFERENCES

1. Hendrickson DA. History and instrumentation of laparoscopic surgery. In: Hendrickson DA, editor, Endoscopic surgery, veterinary clinics of North America: equine practice, vol. 16. Philadelphia: W.B. Saunders; 2000. p. 233–49.
2. Williams PP. Avoiding laparoscopy complications. Fertil Steril 1974;25(3):280–6.

3. Philosophe R. Avoiding complications of laparoscopic surgery. Sexuality, Reproduction & Menopause 2003;1(1):30–9.

4. Wadlund DL. Laparoscopy: risk, benefits and complications. In: Nursing clinics of North America, vol. 41. Philadelphia: Elsevier Saunders; 2006. p. 219–29.

5. Shettko DL. Complications in laparoscopic surgery. In: Hendrickson DA, editor, Endoscopic surgery, veterinary clinics of North America: equine practice, vol. 16. Philadelphia: W.B. Saunders; 2000. p. 377–83.

6. Walmsley JP. Review of equine laparoscopy and an analysis of 158 laparoscopies in the horse. The Sir Frederick Hobday Memorial Lecture. Equine Vet J 1999;31:456–64.

7. Skarda RT, Muir WW. Caudal analgesia induced by epidural or subarachnoid administration of detomidine hydrochloride solution in mares. Am J Vet Res 1994;55:670–80.

8. Wittern C, Hendrickson DA, Trumble T, et al. Complications associated with administration of detomidine into the caudal epidural space in a horse. J Am Vet Med Assoc 1998;213:516–8.

9. Safran DB, Orlando R. Physiologic effects of pneumoperitoneum, Am J Surg 1994:167:281–6

10. Donaldson LL, Trostle SS, White NA. Cardiopulmonary changes associated with abdominal insufflation of carbon dioxide in mechanically ventilated, dorsally recumbent, halothane anaesthetized horses. Equine Vet J 1998;30:144–51.

11. Latimer FG, Eades SC, Pettifer G, et al. Cardiopulmonary, blood and peritoneal fluid alterations associated with abdominal insufflation of carbon dioxide in standing horses. Equine Vet J 2003;35:283–90.

12. Desmaizieres LM, Martinot S, Lepage OM, et al. Complications associated with cannula insertion techniques used for laparoscopy in standing horses. Vet Surg 2003;32:501–6.

13. Olmi S, Scaini A, Erba L, et al. Use of fibrin glue (Tissucol) as a hemostatic in laparoscopic conservative treatment of spleen trauma. Surg Endosc 2007;21:2051–4.

14. Wilson DG, Hendrickson DA, Cooley AJ, et al. Laparoscopic methods for castration of equids. J Am Vet Med Assoc 1996;209:112–4.

15. Bergeron JA, Hendrickson DA, McCue PM. Viability of an inguinal testis after laparoscopic cauterization and transection of its blood supply. J Am Vet Med Assoc 1998;213:1303–4.

16. Voermans M, van der Velden MA. Unsuccessful laparoscopic castration in a cryptorchid Frisian stallion. Tijdschr Diergeneeskd 2006;131:774–7.

17. voermans M, Rijkenhuizen AB, van der Velden MA. The complex blood supply to the equine testis as a cause of failure in laparoscopic castration. Equine Vet J 2006;38:35–9.

18. Joyce J, Hendrickson DA. Comparison of intraoperative pain responses following intratesticular or mesorchial injection of lidocaine in standing horses undergoing laparoscopic cryptorchidectomy. J Am Vet Med Assoc 2006;229:1779–83.

19. Rodgerson DH, Hanson RR. Ligature slippage during standing laparoscopic ovariectomy in a mare. Can Vet J 2000;41:395–7.

20. Alldredge JG, Hendrickson DA. Use of high-power ultrasonic shears for laparoscopic ovariectomy in mares. J Am Vet Med Assoc 2004;225:1578–80.

21. Shoemaker RW, Read EK, Duke T, et al. In situ coagulation and transection of the ovarian pedicle; and alternative to laparoscopic ovariectomy in juvenile horses. Can J Vet Res 2004;68:27–32.

22. Farstvedt EG, Hendrickson DA. Intraoperative pain responses following intraovarian versus mesovarian injection of lidocaine in mares undergoing laparoscopic ovariectomy. J Am Vet Med Assoc 2005;227:593–6.

23. Silva LC, Zoppa ALV, Hendrickson DA. Equine diagnostic laparoscopy. J Equine Vet Sci 2008;28:247–54.

24. Farstvedt EG, Hendrickson DA. Laparoscopic closure of the nephrosplenic space for prevention of recurrent nephrosplenic entrapment of the ascending colon. Vet Surg 2005;34:642–5.

25. Edwards RB 3rd, Ducharme NG, Hackett RP. Laparoscopic repair of a bladder rupture in a foal. Vet Surg 1995;24:60–3.

26. Boni L, Benevento A, Rovera F, et al. Infective complications in laparoscopic surgery. Surg Infect (Larchmt) 2006;7(Suppl 2):S109–11.

27. Gupta R, Sample S, Bamehriz F, et al. Infectious complications following laparo-scopic appendectomy. Can J Surg 2006;49:397–400.

28. Boure LP, Pearce SG, Kerr CL, et al. Evaluation of laparoscopic adhesiolysis for the treatment of experimentally induced adhesions in pony foals. Am J Vet Res 2002;63:289–94.

29. Klohnen A, Peroni JF. Thoracoscopy in horses. In: Hendrickson DA, editor. Endoscopic surgery, veterinary clinics of North America: equine practice. vol.16. Philadelphia: W.B. Saunders; 2000. p. 351–62.

Complications Associated with Equine Arthroscopy

Laurie R. Goodrich, DVM, MS, PhD[a],*, C. Wayne McIlwraith, MS, PhD[b]

KEYWORDS

• Arthroscopy • Horse • Complications

Arthroscopic surgery in the horse generally is accepted to be a low risk procedure. It is the treatment of choice for most joint diseases or conditions in which surgery is deemed necessary. Although complications associated with arthroscopy are infrequent, they can be significant when they do occur. In a review of the literature, currently only two peer-reviewed manuscripts exist in the horse regarding complications, one of which is a case report.[1,2] There are also two chapters in textbooks that review some of the more common complications.[3,4] This article reviews some of the common and uncommon complications that may occur during and after arthroscopy so that the reader may be aware of, and more importantly avoid, the pitfalls that may arise during and after arthroscopic surgery.

A REVIEW OF THE COMPLICATIONS OF ARTHROSCOPY IN PEOPLE

The knee is the most common joint subjected to arthroscopic procedures. Arthroscopy of the knee has been found to account for 50% of outpatient orthopedic surgery, and up to 650,000 are performed yearly.[5] Other joints that commonly have arthroscopic surgery performed are the shoulder, hip, ankle, and wrist. Various surveys of complications have been reported, with earlier surveys in the 1980s quoting complication rates ranging from 0.5% to 1.7%.[6,7] More recently, complication rates reported tend to be higher, with overall rates ranging from 6% to 16% depending on the joint operated and the difficulty of the procedure.[5,8–11] A recent paper described the overall complication rate of knee arthroscopies to be 5%, with only 0.68% having therapeutic consequences.[5] Arthroscopic complications vary with the joint and procedure performed. A paper reporting on the complications of anterior cruciate ligament reconstruction reported a complication rate up to 13.5%.[9] Kelly reported a 12% complication rate following elbow arthroscopy.[12] Brislin and colleagues[13] reported a 10.6% complication rate following shoulder arthroscopy. Foot and ankle surgeries

[a] Department of Clinical Sciences, College of Veterinary Medicine and Biomedical Sciences, Colorado State University, 300 West Drake Road, Fort Collins, CO 80523, USA
[b] Department of Clinical Sciences, Colorado State University, 300 West Drake Road, Fort Collins, CO 80523, USA
* Corresponding author.
E-mail address: Laurie.Goodrich@colostate.edu (L.R. Goodrich).

Vet Clin Equine 24 (2009) 573–589
doi:10.1016/j.cveq.2008.10.009
0749-0739/08/$ – see front matter © 2009 Elsevier Inc. All rights reserved.

vetequine.theclinics.com

comparatively have similar complication rates at 9% to 10%.[14] Reports associated with arthroscopic surgery of the hip range from 0.5% to 6%.[15]

The most common complications in people associated with knee arthroscopy are broken down into perioperative and postoperative complications. Common perioperative complications appear to be related to anesthesia, instrument breakage, prolonged tourniquet application, injurious use of leg holders, compartment syndrome, intra-articular damage, neurologic or vascular injury, and diagnostic errors.[7,10,16–19] Postoperative complications include hemarthrosis, thromboembolism, infection, effusion and synovitis, synovial fistula, and complex regional pain syndrome.[7,10,16,17,20–24]

Not surprisingly, the more complex arthroscopic procedures such as meniscal repairs, anterior cruciate ligament reconstructions, and transplant procedures such as osteochondral transplants have greater risk of complications.[10,11] Interestingly, experience of the surgeon has not been found to be related to complication rate; however, length of surgery, length of time tourniquets were applied, and age of patient (greater than 50 years) all have had relevance to increased complication rates.[10,16]

In summarizing recommendations to avoid surgical complications associated with arthroscopy of the knee, Allum recommended:

Use of a sharp trocar should be avoided.
Instruments should be used only when they can be observed clearly.
Tissues only should be cut under direct visualization.
Great care should be exercised with power instruments, especially with use of suction, as compromised visibility can result rapidly.[10]

Allum further warned new surgeons that visualization might be the greatest challenge because of poor technique. He stressed the importance of adequate supervision in the early stages of learning so that the important technical aspects of the operation are addressed. These include, but are not limited to, portal placement, positioning, triangulation, and adequate irrigation.[10]

Postoperative infection rates in people following arthroscopy have been reported to range from 0.08% to 1.4%.[6,17,21,25] Factors associated with increased risk of infection were longer operating times, corticosteroid use, prior surgical procedures, and soft tissue debridement.[12,26] The use of perioperative antibiotics varies depending on the surgeon and the joint undergoing surgery; however, Allum reports that most surgeons do not use antimicrobial drugs routinely except for complex procedures such as anterior cruciate ligament reconstructions.[10]

Instrument breakage and loose fragments associated with instruments have been reported as infrequent occurences.[27] In most cases, pieces are retrieved without incident by inhibiting fluid lavage and removal with forceps. An occasional report, however, has been published on long-term foreign body retention causing chronic pain.[19,28]

Pain and joint stiffness are uncommon complications associated with arthroscopic surgery; however, when they occur, significant morbidity to the patient may result.[10,29] As expected, pain can be more severe with extensive procedures such as intra-articular reconstruction of ligaments or extensive debridement of synovia or menisci.[10] Regional blocks, epidural anesthesia, intra-articular opiates, and local analgesics have been utilized to control or prevent associated pain.[30] A complex regional pain syndrome (CRPS) occurs infrequently in people, but it can lead to significant negative outcomes.[10] Fortunately, this syndrome has not been recognized to occur in the horse.

Iatrogenic damage to articular cartilage has been reported to be the most frequently unreported complication of all arthroscopic surgeries.[3,14] The use of conical obturators and careful use of sharp instruments have been recommended to avoid damage.[10]

Neurovascular injuries have been reported to occur infrequently and most commonly are associated with inappropriate portal placement or tourniquet application beyond 2 hours.[10,12,14,31] Compartment syndrome also may cause neural injury because of extrasynovial extravasation of fluid.[32] The most commonly reported nerve injury appears to be the peroneal nerve associated with knee arthroscopy.[33] Likewise, the most common vascular injury was popliteal puncture secondary to knee arthroscopy.[10]

Lastly, hemarthrosis, postoperative effusion, and skin suture abscesses occasionally occur but rarely cause a problem.[10] Hemarthrosis usually is treated by lavage and instillation of local analgesics. Effusion and synovitis usually is treated with anti-inflammatories, cold packs, elevation of the limb, and nonsteroidal drugs. If recalcitrant, however, the condition may be difficult to treat or may be a sign of ongoing or unresolved joint disease.[10] The use of sutures or adhesive tape has been compared and has not shown a difference in complication rates with the exception of the foot and ankle.[34] Use of sutures has been shown to be associated with reduced complications in the foot and ankle.[14]

INTRAOPERATIVE COMPLICATIONS IN THE HORSE
Hemarthrosis

Hemarthrosis during arthroscopy is usually more of an annoyance than a serious complication. It is more likely in those cases that prolonged surgical time is the resultant complication. In cases where the horse is in dorsal recumbency, hemarthrosis is reduced because of gravity compared to lateral recumbency. Cases where hemarthrosis seem to be the most common are in the tibiotarsal joint with extensive synovial proliferation, a septic joint where the synovium is prolific and inflamed and in tendon sheaths (**Fig. 1**). An important point to note is that bleeding can be minimized with adequate distension and that after a period of lavage, closing the egress cannula allows good visualization. When hemarthrosis occurs, the surgeon must use copious lavage utilizing an egress cannula to provide better visualization of the joint. In tendon sheaths, especially with the horse in lateral, tourniquets almost always are used to control bleeding. One of the authors (LG) also has used ephedrine occasionally in the fluids during lavage of both tendon sheaths and joints, and this has seemed to reduce the amount of bleeding.

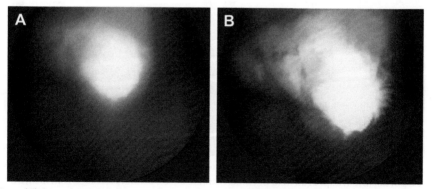

Fig.1. (*A*) An arthroscopic image of a carpal sheath in which hemarthrosis has obstructed the visualization of a distal radial exostosis. (*B*) Improved visualization of the distal radial exostosis after copious lavage of the sheath and increased fluid pressure within the sheath.

Obstruction of View by Synovial Villi

Each joint has areas of synovial villi that are more prolific than others. When obstruction of visualization occurs, it most frequently is associated with areas of the joint that are highly villous. If the visualization throughout the joint seems impaired by villous obstruction, then inadequate distension is most likely the cause. If distension cannot be accomplished, there may be capsular fibrosis present or, more commonly, extravasation of fluid causing collapse of the joint capsule. Excessive fluid movement through the joint also may result in synovial villi to obstruct the field of vision, which is usually the most common reason (**Fig. 2**). This can occur with an open outflow portal such as an open egress cannula or an excessively large and a patent instrument portal.[3] Large instrument portals can be a technical error or the result of removing a large intra-articular fragment(s). To minimize this problem, the initial arthroscopic examination should be performed with a closed egress cannula, and smaller fragments should be removed prior to large fragments.[3] Current fluid pumps will provide up to 1 liter/minute, which will compensate to some degree for a large outflow; however, at higher rates of fluid flow, bubbles may form, which also may result in diminished visualization.[3] Fluid flow from the arthroscopic portal additionally may be reduced by retaining an instrument in the portal. The surgeon, however, should not attempt to reduce fluid flow from the portal by placing a finger over the portal, as this will result in rapid fluid extravasation.[3]

Certain areas of joints are associated with greater obstruction of view compared with the other areas. Examples of areas that can be particularly troublesome are the dorsal and palmar/planter articular margins of the proximal phalanges, osteochondritis dissecans of the lateral trochlear ridge of the femur, and the lateral trochlear ridge of the talus.[3] A probe or an egress cannula often may be used to assess the lesions by displacing the synovial villi; however, a synovial resector often is required to adequately shave the synovium and allow necessary visualization. A motorized synovial resector and a manual resector for minor resecting are useful tools to accomplish this. Both should have a suction option to remove the tissue that is resected within the joint (**Fig. 3**). Because studies have proven that synovium does not regenerate,[35,36] overzealous use of these instruments should be avoided; joint capsule fibrosis may result.[3] The use of gas arthroscopy obviates many of the problems associated with the view being obscured by the synovium.

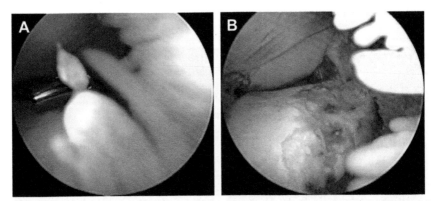

Fig. 2. (A) Synovial villi obstructing the field of vision due to extensive fluid flow through the egress portal. (B) An improved field of vision with the egress cannula closed. (*From* McIlwraith CW, Nixon AJ, Wright IM, et al. Problems and complications of diagnostic and surgical arthroscopy. In: McIlwraith CW, Nixon AJ, Wright IM, et al, editors. Diagnostic and surgical arthroscopy in the horse. 3rd edition. Philadelphia: Elsevier; 2005. p. 448–54; with permission.)

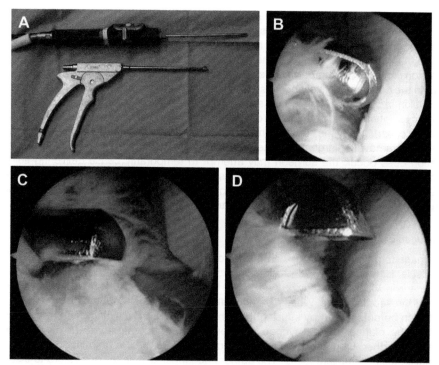

Fig. 3. (*A*) A motorized synovial resector (*top*) and a manual synovial resector (*bottom*). (*B*) A motorized synovial resector before resection of villi. (*C*) Resectioned synovial villi following use of the motorized resector. (*D*) A manual resector in which negative suction is created when the jaws are open. Note the villi being pulled into the jaws of the resector. Upon closing the jaws, villi are cut, and when jaws are opened, negative pressure forces cut tissue and fluid out through the shaft of the resector.

Extrasynovial Extravasation of Fluid

Extravasation of fluid between the joint capsule and skin or along facial planes is a commonly encountered problem for new arthroscopists; however, even experienced arthroscopic surgeons occasionally encounter this problem. The prevailing factors associated with this problem are the shape of the instrument portals (skin incision smaller than capsular incision), excessive intra-articular pressure, and excessive instrument manipulation through the portals.[3]

Shape of portals can play an important role in minimizing extravasation of fluid. It is important for beginning arthroscopists to attempt to complete the skin incision before the synovial capsule. One always should use a number 11 blade also, because the wedge shape of the blade ensures that the skin incision remains larger than the capsule. If a number 15 blade is used to create an arthroscopic portal, the surgeon should ensure the blade is angled appropriately during incision creation so that the skin portion of the portal is slightly larger than the capsule.

Removal of large intra-articular fragments while there is a high ingress fluid pressure into the joint often will lead to fluid extravasation. The risk of this occurring can be reduced by removing the smallest fragments first and reducing fluid flow during the removal of the large fragment through the arthroscopic portal.[3] Repeated entry of instruments through fluid portals or excessive instrument manipulation with force applied to the portal edges also weakens fascial planes and can result in extracapsular fluid.[3] Regardless of the cause, it is important to note that good articular visualization will be reduced when this occurs, leading to reduced surgical access, which can be quite frustrating to the surgeon if the lesion remains. In people, excessive fluid extravasation can result in compartment syndrome.[10] Fortunately, this does not seem to occur in the horse, most likely because of fewer tissue planes between the joint capsule and skin in the horse. Joints that seem to be more prone to fluid extravasation are the scapulohumeral joint, because of the complex muscle and facial planes that exist, the stifle, particularly the caudal compartments, and the tibiotarsal joint because of the frequent removal of large distal intermediate ridge lesions. If excessive fluid extravasation does occur, the surgeon may attempt to temporarily cease delivering fluids and apply firm massage to the skin portals and then recommence surgery. If a large quantity of fluid remains in the skin causing excessive tension on skin sutures, simple massage of the area usually can ameliorate the tension.[3]

Iatrogenic Damage to Articular Cartilage

Damage to articular cartilage can result from poor technique when entering the joint capsule. Either partial- or full-thickness articular lesions may result. The most common scenario in which this occurs is inadequate fluid distension of the joint prior to inserting the arthroscopic sleeve. When distending the joint capsule, adequate distension usually can be determined by infusing the joint with fluid from a syringe and monitoring when the plunger of the syringe requires mild-to-moderate force to distend the capsule further. Large synovial joints obviously require greater amounts of fluid than smaller, less- compliant joints. The authors no longer use sharp obturators to insert the arthroscopic sleeve because of the likelihood of damaging cartilage with the sharp end. The sleeve can be inserted easily with a conical obturator if a stab incision initially is made with a number 11 blade. Surgeons also should angle the blunt obturator and sleeve away from the articular cartilage. For instance, when entering the middle carpal joint, the obturator and sleeve should angle from side to side rather than dorsal to palmar (**Fig. 4**). Furthermore, when entering the joint capsule, excessive force should not be placed on the sleeve and obturator, because, even when using the conical

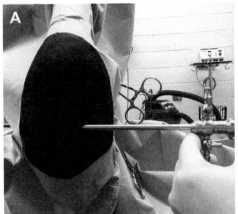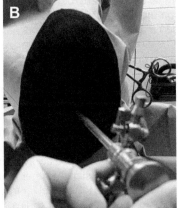

Fig. 4. (A) The arthroscopic sleeve and obturator correctly angled once through the skin and joint capsule to avoid damaging articular cartilage. (B) The arthroscopic sleeve and cannula incorrectly positioned risking damage to the articular cartilage.

obturator, excessive force can result in cartilage damage as a result of the space between the sleeve and cannula scraping across the cartilage surface. In the event of minor scuffing, significant long-term morbidity does not seem to occur.[3,37] When operating, arthroscopic instruments should not be used unless they can be seen clearly, and tissue never should be cut blindly, but always under direct vision.

Iatrogenic Damage to Other Tissues

Neurovascular structures may be damaged inadvertently upon entering the joint capsule depending on the portal sites. Areas where extra care should be taken are the palmar/planter regions of the limbs such as the portals necessary to enter the tendon sheath, caudal proximal and distal phalangeal joints and the navicular bursa, and the tibiotarsal joint (saphenous vein). When an Esmarch bandage or tourniquet is used, these structures become harder to identify and often predispose to injury of these structures.[3] Laceration of the palmar/plantar arteries becomes evident upon release of the tourniquet or by presence of hemorrhage postoperatively. If the saphenous vein is damaged upon creation of the portal, significant hemorrhage can occur intra-operatively which dramatically reduces visualization. In this situation, the authors have used extra-articular suture through the skin and joint capsule during surgery to complete the surgery and then remove the suture at the end of surgery. At that point, direct pressure with bandaging usually suffices to control bleeding. Damage to palmar or plantar nerves can be clinically silent initially; however, a painful neuroma may develop at the site postoperatively.[3]

The sheaths of the extensor carpi radialis and common digital extensor tendons can be penetrated by inappropriate arthroscope or instrument portals when doing carpal arthroscopy. This usually becomes apparent postoperatively and can result in constant and significant effusion of the sheath.[2,3] This usually does not cause lameness but results in very poor cosmesis in which owners are usually unhappy. A case report by Wilson reports communication between the sheath of the extensor carpi radialis and the middle carpal joint secondary to arthroscopy of the middle carpal joint to remove osteochondral fragmentation.[2] Once identified with radiocontrast, the communication was repaired by anesthetizing the horse and resecting and closing the tendon sheath synovial herniation. This incident can be avoided by careful palpation and creation of the skin incisions prior to distension of the joint capsule in this region.

Other soft tissues that potentially can be damaged are the menisci/cranial tibial meniscal ligaments or tendons during tenoscopy. In arthroscopy of the human knee, it is recommended to cut upwards with the blade away from the meniscus rather than downwards to avoid damaging menisci and their associated structures.[10] In the horse, the meniscus and cranial tibial meniscal ligament are more protected by the condyles; however, a needle should be used to ascertain the creation of the instrument portal, and the blade should be visualized with the arthroscope when making the instrument portal (**Fig. 5**). Likewise, when using motorized instruments with suction, tissue resection should not proceed unless the surgeon has a clear view of the resector or burr, especially while suction is applied, because rapid decrease in distension can result in loss of the field of surgical view.

Instrument Breakage

Instrument breakage most commonly occurs because of inappropriate force or using the instrument for an inappropriate task. If an instrument breaks, fluid flow should be stopped or dramatically reduced so that the fragment stays within the visual field. Ferris-Smith ronguers (Stryker Biotech, Hopkinton, Massachusetts) or an appropriate grasping device should be utilized to immediately grasp the fragment (**Fig. 6**). If the

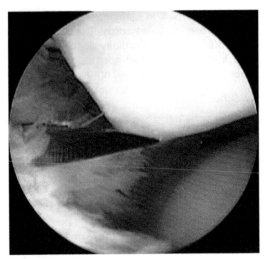

Fig. 5. Visualization of the scalpel tip while the instrument portal is created. Visualization of the blade will prevent injury to the cartilage surface or other structures within the joint.

fragment disappears from view, the surgeon should remain calm, and a systematic search should ensue. If the fragment is metallic, radiographs or fluoroscopy can be used to triangulate (by taking two views) and find the piece.

Surgeons should avoid excessive bending of instruments and use fixed rather than disposable blade cutting instruments within joints.[3] Number 11 or 15 scalpel blades and shafts of small angled spoon curettes are considered to be high risk in breaking under excessive force. If these instruments are used during a procedure, surgeons should be cognizant to check instruments after removing from the joint. Case reports exist in the human literature of unidentified pieces of instruments being left in the joint for several years causing ongoing pain.[19,28]

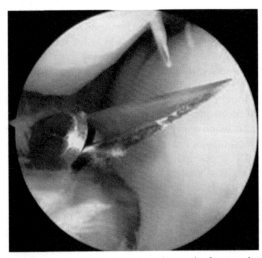

Fig. 6. Use of a Ferris-Smith rongeur in removing the end of a number 11 blade that has broken off in the joint.

Arthroscopic ronguers can break because of inappropriately twisting fragments while significant capsular attachments remain. In this case, the ronguers can break at the pin, and the instrument becomes nonfunctional. Manufacturers usually can replace the pin in these cases.[3]

In institutions where residents are being trained in the field of arthroscopy, scratching of the arthroscopic distal window will occur commonly. This can occur with hand or motorized instruments. Scratches will result in loss of clarity of the visual field. This situation can be avoided mostly by careful technique and only using instruments when they are in clear view. Most manufacturers provide service contracts to repair or replace the lens. These contracts are highly recommended for any institutions that run training programs, as the cost–benefit ratio is met quickly.

Finally, severe instrument damage can result when animals become light under anesthesia (**Fig. 7**). If the surgeon suspects a light plain of anesthesia, it is good practice to immediately withdraw the arthroscope to prevent catastrophic breakage of instruments and avoiding unnecessary damage to intra-articular structures.

Intrasynovial Foreign Material

Small pieces of metallic fragments sometimes can be seen following the impact of instruments on the arthroscopic sleeve or other metal-on-metal contact. This debris, if small, usually will flush out through an egress portal. Occasionally, it may become embedded within the synovium, but this has not been observed to result in morbidity.

When needles are used to distend the synovial cavity or determine portals, small pieces of skin or adhesive drape may be carried into the joint.[3] Adhesive drape fragments should be cut and opened slightly before entering the joint to minimize entrance of debris in the joint. Usually, if this debris gains entrance into the joint, it is easily lavaged out through portals or the egress cannula.

Intra-Articular or Subcutaneous Loss of Osteochondral Fragments

This problem is associated more frequently with the inexperienced surgeon; however, the experienced surgeon occasionally can lose large osteochondral pieces while attempting to pull them through a portal. If an osteochondral fragment becomes lost intrasynovially, as with instrument breakage, it needs to be located; ingress fluids then should be stopped, and the fragment retrieved. Fluid distension is necessary to

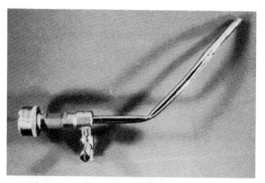

Fig. 7. Picture of a bent arthroscope sleeve incurred in a femoropatellar joint when the horse woke up and flexed the stifle during a light plane of anesthesia. (*From* McIlwraith CW, Nixon AJ, Wright IM, et al. Problems and complications of diagnostic and surgical arthroscopy. In: McIlwraith CW, Nixon AJ, Wright IM, et al, editors. Diagnostic and surgical arthroscopy in the horse. 3rd edition. Philadelphia: Elsevier; 2005. p. 448–54; with permission.)

assist in initial vision, but fluid movement also can displace a fragment rapidly, and the search can be frustrating. Gas arthroscopy also can assist in this situation, if available. If the piece is large enough or has bone, it should be visible radiographically or with the fluoroscope, and this can aid in locating the fragment. This is also the case in which fragments are lost in the subcutaneous tissue; these situations often can be more frustrating. Probably, the most common situation where fragments are lost from the rongeurs is when large distal intermediate ridge lesions of the tibia are removed from the joint. It is important to use large enough rongeurs when removing these fragments that when pulling through the skin portals, they do not slide off of the ends of the rongeur. This can be avoided by grasping the fragments, rolling within the joint (if there is enough space), and then making a larger skin incision. One of the authors (LG) uses the rule of thumb that if mild-to-moderate tension is encountered when the rongeur ends meet the skin edge, a scalpel blade is used to excise the skin over the rongeur ends while gently pulling on the instrument until easy passage is accomplished. Although this often results in a large skin portal, fluids can be increased to maintain distension for debridement of the rest of the joint (**Fig. 8**). Another situation that often leads to dropping a fragment is a lack of sufficient resection of capsular attachments such as in large carpal chip fragments where joint capsular attachment is significant. In these cases, intra-articular blades, synovial resectors, or radiofrequency probes can be used to cut away capsule. Ronguers then should be used to grasp the fragments and then rolled longitudinally to ensure that all attachments have been severed before bringing through the portal. It is also useful to visualize removal of these fragments in the event the piece slides off of the end of the instrument back into the joint.

Poor Portal Placement

Poor portal placement most frequently occurs because of inexperience and lack of familiarity with joint anatomy. It is important for the inexperienced surgeon to have adequate guidance to avoid the pitfalls and frustrations that often accompany poor portal placement that may lead to longer surgical times and difficulty in accomplishing the necessary procedure within the joint. It is the authors' opinion that comfort with arthroscopy of various joints varies with the individual; however, practice on cadavers before proceeding cannot be overemphasized in learning the technical aspects of triangulation. Poor portal placement can be avoided by being familiar with the joint anatomy, palpating structures associated with the joint before proceeding with the

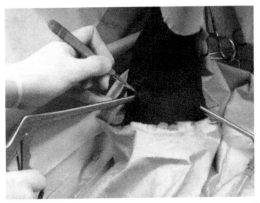

Fig. 8. A technique of incising the skin over the rongeur jaws while applying gentle tension to remove the large fragment from the joint.

surgery, and adequate practice for each joint. Once the arthroscope is placed in the joint, the surgeon should view a needle entering where the instrument portal will be prior to making the incision. Care should be taken to ensure that the needle not only can access the fragment but that the instrument can make all the necessary manipulations, and removal will not be hindered by a curved articular surface.

Occasionally, with flexing or extending the joint, portals may lose their patency. This is not necessarily because of poor portal placement; however, it can be frustrating to get instruments in and out of the portals. The instrument portal should be remade in the same place and direction as before. Switching sticks also can be used through the arthroscopic sleeve before flexion or extension of the joint (**Fig. 9**). The stick can be placed through the sleeve; the sleeve can be slid over the stick, the joint manipulated, and the sleeve slid back over the stick once the joint is flexed or extended appropriately. This maintains the portal and aids in ease of arthroscopic entrance through the portal and avoids separation of facial planes leading to fluid extravasation.

Postoperative Complications

Infection

One retrospective study has been performed on the incidence of infection after arthroscopic surgery in the horse.[1] In a review of 932 joint arthroscopies that were performed in 682 horses, eight joints became infected (0.9%). Factors evaluated for prevalence of infection included breed, sex, joint, preoperative intravenous antimicrobial administration, and intra-articular antibiotic administration. Of all factors evaluated, breed and joint operated were the only significant risks with draft breeds and tibiotarsal joints more likely than others to become infected. Of note was that antimicrobial administration did not influence risk, with 40% of the horses in the study receiving preoperative antibiotics. Most horses in the study that received antibiotics were administered some formulation of penicillin that was administered alone or concurrently with gentamicin. Several others received trimethoprim sulfamethoxazole or ceftiofur. Interestingly, most horses first had clinical signs of joint infection several days to weeks after discharge, with the median time of 20 days and a mean of 47 days.

Surgeons should be aware that sepsis can be subclinical for several days to weeks before signs become obvious to owners. This certainly may be influenced by the fact that horses are rehabilitating, and subtle lameness may not be apparent. The bacteria most frequently isolated in the joints in which culture was positive were

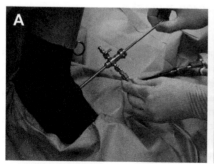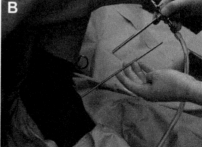

Fig. 9. (A, B) The metal instrument called a switching stick can be placed through the arthroscopic sleeve; the sleeve then is withdrawn over the stick (A) and removed (B). The joint then can be manipulated, and the portal is preserved. The arthroscope then is placed over the stick when the surgeon is satisfied with the new position of the leg.

Staphylococcus species, indicating that iatrogenic contamination from human skin was likely. One study reported that bacteria are more abundant on equine skin over joints close to the ground, but there was no evidence those joints were at higher risk.[38] Another study has been completed comparing skin bacterial flora over various joints of equine limbs, and it did not detect any differences in bacterial species (DA Hendrickson and colleagues, unpublished data). In the study by Olds and colleagues,[1] it was hypothesized that the tibiotarsal joint may be more predisposed to septic arthritis because of a close proximity between skin and the underlying synovial incision, so that leaking joint fluid easily contacts resident dermal bacteria. Furthermore, bone fragments removed from the tibiotarsal joint can be large and require a sizable instrument portal, which may further risk of leakage and infection increase. One of the authors (CWM) recorded five infections in his first 3000 cases, and four were in the tarsus. In all cases, the horse removed the bandage in the first 24 hours after surgery, and incisions were exposed.

Despite the results of the previously mentioned study, some clinicians still use perioperative antibiotics; however, their efficacy is questionable at best. Some clinicians also like to administer perioperative antibiotics to help prevent postoperative respiratory tract infections; however, greater use of antibiotics also increases the likelihood of antibiotic-induced diarrhea. Therefore, they should be used judiciously and the length of time administered should be kept at a minimum. The second author (CWM) does not use perioperative antibiotics if there is no implant insertion or no history of recent intra-articular injection.

In the event that a horse becomes lamer than expected following surgery, it is imperative for the clinician to investigate by aspirating joint fluid and obtaining a bacterial culture. Management should ensue quickly by copious lavage of the joint by either arthroscopic means or large bore needle lavage, with the first method preferable. Intra-articular, regional or intravenous administration should begin and consist of broad-spectrum antibiotics. Of the seven horses that had septic arthritis secondary to arthroscopy, all responded initially to intra-articular and systemic antibiotics; however, two horses became severely lame after antibiotics were discontinued and were euthanized.

Occasionally, infected cellulitis or fasciitis may occur as an uncommon sequela to arthroscopic surgery.[3] Most cases appear to resolve following systemic administration of antibiotics. Furthermore, infrequently, small skin abscesses or suture sinuses may occur following arthroscopy.[3] With removal of sutures, resolution of this complication ensues. If sutures are not removed in their entirety, a small fibrous lump may persist at the site or be associated with drainage at the skin.

Postoperative joint distention/synovitis

Postoperative distension may be a sign of ongoing disease but also may be a result of long-standing distension caused by chronic osteochondritis dissecans or inflammation related to osteochondral fragmentation present preoperatively. It is important for the clinician to ascertain the length of time capsular distension has been present so as to caution the owner preoperatively that distension may not resolve or only minimally decrease following arthroscopic surgery. Clinicians often use the 6- to 8-week time frame as a reference to whether resolution of distension will occur postoperatively. Distension also may occur with ongoing disease, or failure to remove loose bodies, so it is important for the surgeon to investigate with imaging modalities to ensure this is not the case. If all disease has been ruled out, ongoing distension can persist without clinical significance. Recently, Bergin and colleagues[39] reported oral hyaluronan gel significantly reduced postoperative tarsocrural effusion in the yearling Thoroughbred.

Failure to remove fragments

Joints presenting with multiple fragments present within a joint are particularly at increased risk of having a fragment left within a joint. It can be quite frustrating to the surgeon and embarrassing to explain to an owner that another arthroscopy is necessary to remove fragments left in the joint. In addition to joints where multiple fragments are present, large joints also can be at higher risk because of the extensive movement fragments can undergo within the joint when loose such as within femoropatellar joint. The following are recommended to prevent failure to remove fragments:

Try to identify all fragmentation preoperatively. This may include taking more than one radiograph of a standard view such as an oblique view of a palmar or plantar proximal phalangeal fragment to ensure identification of the osteochondral piece.

Adequate resection of synovium to expose any area of question where fragments may lodge and be obscured by proliferated synovium.

If unsure that the fragments are gone during surgery, take intraoperative radiographs before recovering the horse to ensure removal of all pieces.

Areas that seem to be prone to having migration of fragments are: the suprapatellar joint pouch, the intercondylar fossa of the medial femorotibial joint, and the palmar or planter pouches of the fetlock joint. When radiographing areas such as the suprapatellar pouch, the surgeon should ensure the very proximal recess is within the radiographic image. The proximal extent of that pouch is quite proximal, and the entire area can be easy to miss on radiographs, which could lead to missing a fragment(s) present. The authors routinely take intraoperative radiographs at the completion of surgery.

Enthesous new bone formation/soft tissue mineralization

In some cases where there is extensive tearing of the joint capsule preoperatively or because of large fragments being present at the joint capsule, the attachment is disrupted intraoperatively, and enthesous new bone can form (**Fig. 10**). This also seems to be more common in middle-aged to older horses; therefore, care should be practiced at these areas of the joint in any horse but especially in older horses. Enthesophytes in the dorsal carpus is common and not usually of consequence. The most critical intraoperative rule to avoid any postoperative capsular mineralization is to avoid trauma to the fibrous joint capsule. The authors feel that use of a local nonsteroidal anti-inflammatory applied to the joint capsule (Surpass, Idexx) may provide analgesia and reduce inflammation in these cases.

Synovial herniation

This was covered in the intraoperative complications section. It is associated with the extensor carpi radialis tendon sheath when arthroscopy of the radial or middle carpal joint is performed. If distension of this sheath is recognized postoperatively, entrance of the sheath and establishment of communication should be investigated.[2]

Neuropathy/myopathy

Neuropathy and myopathy are seen more commonly in people secondary to arthroscopic complications.[10] They usually are caused by prolonged tourniquet application or overzealous use of leg positioning devices. This does not seem to occur in horses. The more common paralysis secondary to arthroscopy seems to be associated with leaving both hind limbs in extension when operating the femoropatellar joints. These horses tend to be unable to bear weight adequately on one or both hind limbs and may have difficulty locking the patella. This may be caused by femoral neuropathy or neuromyopathy involving the quadriceps muscles. With either, the condition usually

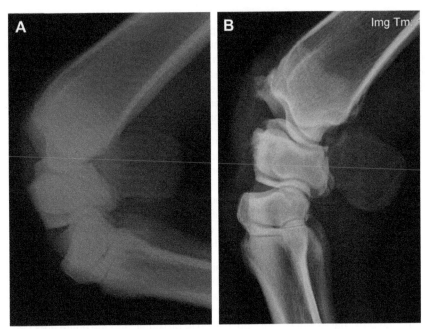

Fig. 10. (*A*) Radiographic image of a carpal joint of a 15-year-old Arabian that had mild osteochondral defects within the radiocarpal joint and small fragmentation on the dorsal aspect of the distal radius. (*B*) 6 months after arthroscopy, where tearing of the joint capsule created enthesophyte formation.

resolves quickly with rest and nonsteroidal therapy. It is important for the surgeon to be aware of positioning of the hind limbs when the stifles are being clipped, prepared, and positioned (**Fig. 11**). When surgery begins, it is important to flex the contralateral stifle that is not being operated on. When performing arthroscopy in lateral recumbency for joints such as the elbow or shoulder or tendon sheaths, radial nerve

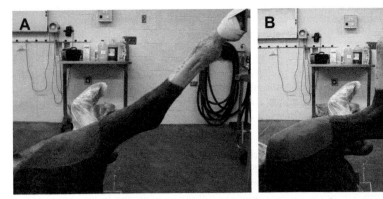

Fig. 11. It is important to flex the contralateral hind limb when the femoropatellar joint is explored with the arthroscope. (*A*) Exhibits the position of the leg for femoropatellar arthroscopy. (*B*) Exhibits how the contralateral limb should be positioned to avoid neuromuscular paralysis. If left in extension for the entire surgery, these horses often will attempt to bear weight on the toe but cannot support the weight of the limb.

paralysis and triceps myopathy may result from inadequate padding. Further discussion of anesthetic complications is found in Wagner's article elsewhere in this issue.

Pain

By virtue of entering the joint and performing copious lavage in arthroscopic procedures, often surgery will reduce inflammatory mediators associated with inflammation in the joint. Frequently, however, more joint manipulation needs to be performed than just fragment removal and, in situations where synovium and joint capsule will be cut and subchondral bone will be debrided, adequate pain management is necessary and important to decrease tissue morbidity and improve the welfare of the horse.

The best way to prevent postoperative pain is to treat it preemptively. This can be done by performing a perineural block preoperatively if the surgeon anticipates a moderate degree of pain caused by fragment removal or debridement. Furthermore, the use of Carbocaine or bupivicaine also can be utilized for distending the joint before creation of the portals.[3] It should be recognized that short procedures involving small fragments or minimal time in the joint may require minimal perioperative pain management. One of the authors (LG) currently performs epidurals using 0.1 mg/kg of morphine and 0.03 mg/kg of detomidine aliquoted up to 20 mL with saline for any procedures that are predicted to cause moderate or severe postoperative pain of the joints in the hind limbs. Procedures such as osteochondral fragment removal and subchondral bone debridement of large areas caused by osteochondritis dessicans lesions or femorocondylar cysts (that will undergo debridement) would be examples where this management would be utilized. A study by Goodrich and colleagues[40] proved significant analgesia following stifle arthroscopy using this method of pain control. Horses seem to be able to be maintained under a lighter plane of anesthesia and have improved recoveries with pre-emptive pain management. Furthermore, preoperative epidurals using morphine and detomidine do not decrease the quality of recovery from anesthesia, because only sensory (and not motor) nerves are affected.[41] Postoperatively, most horses are administered phenylbutazone intravenously or orally for 3 to 7 days depending on the procedure. The second author of this article (CWM) limits pain management to perioperative phenylbutazone and gives flunixin meglumine at the end of surgery unless there are extenuating circumstances. Recently, topical nonsteroidal therapy has been investigated, and (Surpass, Idexx) seems to be a beneficial adjunctive therapy to oral nonsteroidal drugs when capsulitis occurs secondary to the procedure.

SUMMARY

The incidence of complications associated with equine arthroscopy is low. This, however, does not obviate the importance of preventing and recognizing those complications when they occur. It is the responsibility of the surgeon to be aware of the pitfalls and know how to manage them when they arise. Many of the complications of arthroscopy can be avoided by good technique, being familiar with anatomy, and having ample experience with triangulation and arthroscopic instrument usage. New arthroscopists should spend the time necessary to be familiar with the techniques and instrumentation through ample practice on cadaver legs and under supervision of an experienced surgeon.

REFERENCES

1. Olds AM, Stewart AA, Freeman DE, et al. Evaluation of the rate of development of septic arthritis after elective arthroscopy in horses: 7 cases (1994–2003). J Am Vet Med Assoc 2006;229:1949–54.

2. Wilson DG. Synovial hernia as a possible complication of arthroscopic surgery in a horse. J Am Vet Med Assoc 1989;194:1071–2.

3. McIlwraith CW, Nixon AJ, Wright IM, et al. Problems and complications of diagnostic and surgical arthroscopy. In: McIlwraith CW, Nixon AJ, Wright IM, et al, editors. Diagnostic and surgical arthroscopy in the horse. 3rd edition. Elsevier; 2005. p. 448–54.

4. McIlwraith CW. Diagnostic and surgical arthroscopy in the horse. 2nd edition. Philadelphia: Lea and Febiger; 1990.

5. Reigstad O, Grimsgaard C. Complications in knee arthroscopy. Knee Surg Sports Traumatol Arthrosc 2006;14:473–7.

6. Delee JC. Complications of arthroscopy and arthroscopic surgery: results of a national survey. Committee on Complications of Arthroscopy Association of North America. Arthroscopy 1985;1:214–20.

7. Small NC. Complications in arthroscopic surgery performed by experienced arthroscopists. Arthroscopy 1988;4:215–21.

8. Michot M, Conen D, Holtz D, et al. Prevention of deep-vein thrombosis in ambulatory arthroscopic knee surgery: a randomized trial of prophylaxis with low molecular weight heparin. Arthroscopy 2002;18:257–63.

9. Almazan A, Miguel A, Odor A, et al. Intraoperative incidents and complications in primary arthroscopic anterior cruciate ligament reconstruction. Arthroscopy 2006; 22:1211–7.

10. Allum R. Complications of arthroscopy of the knee. J Bone Joint Surg Br 2002;84: 937–45.

11. Allum R. Complications of arthroscopic reconstruction of the anterior cruciate ligament. J Bone Joint Surg Br 2003;85:12–6.

12. Kelly EW, Morrey BF, O'Driscoll SW. Complications of elbow arthroscopy. J Bone Joint Surg Am 2001;83-A:25–34.

13. Brislin KJ, Field LD, Savoie FH III. Complications after arthroscopic rotator cuff repair. Arthroscopy 2007;23:124–8.

14. Ferkel RD, Small HN, Gittins JE. Complications in foot and ankle arthroscopy. Clin Orthop Relat Res 2001;391:89–104.

15. Smart LR, Oetgen M, Noonan B, et al. Beginning hip arthroscopy: indications, positioning, portals, basic techniques, and complications. Arthroscopy 2007;23: 1348–53.

16. Small NC. Complications in arthroscopy: the knee and other joints. Committee on complications of the Arthroscopy Association of North America. Arthroscopy 1986;2:253–8.

17. Sherman OH, Fox JM, Snyder SJ, et al. Arthroscopy—no problem surgery. An analysis of complications in two thousand six hundred and forty cases. J Bone Joint Surg Am 1986;68:256–65.

18. Gambardella RA, Tibone JE. Knife blade in the knee joint: a complication of arthroscopic surgery. A case report. Am J Sports Med 1983;11:267–8.

19. Rajadhyaksha AD, Mont MA, Becker L. An unusual cause of knee pain 10 years after arthroscopy. Arthroscopy 2006;22:E1–3.

20. Dandy DJ, O'Carroll PF. Arthroscopic surgery of the knee. Br Med J 1982;285: 1256–8.

21. D'Angelo GL, Ogilvie-Harris DJ. Septic arthritis following arthroscopy, with cost/benefit analysis of antibiotic prophylaxis. Arthroscopy 1988;4:10–4.

22. Dandy DJ. Complications and technical problems. In: Dandy DJ, editor. Arthroscopic managment of the knee. 2nd edition. Edinburgh: Churchill Livingstone; 1987. p. 64–71.

23. Proffer DS, Drez D Jr, Daus GP. Synovial fistula of the knee: a complication of arthroscopy. Arthroscopy 1991;7:98–100.
24. O'Brien SJ, Ngeow J, Gibney MA, et al. Reflex sympathetic dystrophy of the knee. Causes, diagnosis, and treatment. Am J Sports Med 1995;23:655–9.
25. Barber FA, Click J, Britt BT. Complications of ankle arthroscopy. Foot Ankle 1990; 10:263–6.
26. Armstrong RW, Bolding F, Joseph R. Septic arthritis following arthroscopy: clinical syndromes and analysis of risk factors. Arthroscopy 1992;8:213–23.
27. Gruson KI, Ilalov K, Youm T. A broken scalpel blade tip: an unusual complication of knee arthroscopy. Bull NYU Hosp Jt Dis 2008;66:54–6.
28. Oldenburg M, Mueller RT. Intra-articular foreign body after arthroscopy. Arthroscopy 2003;19:1012–4.
29. Beredjiklian PK, Bozentka DJ, Leung YL, et al. Complications of wrist arthroscopy. J Hand Surg [Am] 2004;29:406–11.
30. Chakravarthy V, Arya VK, Dhillon MS, et al. Comparison of regional nerve block to epidural anaesthesia in day care arthroscopic surgery of the knee. Acta Orthop Belg 2004;70:551–9.
31. Kornbluth ID, Freedman MK, Sher L, et al. Femoral, saphenous nerve palsy after tourniquet use: a case report. Arch Phys Med Rehabil 2003;84:909–11.
32. Kim TK, Savino RM, McFarland EG, et al. Neurovascular complications of knee arthroscopy. Am J Sports Med 2002;30:619–29.
33. Krivic A, Stanec S, Zic R, et al. Lesion of the common peroneal nerve during arthroscopy. Arthroscopy 2003;19:1015–8.
34. Hussein R, Southgate GW. Management of knee arthroscopy portals. Knee 2001; 8:329–31.
35. Theoret CL, Barber SM, Moyana T, et al. Repair and function of synovium after arthroscopic synovectomy of the dorsal compartment of the equine antebrachiocarpal joint. Vet Surg 1996;25:142–53.
36. Doyle-Jones PS, Sullins KE, Saunders GK. Synovial regeneration in the equine carpus after arthroscopic mechanical or carbon dioxide laser synovectomy. Vet Surg 2002;31:331–43.
37. McIlwraith CW, Fessler JF. Arthroscopy in the diagnosis of equine joint disease. J Am Vet Med Assoc 1978;172:263–8.
38. Hague BA, Honnas CM, Simpson RB, et al. Evaluation of skin bacterial flora before and after aseptic preparation of clipped and nonclipped arthrocentesis sites in horses. Vet Surg 1997;26:121–5.
39. Bergin BJ, Pierce SW, Bramlage LR, et al. Oral hyaluronan gel reduces post operative tarsocrural effusion in the yearling Thoroughbred. Equine Vet J 2006; 38:375–8.
40. Goodrich LR, Nixon AJ, Fubini SL, et al. Epidural morphine and detomidine decreases postoperative hindlimb lameness in horses after bilateral stifle arthroscopy. Vet Surg 2002;31:232–9.
41. Goodrich LR, Butler E, Donaldson L, et al. The efficacy of epidurally administered morphine and detomidine in decreasing stress levels under general anesthesia and the effect on anesthetic recoveries. Vet Surg 2000;29:463.

Complications of Orthopaedic Surgery in Horses

Dean W. Richardson, DVM

KEYWORDS

- Horse • Fracture repair • Complications • Infection
- Technical errors • Internal fixation

The definition of a "complication" in surgery is, itself, complicated. To the surgeon, a complication would probably be best defined as an untoward event of any type that adversely affects the expected outcome of the case. To an owner, the definition might tend toward meaning anything that affects the expense by a single dollar. Most surgeons would probably agree that the major complications of orthopaedic surgery are infection and implant failure/instability, but technical errors leading to functional impairment are probably the most preventable complication. Inadequate reduction of articular fractures, iatrogenic damage to important structures (articular cartilage, ligaments, tendons, nerves), cast sores, fractures distant from the original injury, and anesthetic recovery catastrophes are only a few of the reasons why an equine orthopaedist needs to be resilient. Perhaps the most unnerving complication is contralateral laminitis because it can be so unpredictable. One horse can stand on three legs for months and another horse will fall through its foot in a matter of days when that horse doesn't even appear all that uncomfortable.

INTRAOPERATIVE COMPLICATIONS

Technical errors associated with internal fixation are probably no more common in horses than in other species, but there is little doubt that the margin for technical error is especially slim in horses. The essential premise of equine fracture repair is that the patient must be able to bear weight comfortably and immediately to consistently avoid problems in the contralateral limb (see chapter by Baxter and Morrison). The best single means of preventing laminitis in the fracture patient is to make the horse bear weight on all four limbs as soon as possible. Slings and/or prolonged recumbency can be successfully used in some horses but certainly not all and such intensive nursing efforts are extremely expensive. Although laminitis is rare in foals and yearlings, weight-bearing comfort is essential if plastic deformation of the contralateral limb is to be

New Bolton Center School of Veterinary Medicine, University of Pennsylvania, 382 West Street Road, Kennett Square, PA 19348-1692, USA
E-mail address: dwr@vet.upenn.edu

Vet Clin Equine 24 (2009) 591–610
doi:10.1016/j.cveq.2008.11.001
0749-0739/08/$ – see front matter © 2009 Elsevier Inc. All rights reserved.

avoided. The development of permanent damage to joints and long bones of the opposite limb can be amazingly insidious in young horses. Fractures can heal with great success only to have an unsound horse at a much later date. The bottom line is that any technical error in internal fixation that compromises the mechanical integrity of the repair can lead to instability, which is the most common cause of discomfort.

The major complication of bone plating is loss of stability. Although reality (and physics) dictates that clinicians still do not have the technical capacity to achieve stable fixations of all fractures, there are a number of common operative errors that can increase the probability of instability.

Inadequate Reduction

Inadequate reduction is one of the most common and important errors both for biological and mechanical reasons. Mechanically, surgeons are often balanced on the precipice of strength of the metal implants so it is essential to seek load-sharing of the reconstructed fracture whenever possible by accurately re-aligning bone ends. Fracture gaps, even small ones, result in enormous increases in cyclic loads on the implants. It is essential for the surgeon to understand that small fracture gaps in otherwise well-repaired fractures are still a major concern because the strain of the bone-implant construct will be concentrated at that small gap and this may result in fatigue failure or enough motion that comfort and fracture healing are impaired. Large fracture gaps have a different problem because the plates and screws alone have to sustain weight-bearing loads. Angular malalignments of fractures will increase bending moments that may also overwhelm the strength of the implants. Although it is certainly not always possible, the surgeon should always seek optimal reduction. When load-sharing by the bone is not feasible, the use of fixed angle implants such as locking plates becomes more essential.

Inaccurate reduction of major articular fractures, such as displaced lateral condylar fractures, carpal slab fractures and mid-body sesamoid fractures, is a major complication and will always result in suboptimal results. (**Fig. 1**) One must do everything possible to assure alignment of articular fractures if an athletic outcome is desired. Arthroscopic reduction of articular fractures has become a standard technique to assure accurate reduction. With any displaced articular fracture being repaired with

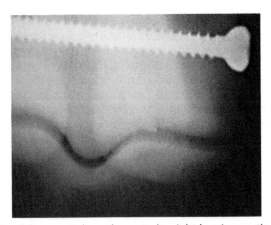

Fig.1. Even a small malalignment along the central weight-bearing portion of the condyle is a major complication of a displaced lateral condylar fracture. This problem can nearly always be avoided by careful arthroscopically monitored reduction and screw fixation.

lag screws, a useful technique is to drill the glide hole accurately fully through to the fracture plane but no farther. The arthroscope is best positioned directly over the proximal margin of the fracture plane. When the drill bit for the glide hole is removed, a smooth pin is dropped in the glide hole and the protective drill guide is removed. The centering insert sleeve is then slid over the pin and fully inserted in the glide hole. With a displaced condylar fracture, fluid will exit the sleeve. (**Fig. 2**A) The centering sleeve (with or without the pin in it) is then used as a "handle" on the fracture fragment until a combination of limb manipulation and fragment manipulation places the fracture edges in perfect alignment. One or more bone clamps are then used to maintain the reduction while the remaining steps of the lag screw technique are completed. (**Fig. 2**B) The arthroscopic view must include the broadest region possible to be certain that the reduction is truly correct. Two curved surfaces can be apparently well aligned in one specific area where they overlap but be badly aligned proximal and distal to that one area.

Inadequate Size or Number of Implants

Inadequate size or number of implants in horses is a problem that cannot be readily overcome by external coaptation or verbal instructions about limited weight-bearing as it might be with a person's injury. Therefore, the tendency of most equine surgeons is to err somewhat on the side of more metal when there is a question. This is not to suggest that experience and increasing confidence can lead toward less aggressive fixations, but it is important to recognize that most long bone fractures in horses absolutely need two plates and that larger diameter screws can be the difference between success and failure. In difficult long bone fractures, longer plates are better because they will increase the overall strength of the repair and lessen stress concentration in the diaphyseal region. The surgeon also needs to consider all of the dimensions of each plate, not just its length.

Incorrect positioning of plates

Incorrect positioning of plates can lead quickly to failure. A plate should optimally be directly on the tension surface of the bone and whenever possible, plates should be placed at right angles to one another (ie, lateral and dorsal or dorsolateral and dorsomedial). When double plating, plates should be staggered exactly one half-hole so that

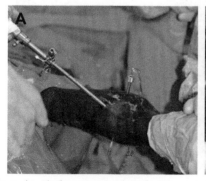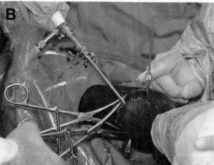

Fig. 2. (A, B) The scope is placed at the proximal edge of the fracture. The centering sleeve is placed through the fragment to the fracture plane and, in a displaced fracture, fluid from the arthroscope sleeve will exit. (A) While observing with the arthsocope, the distal limb is manipulated and the fragment manipulated with the insert sleeve. When proper reduction is achieved, large, pointed, bone-reduction forceps are used to maintain the reduction.

screws from one plate will not interfere with screws in the other. This is absolutely critical in locking plates in which the screws must be inserted exactly 90° to the plate.

Complications of Lag-Screw Fixation

I) Poor placement of screws, (ie, directed into or through an articular surface, too close to the edge of a fragment or angled inappropriately) (**Fig. 3**).

- Drape generously; leave as much of the limb's long axis exposed as is practical by using impervious stockinet and transparent plastic adhesive drapes.
- Palpate well-defined external landmarks that can help with alignment of the drill.
- Stand back away from the patient and look at the drill position from a distance.
- Don't delude yourself. If the bit/screw looks as if it is in the incorrect place, it probably is. Change it.
- Take the appropriate radiographs during surgery before you make a mistake (ie, with needles/small diameter marker drill bits). Fluoroscopy or digital radiography is nearly essential for efficiency.

II) The screw doesn't tighten

- Excessive force was applied by the surgeon. This can only be avoided by developing a "feel." Good practice is to try to strip different size screws in different types of bone from different age cadavers.

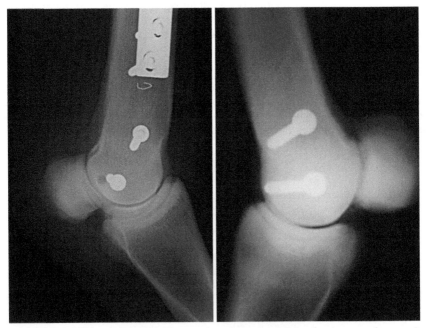

Fig. 3. Incorrect aiming of the distal screw in a lateral condylar fracture can be a serious complication. It is best to remove and reposition the screw (*left*) if the error is recognized. If the surgeon drills perpendicular to the floor even though the horse's limb is externally rotated, the result will be the tip of the screw being too far palmar (*left*). Overcorrection of this tendency can result in the equally bad mistake of directing the screw too far dorsally (*right*).

- The thread hole was improperly tapped. This problem can occur in soft bone is when there is a "bottom" in the hole and the surgeon gives an extra turn with the tap.
- The tapped portion of the hole is too short because of underdrilling the pilot hole or overdrilling the glide hole. Two or three threads are much easier to strip than 10 or 12 threads.
- The hole was improperly measured and too short a screw was used to engage the threads.

Options when this occurs:

- Try a longer screw of the same diameter. This is not recommended unless the error in screw length was significant.
- Try a larger diameter screw. If the screw is intended to lag, be sure to enlarge the glide hole.

III) The fracture doesn't compress when the screw is tightened

- The glide hole didn't reach to or extend across the fracture line (**Fig. 4**). When this happens, the fracture line usually widens slightly as the screw is tightened. If this occurs, carefully redrill the glide hole a small measured amount further.
- The screw is too long for the hole (if the thread hole did not pass entirely through the bone). The screw's tip hits the bottom of the hole before the head engages the outer surface of the bone. Measure again and place a shorter screw.
- The thread hole was incompletely tapped. The screw will tighten before the head engages. If this occurs, carefully re-insert the tap and rethread after measuring

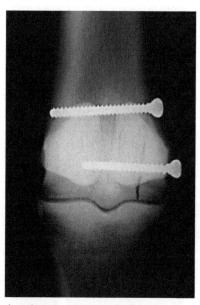

Fig. 4. If a screw feels tight but doesn't compress the fracture, the most likely technical errors are: not tapping the full depth of the hole; not drilling a long enough thread hole; or inserting too long a screw in a hole with a "bottom." In such a case, the easiest solution is to remove the screw, drill farther out the far side, retap and place a longer screw.

the hole again. Compare the depth of the hole to the length of the tap inserted or check with radiographic guidance that the tap extends the length of the hole.

- Debris is in the fracture plane. Loosen the screw (or screws) and debride.

IV) The screw bends or breaks

- Inadequate countersinking in a highly contoured bone such as proximal lateral P1. Remove the screw, countersink again and place a new screw. Check the length because the second countersinking may necessitate a slightly shorter screw.
- Excessive tightening. This is a problem in the extremely dense cortical bone of horses (**Fig. 5**). In most bone in other species, the screw will strip before it breaks.
- Poor reduction of fracture can result in shifting of the fragments and postoperative bending or breakage of implants (**Fig. 6**) If this occurs, the decision whether or not to replace a bent or broken implant is usually dependent on the clinical progression (ie, comfort) of the patient. See comments below regarding broken implant removal.

V) Broken bits or taps

- Lubricate constantly with sterile fluids when drilling and tapping. Use your arthroscopic fluid delivery system.
- Clean drill bit flutes frequently, especially in dense bone. Cleaning of bits needs to be done more frequently in smaller diameter bits.
- Use sharp bits and taps. This is especially critical when doing standing procedures.
- When tapping dense bone, always make one turn backward for every two or three forward turns.
- Watch the drill bit to avoid bowing (bending) while drilling.
- Do not power tap a critical hole (ie, a juxta-articular one) unless you are very experienced. Especially be careful if there is a "bottom" to the hole.
- Drill round holes. Minimize drill wobble. Use drill guides.
- Drill straight holes. Don't let the bit slide up or down the endosteal side of the far (trans-) cortex.
- Think three-dimensionally to avoid other screws if it is a complex reconstruction.

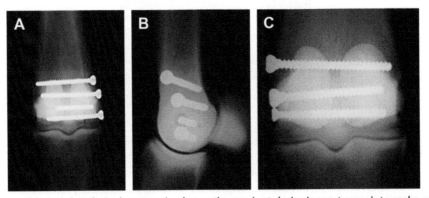

Fig. 5. If a screw breaks in dense equine bone, the prudent choice in most cases is to make no effort to remove it. Instead, place a screw adjacent to it (*A, B*). This can be the same size screw if there is adequate room. If not, use a smaller screw (*C*).

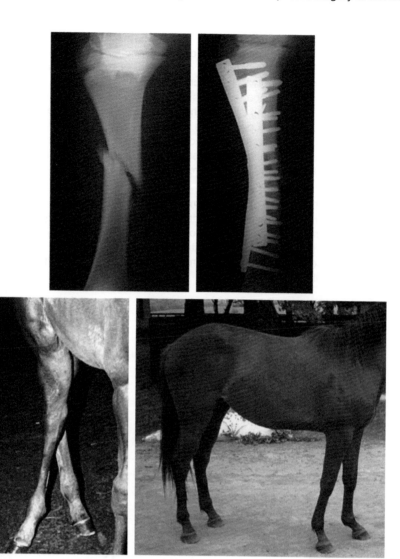

Fig. 6. A poorly repaired tibial fracture in which the reduction was imperfect and the end of the oblique fracture was not supported by a plate. The inevitable consequence is bending of the plate and eventual failure of the repair. The plates were removed, the fracture replated, and, 2 years later, the filly had a functional hindlimb. Mechanical errors need to be recognized and repaired when it is feasible.

It is useful to know how to remove broken drills, taps and screws. Drills and taps are most often broken intraoperatively and the prudent decision, especially in a complex double-plating procedure, is usually to leave them in the bone and work around them. Always think about the limited benefit afforded by removing a broken bit, tap or screw in a complex repair; it usually is simply not worth the time and trauma. A high-quality pair of locking pliers is an invaluable instrument; hardware store locking pliers simply do not work as well in tight spaces. Bits are usually removed by removing enough bone such that they can be grasped and pulled. Broken taps are removed similarly to screws. There are three basic ways that a screw can fail and be difficult to remove. If the hex-recess or star-recess is stripped, a conical counterthreaded hardened steel screw (Synthes 309.5 this needs to be completed) of the correct size can be used to remove the stripped implant. If the screw is broken in the near cortex, it is usually possible to use a narrow gouge or small drill holes around it until the broken shaft can be grasped with locking pliers (Synthes 359.204) and extracted (**Fig. 7**). If the screw is broken and is too deep to be adequately exposed, a hollow reamer with a centering pin is used to ream a larger hole directly over the broken screw. An extraction bolt that is turned onto the broken screw threads is attached. The broken screw can then simply be removed by counterclockwise effort (**Fig. 8**).

VI) Thermal Injury (usually recognized by ring sequestra)
- Clean bits frequently when drilling dense, thick equine bones (**Fig. 9**). You should not try to drill across an adult cannon bone without removing the bit a few times to remove the cuttings from the flutes of the bit.
- Lubricate copiously. Use your arthroscopic fluid delivery system.
- Discard dull drill bits.

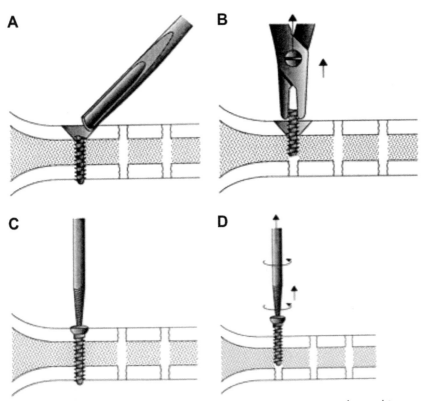

Fig. 7. (*A*) If the screw breaks in the near cortex, a gouge or curette can be used to expose enough of the screw that (*B*) extraction pliers can remove it. (*C*) If the screw head recess strips, a counterthreaded screw extractor can be drilled into the screw head. (*D*) It is critical that the extraction bit is drilled very carefully in the center of the screw head. (This tool is essentially identical to "easy-out" screw extraction bits in machine shops.) (*Courtesy of Synthes, Inc., Paoli, PA. Copyright 2008, Synthes, Inc. or its affiliates. All rights reserved.*)

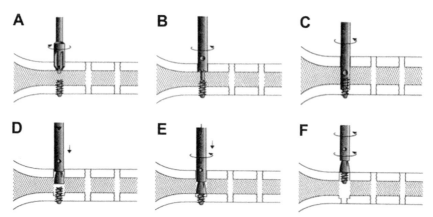

Fig. 8. If a screw breaks deep in the bone or far cortex and it is necessary to remove the broken screw, specialized instrumentation can prove helpful. (*A*) A countersink (*shown*) or larger drill bit can be used to enlarge the hole in the near cortex. (*B*) A hollow reaming tool is used in a counterclockwise direction. A centering pin is used to help align the reamer with the end of the broken screw. The reamer is then removed and the centering pin removed (not shown). (*C*) The reamer is reinserted and counterclockwise drilling continued several millimeters to expose screw threads. (*D*) The reamer is removed and replaced with an internally threaded extraction tool. (*E*) The extraction tool is pushed down and turned counterclockwise to engage the broken screw threads. (*F*) With continued counterclockwise rotation, the screw backs out of the bone. (*Courtesy of* Synthes, Paoli, PA; with permission.)

Postoperative Complications

Instability of a major fracture repair is probably the most challenging postoperative complication because it demands that the clinician make a number of important decisions, none of which are easy. Instability nearly always results in diminished comfort

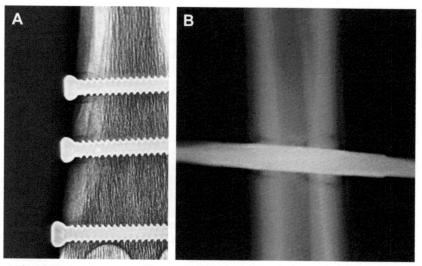

Fig. 9. (*A, B*) Ring sequestra readily occur when drilling extremely dense cortical bone. It is essential to use copious fluid irrigation, sharp drill bits, frequent removal and cleaning of drill bits and patience if they are to be avoided.

for the patient. Increasing analgesia of an inherently unstable repair generally doesn't help that much in an adult horse because the repair usually progresses toward failure. In a very young horse, callus formation may be rapid enough to stabilize the fracture before major disruption of the fracture or breakdown of the contralateral limb occurs. In most cases with apparent instability, the first step is usually to maximize external coaptation; if it is in a bandage, put it in a cast and if it is in a cast, put it in a transfixation cast. The most critical decision is whether or not to make an effort at a complete second repair. This is an enormous financial commitment, but if the surgeon is confident that they are gazing at inevitable failure, another attempt is probably justified. The only justification to consider re-operation would be if the surgeon honestly believes that a second effort will make a difference. Usually, returning to surgery to do the same procedure is not worthwhile unless a correctable technical error was recognized postoperatively, such as removing or replacing a seriously malpositioned screw.

The loosening or breakage of screws are not always indications to replace the implant. This decision must be made after considering the clinical progression of the case. It is fairly uncommon that simple replacement of a loose screw or two will really make a difference.

Common Complications of Common Procedures

Medial condylar fractures

Medial condylar fractures are the most common challenging fracture in racehorses. Unlike lateral condylar fractures, they tend to either spiral up the length of the bone or split in their mid-diaphysis in a "y" configuration. If they propagate proximally, they are prone to catastrophic dehiscence during recovery from general anesthesia or even for weeks after repair (**Fig. 10**). Medial MT3 fractures are particularly dangerous. The surgical options are: standing repair with a few distal lag screws to reduce the articular component; multiple screws placed perpendicular to the spiraling fracture plane (preferably discerned by open exposure or computed tomography); or plate fixation. If general anesthesia is performed, any available special recovery system (eg, pool, sling) should be used. If special recovery systems are not available, many surgeons use full limb casts during recovery. If plate or multiple screw fixation is used for repair, the major concern is entering the fracture plane with one or more screws. In the author's opinion, this concern is less significant if a locking plate is used but it still should be avoided. Another complication to avoid is damage to MC2 by a penetrating screw because the plate is usually placed on the dorsolateral surface (**Fig. 11**).

Third carpal slab fractures

Third carpal slab fractures have a variety of configurations and accompanying complications. The most common complication with frontal plane C3 slab fractures is the presence of a wedge-shaped fragment on the proximal articular surface along the fracture plane. In a small percentage of cases, the fragment can be "trapped" in position when the lag screw or screws are tightened, but usually it has to be removed and a decision made about removal of the proximal margin of the fragment. There is no real "rule" on this decision, but removal of that rim of bone and cartilage is probably indicated in smaller slab fractures with deeper troughs. The most common technical error is failure to center the screw in the middle of the fragment; eccentric placement sometimes will not be an issue, but in other cases, the fragment will crack or the fragment will "spin" as the screw is tightened. If the latter occurs, the screw should be loosened and a second screw placed. If the fragment cracks and the unstable fragment is too

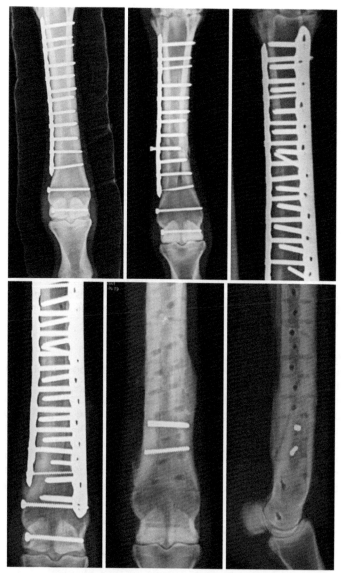

Fig. 10. A medial condylar fracture of MT3 repaired with distal lag screws and a locking compression plate. The horse developed severe colic a few days after surgery and fractured in the mid-diaphysis. The complication was managed by replacing the loose screws in the lateral plate and applying a second dorsomedial plate. Both plates were placed with a minimally invasive technique. The fracture healed, the plates were removed sequentially, and the horse raced successfully.

small to repair, it should be removed. The major complication with sagittal slab fractures is impingement of the screw head on C2. Sagittal C3 fractures are easiest to repair with 3.5 mm screws because the screw head is easier to fit in the narrow space just dorsal to C2.

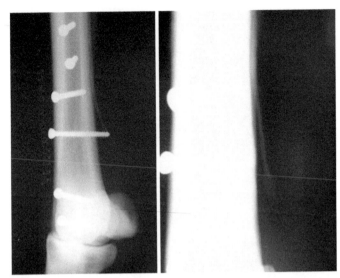

Fig. 11. Whenever a screw is placed obliquely across the metacarpus or metatarsus, care must be taken not to damage the contralateral splint bone (*left*). In this case the splint was fortunately not broken and returned to its normal position when the offending screw was replaced (*right*).

Ulnar fractures

Ulnar fractures are generally considered the easiest of long bone fractures to repair in horses, but they still have some common complications. In young horses (< 6 months), screws that engage the radius distal to the proximal radial growth plate can result in elbow incongruity. In the youngest patients, therefore, the surgeon should try to engage only the ulna with the screws or, preferably in this author's opinion, use a tension band wiring technique. If the radius has to be engaged for some reason, the surgeon should plan to remove the plate as soon as possible. Another major complication of ulnar fractures is comminution involving the proximal aspect of the anconeal notch (**Fig. 12**). If this occurs, the dissection of the lateral aspect of the proximal

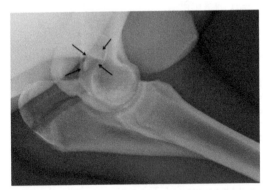

Fig. 12. Comminution of the proximal articular margin of the ulna is a serious potential complication if it is not recognized. The surgical dissection over the proximal fragment can be extended cranially so that fingers and instruments can be used to find and remove the fragment.

fragment can easily be extended cranially far enough to enter the joint and remove the unstable fragment. The most common pure technical error in ulnar fractures is not placing the plate exactly on the caudal ulna. If the plate is applied too laterally, it is difficult to fully engage the proximal fragment because the medial side of the olecranon is concave. Another common technical error is to inadvertently enter the joint with screws placed through the proximal part of the plate. This problem is avoidable by using a tension band wiring technique, especially in smaller horses or foals.

Sagittal fractures of the proximal phalanx
Sagittal fractures of the proximal phalanx should be easy to repair, but it is important for the surgeon to keep in mind that the cortices are relatively thin where the second most proximal screw is placed. It is remarkably common to strip this screw because of an inaccurately short screw or overtightening of the few threads on the far cortex. The surgeon should be prepared to replace the screw with a larger screw or place an adjacent functional screw.

Metacarpophalangeal arthrodeses are fairly complex and there are numerous potential complications. The most common serious technical error is to attach the plate to the proximal phalanx at a slight angle. Even a slight angle will result in the most proximal part of the plate not being centrally aligned on the dorsal surface of MC3. It is absolutely essential to check the alignment of the plate before the second screw is placed in P1. If malalignment occurs, the only option is to remove the plate and use twisting irons to shape it to fit MC3. Another common technical error with MCP arthrodesis is to fuse the joint in a over extended position or an excessively flexed position. An overly upright fetlock will result in more of a tendency for pastern subluxation and an overly flexed fetlock will put the implants at much higher risk of mechanical failure.

Another complication with fetlock arthrodesis is inadvertently breaking the tension band wire while drilling and placing the plate screws. This is difficult to avoid and, as a result, many surgeons choose to place two wires to minimize the loss of palmar fetlock stability.

Pastern arthrodesis
Pastern arthrodesis is technically straightforward, but because horses are expected to be athletic after healing, minor technical mistakes that go unnoticed in salvage surgeries can lead to clinical failure. The most common mistake is to drill too close to the navicular bone when placing the transarticular screws. This problem can be avoided by simply paying careful attention to the drill angle and by taking appropriate intraoperative images. The transarticular screws should engage the palmar portion of the middle phalanx. If the screws are not compressing the palmar joint, tension applied by the dorsal plate will result in gapping of the palmar pastern and an inherently less stable fixation. If a central dorsal plate technique is used, no more than one screw should be placed in the middle phalanx; more distal placement has too high a risk of interfering with the extensor process of P3 and consequent distal interphalangeal joint pain (**Fig. 13**).

Physeal fractures all have the potential complication of future deformity. The surgeon must recognize the risk of growth retardation of the specific anatomic location. If implants have crossed a physis in a vulnerable location or age, the bridging implant(s) should be removed as soon as possible. Because physeal fractures heal so quickly, it is often possible to remove bridging implants within 3 to 4 weeks in the youngest foals. Unfortunately, growth retardation of long bones, such as the radius and tibia, may not be clinically obvious immediately. A small limb length difference will

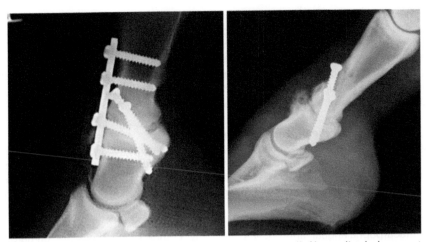

Fig. 13. Two major errors to avoid in a pastern arthrodesis are (*left*) too distal placement of the central dorsal plate resulting in possible impingement on the extensor process of the distal phalanx and (*right*) an excessively vertical placement of transarticular screws that results in the drill bit/tap/screw possibly injuring the navicular bone or its attachments.

often result in a nonathletic horse and a major disparity will result in more serious complications, such as an excessively upright fetlock that "knuckles forward" (**Fig. 14**).

Another predictable complication associated with growth follows engagement of the proximal radial metaphysis when placing a bone plate on the caudal ulna in a foal. This placement can result in serious subluxation of the elbow as the ulna is distracted distally by the continued growth of the proximal ulna (**Fig. 15**). This complication can be avoided by: 1) placing the distal screws in the plate only in the ulna; 2) repairing the ulnar fracture with a tension band wiring technique; or 3) early removal of the plate or the screws in the radius (usually ~45 days post-operative in a young foal).

Cast coaptation

Cast coaptation in horses probably fits in the category of a "necessary evil." If you place enough casts, you will have complications. Every clinician develops techniques that help to minimize complications, but there are many interdependent variables and it is truly difficult to tell someone how to apply a cast in a way that minimizes their risk of rub sores. An important axiom is to recognize the risk and change the cast if there are signs of diminishing comfort, focal heat, odor or discharge. A cast causing a proximal dorsal cannon bone rub sore can often have its function prolonged by placing a heel wedge, but the cast should still be changed within a week or two. In this author's opinion, it is easiest to place a long-term cast on a horse in the standing position, but this approach is particularly difficult in hindlimbs or in horses that are not comfortable enough to bear full weight for a long enough time on that limb. If you absolutely need to keep a cast on and severe rub sores are developing, transfixation pins will limit motion of the limb within the cast and mitigate rubs.

Broken casts should usually be changed completely, but it is possible to successfully "patch" them if the hinging at the break is minor. The key to patching casts is to apply 90% of the material longitudinally on the palmar and dorsal surfaces over the break. Most casts break directly over a joint and the bulk of the material should be

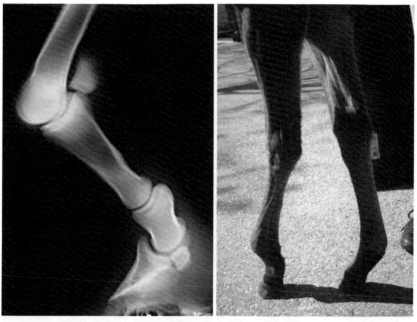

Fig. 14. This yearling suffered a physeal fracture of the distal radius as a young foal that resulted in a shortened limb. A limb initially can adapt to this by straightening the fetlock angle but eventually some will collapse dorsally as they bear weight. A treatment goal in any physeal fracture is to avoid closing the physis prematurely.

on the compression side (ie, dorsal fetlock and hock). Simply applying more circumferential cast tape consistently fails.

Transfixation casts have predictable complications: pin tract infection, ring sequestra, pin breakage, and catastrophic fracture through the pin-hole. Thermal injury causing ring sequestra can be avoided by meticulous drilling of graduated holes before placing the pin, copious irrigation, and slow insertion of threaded pins. The pin should not be hot to the touch when it exits the far cortex. Pin breakage is less likely if appropriately sized pins are used; the risk of fracture is minimized by placing pins as far as possible from the proximal margin of the cast. In a typical distal limb transfixation cast, the pins should ideally be kept in the distal 1/3 of the cannon bone.

Cast removal can also result in serious complications. If an oscillating saw is used palmarly, a deep cut can result in serious injury to the flexor tendon. Cutting directly over an incision or an implant also carries additional risk. A trivial looking oscillating saw cut can result in a deep infection if it contaminates an area that communicates with the implant. The other important complications of cast removal are serious injuries that may occur when the cast is partially removed. Horses may panic if they have their skin pinched by the split cast edges or they suddenly feel a flapping, unstable cast on their lower limb. During standing cast removal, it is critical to have the horse heavily sedated and to be sure that the cast is cut far enough distally before spreaders are used.

Soft tissue laxity in foals after cast coaptation can be a serious enough complication that many surgeons avoid casts in young foals even at the risk of losing stability of the

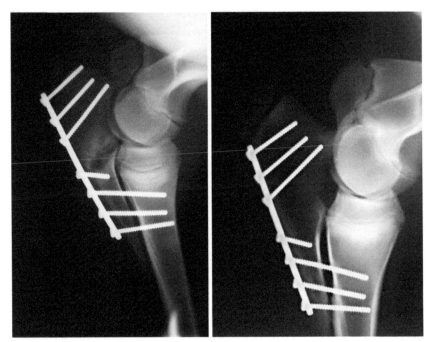

Fig. 15. A simple chronic ulnar fracture in a foal that was repaired with a bone plate engaging the radial metaphysis may result in a severe incongruity of the humero-ulnar artic-ulation (*right*) as the ulna is pulled distally by continued growth of the proximal radial physis.

fracture. The benefit-to-risk ratio for a cast in a foal always involves difficult decision making, but sometimes prolonged coaptation is the only realistic option. Post-coap-tation laxity in foals can be very dramatic, but patience and careful nursing care often yield success. The key points are to gradually decrease the rigidity of coaptation with progressively lighter bandages and to use shoes and splints as indicated. Simple heel extensions can make an enormous difference (**Fig. 16**) and although the foal's feet may become contracted with the appliance in place, the feet also will recover their normal size over the long run. Simple splints (eg, PVC staves) are effective interme-diate "step-down" coaptation in foals with post-casting laxity.

Infection

Infection is, without question, the single most important complication of orthopaedic surgery in horses. An infection at the surgical site, even if it is successfully treated, will have enormous adverse effects on the costs of the case and usually on the cosmetic and functional outcome.

Treatment of orthopaedic infection in horses has improved markedly over the last decade primarily because of improved local delivery of antibiotics. There is little doubt that improved outcomes are possible when extremely high doses of appro-priate antimicrobials can be instilled and maintained in proximity to the infected tissues and implants. Systemically administered antimicrobials even combined with drainage and lavage failed so frequently that equine surgeons have enthusias-tically embraced local delivery techniques. The obvious advantages of local antimi-crobial therapy include the ability to expose the pathogens to extremely high

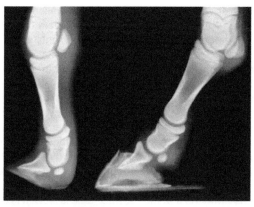

Fig. 16. An extended heel glue-on shoe can markedly improve foals with severe deep digital flexor laxity. The key to dealing with most foal flexor laxity is patience.

concentrations of the drug, the avoidance of adverse side effects (renal, liver, gut and other) from high doses of systemic antimicrobials and, very importantly, the ability to deliver high doses of antimicrobials that would otherwise be economically unfeasible in a large animal.

Although local delivery techniques improve results, basic principles of treating infection must still be followed. If possible, drainage of infected tissues should always be considered. If there is significant exudate visible ultrasonographically or otherwise obvious, open the most ventral aspect of the incision or incise the intact skin in a gravitationally dependent location. Even though local delivery allows clinicians to use otherwise prohibitively expensive antimicrobials, consistent results are only likely to be seen if susceptibility testing is done. Accurate cultures (ie, culturing the depth of a draining tract after proper preparation of the superficial tissues or ultrasound guided needle aspirate) should still be considered the gold standard.

Local antimicrobials: intraosseous, regional perfusion, antibiotic impregnated polymethal methacrylate

The use of antibiotic impregnated polymethylmethacrylate (PMMA) has been popular for years and remains one of the best tools for delivering high levels of local antibiotics to a site of orthopedic infection. The advantages of PMMA as an antibiotic delivery device are: that its biocompatibility has been well studied; elution profiles for many antibiotics from the cement have been documented; and the material is readily available to the surgeon in a sterile, easily used form. The major disadvantages of PMMA are that it is not absorbable and heat labile antibiotics cannot be incorporated within it.

Although it is easier to mix a powdered antibiotic with the PMMA, liquid injectable forms can also be used. Typically 1–2 g of antibiotic are used for each 10 g of PMMA. If a liquid antibiotic is used, the volume of liquid methylmethacrylate is decreased by 1/2 the volume of the added antibiotic. The materials are mixed routinely and formed into cylinders or beads as the material becomes clay-like. The ambient temperature of the room will affect the speed of this process. For plate luting, the screws and plate must be loosened before mixing. If the PMMA is to be put on a suture to facilitate later removal, that suture should be prepared before mixing. The author prefers to use #2 monofilament nylon in which multiple bulky knots are tied intermittently over its length. The PMMA is then fashioned into slender beads between the knots. The latter hold the beads in place and make removal easier. Another alternative that is frequently used is to simply make beads or cylinders that are not attached to suture and pack them in position. Tapered cylindric implants are often used because they are easier to insert and remove than spherical implants. There is also a commercially available mold for making antibiotic impregnated beads (University of Vermont, Instrument and Mold Facility, Burlington, Vermont, USA.) Later removal of the PMMA is not necessary unless the plastic is interfering with function. Antibiotics that have been successfully used include gentamicin (by far the most common), amikacin, tobramycin, multiple cephalosporins, and enrofloxacin. Premade beads can be re-sterilized by ethylene oxide (gas) sterilization. In some situations where removal of PMMA will be particularly problematic, antibiotic impregnated plaster of Paris (POP) can be used. The plaster is slowly degraded and absorbed by the body. The antibiotics leach at a reasonable rate, however, and the material is very inexpensive. The major disadvantage of POP versus PMMA is that the "set-up" time is slow. It is easiest to make the beads up aseptically well in advance and then keep them in a sterile container. They also can be ethylene oxide (ETO) sterilized, but they become more brittle. Antibiotic impregnated POP can also be mixed with a cancellous autograft.

Other products have been used and newer, improved materials will undoubtedly replace PMMA and POP. Polylactide derivatives, alginates, polyanhydrides, calcium sulfate, chitosan and fibrin are all being studied for the local delivery of antimicrobials. It seems likely that a variety of products with different mechanical properties, elution profiles and absorption will eventually be available to clinicians.

Regional limb perfusion with antimicrobials is strongly advocated in situations where a peripheral vessel is accessible and an effective tourniquet can be applied to isolate the infected region. The major disadvantage of regional perfusion in postoperative cases is the condition of the tissues and the need to avoid vascular damage near the surgical site. Some antibiotics, notably enrofloxacin, seem to induce significant vasculitis when used for regional perfusions.

If possible, a tourniquet is placed above and below the area to be treated, but the only absolute necessity is an accessible peripheral vein distal to the proximal tourniquet. It is important to use a good pneumatic tourniquet or a strong wide rubber tourniquet and to use enough sedation to avoid any movement after the infusion is started. If necessary, regional analgesia is used, but most horses will stand with adequate sedation. The smallest possible catheter should be used for the perfusions to minimize trauma to the vessel. A 25–27 gauge butterfly catheter has been optimal in the author's experience. Because repeated treatments are usually desirable, it is imperative to keep the vessel in the best possible condition. Dosage varies, but approximately one third of a systemic dose diluted to about 30–60 mL is typical for the distal limb. Larger volume areas like the tarsus probably can accommodate larger volumes. The injection is done slowly primarily because the needle diameter is so small. The tourniquet is left in place for approximately 30 minutes. The site of the injection is treated with a topical anti-inflammatory, such as Surpass or a glucocorticoid, mixed with dimethyl sulfoxide and then placed under a good compression bandage. Some surgeons will regionally perfuse broad-spectrum antibiotics to a limb just before surgery so that high levels of antibiotics are present at the time the incision is made.

Intra-osseous and intra-articular antibiotic administration are also both used to maximize antibiotic levels at the desired site of action. Commercial intra-osseous catheters (Cook) as well as homemade cannulated screws can be inserted for repeated intra-osseous treatments. An even simpler technique is to drill a 4.0-mm hole into the medullary cavity at the desired location. The male end of a Luer-tipped extension set will fit snugly into the hole, allowing direct injection. Both intraosseous and intra-articular perfusions should ideally be done under tourniquet for 30 minutes to maximize tissue levels.

RECOGNITION OF POSTOPERATIVE INFECTION

Postoperative infection remains the most common and devastating complication of orthopedic surgery. An infection will often compound the cost of treatment by 10-fold or more and if the infection is coupled with instability of an internal fixation, mechanical failure and/or delayed/nonunion are frustratingly common outcomes. Despite all efforts at minimizing orthopedic infections, however, they still occur and better techniques for their management are necessary. The most important key in recognizing acute postoperative infection is simply to truly believe that sepsis is both the most prevalent and most important postoperative complication in orthopedic cases. If you suspect an internal fixation case is infected, you can bet that it is infected. The earlier the intervention, the better the chance of cure.

- A fever that cannot definitively be otherwise explained should be considered a strong indicator of possible surgical infection.
- A decrease in comfort in spite of apparently intact internal fixation is a very strong indicator of infection.
- A failure of routine diminution of postoperative swelling or any increase in swelling of the affected area should be investigated with radiographs and ultrasound.
- Drainage of any nature should be considered evidence of underlying infection.

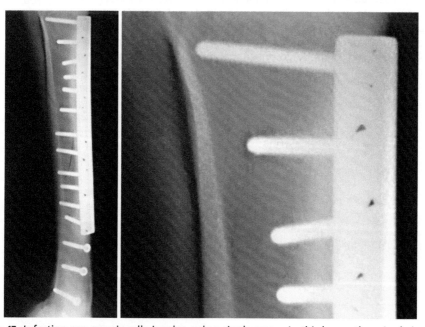

Fig. 17. Infection can occasionally involve only a single screw. In this horse, there is obvious bony lysis around the infected screw. The single screw was removed, the hole curetted, packed with antimicrobial impregnated collagen sponge and no further complications ensued. The plate was later removed on schedule around 3 ½ months postoperatively.

- Failure of the incision to heal normally and/or development of a pink, shiny hairless area in the injured area indicate at least a subcutaneous abscess.
- Leukocytosis is not conclusive evidence of infection: many horses with obvious infections have normal white counts. Plasma fibrinogen is a more reliable indicator.

Specific diagnosis of postoperative infection is typically based on radiographs, ultrasound and microbial culture.

Radiographic signs of acute infection are limited to increased soft tissue swelling and/or possibly separation of tissue planes. Later signs are radiolucency developing adjacent to metal implants (**Fig. 17**) and periosteal proliferative change unassociated with fracture healing. An even later radiographic sign is lysis extending into cancellous bone and/or medullary cavity.

Ultrasound is a particularly useful diagnostic modality for the recognition of early infection if the ultrasound is performed by an experienced examiner. The accumulation of exudate adjacent to a bone or implant can be identified and early accurate aspirates obtained for culture.

Treatment of early postoperative orthopedic sepsis should include:

1) Drainage. If there is significant exudate visible ultrasonographically or otherwise obvious, open the most ventral aspect of the incision or incise intact skin in a dependent location. Accurate culture: culture the depth of a draining tract (after proper preparation of the superficial) or perform an aspirate directed by ultrasound.

2) Antimicrobials. The systemically administered drug, dose, route must be optimal and, most importantly, local antibiotics are essential.

Complications are a price all surgeons eventually pay. Experience and increasing skill will decrease many of them but certainly not all. The most important thing is for the surgeon to react correctly to a complication. Acknowledge the mistake (or bad luck) quickly and take whatever steps you can to correct the problem. Because so many equine orthopaedic cases have the potential for complications, recognizing and responding properly to these complications are imperative for successful outcomes.

Strategies for Reducing the Complication of Orthopedic Pain Perioperatively

Laurie R. Goodrich, DVM, MS, PhD

KEYWORDS

• Orthopedic pain • Horse • Pain management

Equine analgesia has been a neglected subject, lagging behind the progress made in small animals.[1] Various arguments exist against pain relief for horses. One common argument is that if an injured body part does not hurt, further damage will ensue due to overuse.[1] This view has little foundation and can result in the horse having to withstand excessive pain that is inhumane. Pain that is controlled results in a nondepressed horse that maintains a good appetite and has a normal functioning immune system, which results in normal tissue healing. Another benefit that applies to the successful management of perioperative orthopedic pain in the horse is the potential to reduce the risk of support-limb laminitis, an unfortunate sequela that can render all implants and prior surgery needless and that often leads to the demise of the patient. Additionally, the reduction of stress associated with ongoing chronic pain may decrease the risk of gastric ulceration, colitis, and generalized depression associated with continued pain. Lastly, it is the responsibility of the surgeon in conjunction with the anesthesiologist to provide adequate pain management to ensure the best outcome of the surgical procedure to be performed. Poorly planned pain management may obviate the best and most elegant orthopedic surgical procedure.

CONSEQUENCES OF PAIN

One of the most important reasons to control pain is to avoid the consequences of the "wind-up" phenomenon.[2] Pain is usually the first and most dominant clinical sign in horses sustaining orthopedic injury. Pain and inflammatory responses induced by surgical procedures and anesthesia-related ischemia produce a series of behavioral, neurophysiologic, endocrine, and metabolic and cellular responses (stress response) that initiate, maintain, and amplify the release of pain and inflammatory mediators (**Fig. 1**).[2] Pain is normally produced by the mechanical, chemical, or thermal activation

Department of Clinical Sciences, College of Veterinary Medicine and Biomedical Sciences, Colorado State University, 300 West Drake, Fort Collins, CO 80523, USA
E-mail address: laurie.goodrich@colostate.edu

Vet Clin Equine 24 (2009) 611–620
doi:10.1016/j.cveq.2008.10.008
0749-0739/08/$ – see front matter © 2009 Elsevier Inc. All rights reserved.

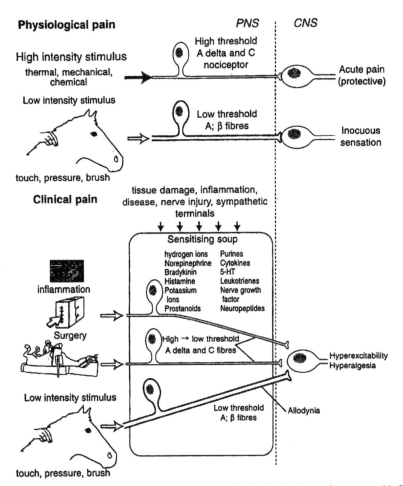

Fig.1. The differences between physiologic pain and clinical pain. Tissue damage and inflammation can lead to hypersensitivity to mechanical, chemical, and thermal stimuli resulting in increased sensation or "hyperalgesia." (*From* Muir WW. Anesthesia and pain management in horses. Equine Veterinary Education 1998;10:336; with permission.)

of small diameter high-threshold sensory nerve fibers.[2] When pain is uncontrolled, inflammation increases the sensitivity of peripheral nerve fibers and stimulates the synthesis and release of nerve growth factor, substance P, and calcitonin gene-related peptide, all of which contribute to the development of sensory hyperexcitability and hyperalgesia. Cumulative increases in positive feedback loops and neural sensitivity result in increases in the excitability of spinal cord neurons and central nervous system wind-up (**Fig. 2**).[2] Uncontrolled pain produces a catabolic state, suppresses the immune response, and promotes inflammation, which delays wound healing and predisposes the patient to infection and intensified medical care.

Although the clinician cannot control the degree of pain that the horse presents with, most commonly, the procedure performed to treat the condition will often cause similar or potentially worse pain until the tissues or bones heal. Pre-emptive analgesia is a term used to denote the administration of analgesic drugs before extensive soft tissue or orthopedic surgery in an attempt to minimize the response to pain,

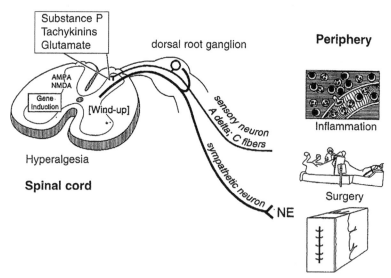

Fig. 2. The result of chronic input of pain centrally causing up-regulation of gene induction and central nervous system wind-up. (*From* Muir WW. Anesthesia and pain management in horses. Equine Veterinary Education 1998;10:338; with permission.)

particularly the development of central nervous system hypersensitivity and resultant hyperalgesia and allodynia.[3]

PREOPERATIVE ANALGESIA
Nonsteroidal Drugs

Nonsteroidal anti-inflammatory drugs (NSAIDs) are some of the most commonly used analgesics. They reduce inflammation by inhibiting the production of prostaglandins and, as a result, are only effective in an inflammatory process.[4] The acidic nature of these compounds allows them to accumulate in inflamed tissues, which are also acidic. They are highly protein bound; therefore, higher concentrations are found in the serum, although inflamed synovial joints have higher concentrations due to increased blood flow and vascular permeability induced during inflammation.[5] At the site of injury, they inhibit the cyclooxygenase pathway (COX) and prevent the formation of prostaglandins. The two enzymes that make up this pathway are COX-1 and COX-2. COX-1 is responsible for normal functions of the mucosa in the gastric stomach by increasing blood flow, decreasing acid production, and increasing mucus production. COX-2 is usually not present in most tissues but is inducible in injured tissues, which results in prostaglandin production and inflammation. NSAIDs that are currently used block both COX-1 and COX-2 and can sometime result in toxicity.

The toxic effects associated with NSAID administration are oral, gastric, duodenal, and colonic ulceration and necrosis, renal papillary necrosis, altered clotting times, a decrease in plasma total protein, diarrhea, and perivascular irritation and necrosis.[6] Early signs of toxicity are depression, anorexia, oral ulceration, and abdominal edema.[5] Clinicians should be aware of these toxicities and immediately stop NSAID administration if they are noted. A study by McAllister compared the adverse effects of phenylbutazone, flunixin, and ketoprofen and found that phenylbutazone had the greatest toxic potential, followed by flunixin and ketoprofen.[7]

NSAIDs provide effective analgesia for many orthopedic procedures that cause mild-to-moderate pain.[8] They are often given intravenously before or during anesthesia so that they will be effective in surgery and postoperatively. Because nonsteroidal drugs are protein bound, they may displace other protein-bound drugs and deepen anesthesia.[9] The most common NSAIDs used perioperatively are phenylbutazone, flunixin meglumine, ketoprofen, and, to a lesser extent, carprofen and firocoxib (Equioxx). Specific dosages are listed in **Table 1**.

Phenylbutazone remains the most commonly administered NSAID in the horse. Its efficacy for musculoskeletal pain has stood the test of time. Although it can have toxic effects on the gastrointestinal tract, when used at the appropriate dosage most horses do not seem to exhibit toxic effects. Surgeons should use caution when administering phenylbutazone for horses at high risk of side effects.

A study by Raekallio and colleagues[10] demonstrated improved pain scores measured postoperatively when horses were administered 4 mg/kg intravenously before surgery and 2 mg/kg every 12 hours following surgery. This study proved the intravenous route of administration of phenylbutazone, when used perioperatively for postoperative pain, was effective. The belief among many clinicians is that phenylbutazone is more effective than flunixin and ketoprofen at providing analgesia for musculoskeletal pain. This belief has been substantiated by studies in which a synovitis model was used to test the efficacy of each of these NSAIDs and phenylbutazone provided improved efficacy over the others.[4,11] Although phenylbutazone has the highest risk of toxicity when compared with flunixin and ketoprofen, its efficacy for orthopedic pain is greatest.

Flunixin meglumine is the second most commonly used NSAID in horses. Although the mechanism of action is similar by blocking the COX pathway, its efficacy has been determined to be greater for visceral pain than for musculoskeletal pain. Horses do not seem to be as sensitive to the kidney perfusion problems seen in dogs and cats; therefore, it is used commonly preoperatively. Although it is used orally and intravenously, it should not be used intramuscularly due to its potential to result in clostridial myonecrosis.[12]

Ketoprofen is still used, although its efficacy for musculoskeletal pain is not as good when compared with phenylbutazone.[4] Some of the initial claims of ketoprofen inhibiting the lipoxygenase pathway were not substantiated in studies.[4] Although it is a potent analgesic and has less risk of toxicity when compared with phenylbutazone, it is not used as commonly as phenylbutazone and banamine.

COX-2 inhibitors are emerging in the area of NSAID therapy. They specifically block the COX-2 pathway but do not inhibit the "housekeeping" functions of prostaglandins such as mucus production and blood flow stimulated by COX-1.[13] Theoretically, they

Table 1		
Doses of nonsteroidal anti-inflammatory drugs		
Drug	**Route**	**Dose**
Flunixin meglumine	Oral or intravenous	1.1 mg/kg for up to 5 days
Ketoprofen	Intravenous	2.2 mg/kg for up to 5 days
Phenylbutazone	Oral or intravenous	4.4 mg/kg twice daily for 1 day, then 2.2 mg/kg twice daily for 2–4 days, then 2.2 mg/kg daily
Firocoxib	Oral	1 mg/kg daily for up to 30 days

should minimize the occurrence of NSAID-induced toxicities and could replace the NSAIDs associated with greater risks of toxicities. A COX-2 inhibitor that has recently come on the market is feroxicob (Equioxx) oral paste. Its efficacy has been compared with that of phenylbutazone for musculoskeletal pain and has been found to be comparative in a large field study.[14] Its main disadvantages when compared with phenylbutazone are its expense and the fact that it is only available as an oral paste.

Epidural Analgesia

Epidural analgesia has grown in popularity in the last 10 years.[15–18] The benefit of epidural analgesia is primarily focused on the hind limbs, because front limb pain does not seem to be reduced with even large volumes of drugs delivered through epidural catheters placed at C1-C2.[15] Epidural analgesia is an excellent adjunctive way to provide analgesia and has several benefits when given preoperatively, such as reducing the need for intraoperative drug therapy, reducing the need for higher concentrations of gas anesthetics, and improved recoveries.[19] Many different drug combinations are reported for epidural analgesia, with xylazine, detomidine, and morphine being the most commonly used combinations. Advantages of using these drugs are the finding that there is no loss of motor function to the hind limbs and the excellent analgesia provided.[16] One of the most common combinations reported is morphine at 0.2 mg/kg and detomidine at 0.03 mg/kg, which is brought up to 20 mL with saline if administering through a needle or an epidural catheter.[16,18] Because this dose of morphine may predispose to decreased gut motility, the author currently uses 0.1 mg/kg of morphine combined with detomidine at the previously listed dosage which provides excellent analgesia. When this combination was administered preoperatively to horses undergoing bilateral hind limb arthroscopies, significant analgesia was provided.[18] Furthermore, stress as measured by cortisol levels was significantly reduced intraoperatively.[19] The technique of administration is the standard approach to delivering epidural drugs through a needle placed in between coccygeal vertebrae 1 and 2 and advancing to the epidural space.

Analgesia through Epidural Catheters

If the surgeon expects ongoing pain postoperatively, an epidural catheter can be placed preoperatively and epidural drugs delivered by this route. The author has placed more that 50 catheters preoperatively to deliver analgesic drugs and has not had a problem with the catheters becoming dislodged during or post recovery. Epidural catheter placement is an effective way to continue delivery of drugs postoperatively, and long-term placement of 3 weeks has not resulted in any detrimental effects.[17] Epidural catheter placement is easy, and horses appear to tolerate them well (**Fig. 3**). A detailed description of epidural catheter placement is available.[20]

Many excellent preoperative analgesic drugs (before the commencement of gas anesthetics) are available. The combinations available are also wide in range. Common combinations are opioids such as morphine and alpha-2 agonists such as xylazine or detomidine.[2] These combinations have proved to be excellent for providing good analgesia before general anesthesia. A more in-depth discussion of the use of these drugs perioperatively is available.[21]

OPERATIVE ANALGESIA

Intraoperative methods to reduce pain are important because a horse feeling pain during anesthesia is more likely to have higher catecholamine levels intraoperatively, a poor recovery, and, potentially, added stress to the nociceptive input of the surgical

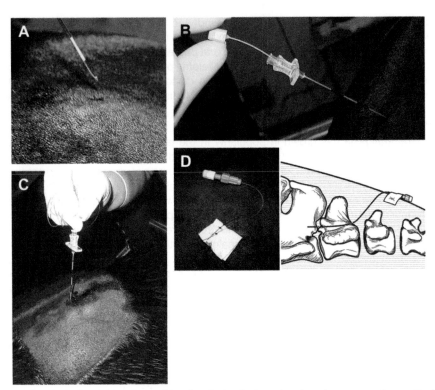

Fig. 3. (A–D) The insertion of an epidural catheter that can be placed pre- or postoperatively to supply excellent analgesia for hind limb orthopedic pain.

procedure. Once the horse is anesthetized, it is the author's preference to regionally anesthetize the limb by using perineural anesthesia with either mepivacaine or bupivacaine. An argument against this practice may be that the horse may not protect the limb on recovery (ie, for fracture repair) if the painful input is lost; however, if adequate coaptation is applied and controlled recovery ensues, adequate fixation should hold up to the forces applied by the horse in the recovery stall.

The mechanism of action is the same as for all local anesthetics, that is, interruption of the propagation of impulses along peripheral nerves preventing noxious stimulation from being transferred and causing complete analgesia in tissues. These agents bind to sodium channels and prevent depolarization.[8] When used operatively, they can decrease the response to painful surgical stimuli and decrease the amount of general anesthesia needed to maintain a desirable plane of anesthesia.[9] If a local block is being performed not only to decrease surgical stimulation but also to assist with recovery and to provide continued analgesia during the postoperative period, bupivacaine should be used based on its extended time of action (6–8 hours).

Intra-articular anesthetics may also be used just before performing arthroscopic procedures. By initially distending the joint capsule with Carbocaine, painful manipulations within the joint may be less perceived by the anesthetized patient. This procedure is commonly practiced in arthroscopy in humans.[22] Recently, toxic effects have been noted due to high concentrations of bupivacaine in human and rat cartilage.[23] These effects have not been studied in horse cartilage. Infusing mepivacaine preoperatively just before arthroscopy should not result in articular toxicity; however, based on bupivacaine studies done in humans, the author would avoid this solution until further effects are studied.

Intra-articular mu receptors have been found in inflamed synovium, which would lend credence to using morphine intra-articularly in the horse;[8] however, no studies have been done to specifically study the efficacy of intra-articular morphine on postoperative orthopedic pain.

If surgery has been long (over 2 hours) and the surgeon believes that moderate orthopedic pain will ensue, NSAIDs administered before moving the patient to the recovery stall appear to be beneficial to some horses in recovery and for postoperative pain (McIlwraith, clinical observation, 2008). In these situations, the dose of NSAID should be taken into consideration when continuation of NSAIDs takes place postoperatively.

POSTOPERATIVE PAIN MANAGEMENT
Nonsteroidal Anti-Inflammatory Drugs

The length and route of administration of NSAIDs depend on the degree of pain and how well the horse is progressing. Every horse seems to have individuality in dealing with pain, with some appearing to need prolonged therapy and others needing much less. The surgeon must be aware that switching the route of NSAIDs from intravenous to oral administration can sometimes reveal pain in the interval, and the efficacy seems to be slightly less when these drugs are administered by the oral route, at least temporarily. In the author's experience, there seems to be a 12- to 24-hour accommodation to the oral route, and, in most cases, the oral route becomes equally beneficial to providing analgesia. In most cases of mild-to-moderate joint pain associated with arthroscopic procedures, NSAIDs are used between 3 and 7 days postoperatively.[8] This use will increase for more chronic situations such as joints presenting for chronic sepsis or when large portions of subchondral bone are exposed.

When NSAIDs are used for more chronic cases of orthopedic implants and when limbs are in casts, NSAIDs are typically used for longer periods of time. In these cases, the author often continues the patient on a low dose of NSAIDs until cast removal to avoid allowing the limb to swell within the cast upon discontinuation of the NSAID. Such continuation of low-dose NSAIDs in horses that are casted does not hide the detection of cast sores and often provides enough analgesia for low but appropriate amounts of movement within the stall.

Continuation of Epidural Analgesia

If an epidural catheter is placed preoperatively, administration of analgesics can be continued for several weeks through this route.[15,17] If a catheter is not placed preoperatively, postoperative placement should be considered for horses with ongoing moderate-to-severe pain of the hind limbs. The author has placed many epidural catheters in horses with fractures, septic joints, and various conditions causing hind limb pain with excellent results. The most common combination used in this situation is morphine (0.1 mg/kg) and either detomidine (0.03 mg/kg) or xylazine (0.17 mg/kg). Administration of either combination usually takes 20 to 30 minutes to have an analgesic effect and can last between 12 to 36 hours depending on the severity of pain. In the author's experience, detomidine and morphine seem to provide greater analgesia and last a longer length of time. The disadvantage with this combination is that the sedative effects of the detomidine are greater and may last approximately 30 to 40 minutes in comparison with the effect of xylazine, which seems to last 10 to 15 minutes.

Fentanyl Patches

Transdermal fentanyl patches have been used extensively in human and small animal patients.[24–26] The efficacy in horses has been tested in the last few years and has shown individual variation.[27–32] The current recommendation for orthopedic pain is to clip the cephalic or saphenous region of the limb and apply two patches each of 10 mg. The time for absorption can vary between 2 and 14 hours and in some horses may not reach serum levels to have an analgesic effect. In the author's experience, there seems to be individual variation with some horses benefiting and some not.

Continuous Peripheral Nerve Block

Methods to provide excellent analgesia to the front limbs continue to evade orthopedic surgeons such that support-limb laminitis continues to be a common sequela to ongoing front limb pain. A method to provide a continuous block with regional anesthesia has been investigated by implanting catheters subcutaneously at the medial and lateral palmar nerves.[33] The continuous infusion appears to be efficacious; however, distal limb swelling associated with the catheters is problematic. Furthermore, if metal implantation is present, the risk of introducing infection subcutaneously may outweigh the benefit of placement of these catheters. Further study is needed in this particular instrumentation to provide analgesia. This method may have a place in future management of orthopedic pain.

Continuous Intravenous Infusions

Continuous rate intravenous infusions of drugs such as ketamine, lidocaine, and butorphanol have been studied to supply analgesia in horses.[34–36] Most studies using these drugs have examined their effects on gastrointestinal pain and not orthopedic pain. These infusions appear to provide some benefit to the equine patient suffering from gastrointestinal pain; however, studies need to be performed on horses with orthopedic pain before they can be recommended.

SUMMARY

In the last decade, pain management has had a larger role in the surgical plan for equine orthopedic procedures. Epidural management of hind limb orthopedic pain has been important in providing analgesic benefits to the equine patient. Furthermore, pre-emptive analgesia has been demonstrated to have beneficial effects on minimizing postoperative pain and some of the complications associated with ongoing pain. Surgeons are becoming aware of the benefits that well-planned analgesia initiated preoperatively can provide to their patients in the recovery stall as well as postoperatively. Further studies on more effective analgesia should be forthcoming and will add more options to providing effective pain management to equine orthopedic patients.

REFERENCES

1. Taylor PM, Pascoe PJ, Mama KR. Diagnosing and treating pain in the horse. Where are we today? Vet Clin North Am Equine Pract 2002;18:1–19.
2. Muir WW. Anaesthesia and pain management in horses. Equine Veterinary Education 1998;10:335–40.
3. Woolf CJ, Chong MS. Preemptive analgesia: treating postoperative pain by preventing the establishment of central sensitization. Anesth Analg 1993;77: 362–79.

4. Owens JG, Kamerling SG, Stanton SR, et al. Effects of pretreatment with ketopro-fen and phenylbutazone on experimentally induced synovitis in horses. Am J Vet Res 1996;57:866–74.
5. Kallings P. Nonsteroidal anti-inflammatory drugs. Vet Clin North Am Equine Pract 1993;9:523–41.
6. Geiser DR. Chemical restraint and analgesia in the horse. Vet Clin North Am Equine Pract 1990;6:495–512.
7. MacAllister CG, Morgan SJ, Borne AT, et al. Comparison of adverse effects of phenylbutazone, flunixin meglumine, and ketoprofen in horses. J Am Vet Med Assoc 1993;202:71–7.
8. Baller LS, Hendrickson DA. Management of equine orthopedic pain. Vet Clin North Am Equine Pract 2002;18:117–31.
9. Nolan AM. Pharmacology of analgesic drugs. In: Flecknell P, Waterman-Pearson A, editors. Pain management in animals. Philadelphia: WB Saunders; 2000. p. 21–52.
10. Raekallio M, Taylor PM, Bennett RC. Preliminary investigations of pain and anal-gesia assessment in horses administered phenylbutazone or placebo after arthroscopic surgery. Vet Surg 1997;26:150–5.
11. McMurphy RM. Providing analgesia. In: White NA, Moore JM, editors. Current techniques in equine surgery and lameness. Philadelphia: WB Saunders; 1998. p. 2–5.
12. Peek SF, Semrad SD, Perkins GA. Clostridial myonecrosis in horses (37 cases 1985–2000). Equine Vet J 2003;35:86–92.
13. Halverson PB. Nonsteroidal anti-inflammatory drugs: benefits, risks, and COX-2 selectivity. Orthop Nurs 1999;18:21–6.
14. Doucet MY, Bertone AL, Hendrickson D, et al. Comparison of efficacy and safety of paste formulations of firocoxib and phenylbutazone in horses with naturally oc-curring osteoarthritis. J Am Vet Med Assoc 2008;232:91–7.
15. Martin CA, Kerr CL, Pearce SG, et al. Outcome of epidural catheterization for de-livery of analgesics in horses: 43 cases (1998–2001). J Am Vet Med Assoc 2003; 222:1394–8.
16. Sysel AM, Pleasant RS, Jacobson JD, et al. Efficacy of an epidural combination of morphine and detomidine in alleviating experimentally induced hind limb lame-ness in horses. Vet Surg 1996;25:511–8.
17. Sysel AM, Pleasant RS, Jacobson JD, et al. Systemic and local effects associated with long-term epidural catheterization and morphine-detomidine administration in horses. Vet Surg 1997;26:141–9.
18. Goodrich LR, Nixon AJ, Fubini SL, et al. Epidural morphine and detomidine decreases postoperative hind limb lameness in horses after bilateral stifle arthroscopy. Vet Surg 2002;31:232–9.
19. Goodrich LR, Butler E, Donaldson L, et al. The efficacy of epidurally administered morphine and detomidine in decreasing stress levels under general anesthesia and the effect on anesthetic recoveries. Vet Surg 2000;29:463.
20. Goodrich LR, Nixon AJ. How to alleviate acute and chronic hindlimb pain. AAEP Proceedings, New Orleans, LA, 2003.
21. Bennett RC, Steffey EP. Use of opioids for pain and anesthetic management in horses. Vet Clin North Am Equine Pract 2002;18:47–60.
22. Hultin J, Hamberg P, Stenstrom A. Knee arthroscopy using local anesthesia. Arthroscopy 1992;8:239–41.
23. Chu CR, Izzo NJ, Coyle CH, et al. The in vitro effects of bupivacaine on articular chondrocytes. J Bone Joint Surg Br 2008;90:814–20.

24. Sandler AN, Baxter AD, Katz J, et al. A double-blind, placebo-controlled trial of transdermal fentanyl after abdominal hysterectomy: analgesic, respiratory, and pharmacokinetic effects. Anesthesiology 1994;81:1169–80.
25. Franks JN, Boothe HW, Taylor L, et al. Evaluation of transdermal fentanyl patches for analgesia in cats undergoing onychectomy. J Am Vet Med Assoc 2000;217: 1013–20.
26. Robinson TM, Kruse-Elliott KT, Markel MD, et al. A comparison of transdermal fentanyl versus epidural morphine for analgesia in dogs undergoing major ortho-pedic surgery. J Am Anim Hosp Assoc 1999;35:95–100.
27. Sanchez LC, Robertson SA, Maxwell LK, et al. Effect of fentanyl on visceral and somatic nociception in conscious horses. J Vet Intern Med 2007;21:1067–75.
28. Orsini JA, Moate PJ, Kuersten K, et al. Pharmacokinetics of fentanyl delivered transdermally in healthy adult horses: variability among horses and its clinical implications. J Vet Pharmacol Ther 2006;29:539–46.
29. Mills PC, Cross SE. Regional differences in transdermal penetration of fentanyl through equine skin. Res Vet Sci 2007;82:252–6.
30. Thomasy SM, Slovis N, Maxwell LK, et al. Transdermal fentanyl combined with nonsteroidal anti-inflammatory drugs for analgesia in horses. J Vet Intern Med 2004;18:550–4.
31. Maxwell LK, Thomasy SM, Slovis N, et al. Pharmacokinetics of fentanyl following intravenous and transdermal administration in horses. Equine Vet J 2003;35: 484–90.
32. Kamerling SG, Weckman TJ, DeQuick DJ, et al. A method for studying cutaneous pain perception and analgesia in horses. J Pharmacol Methods 1985;13:267–74.
33. Driessen B, Scandella M, Zarucco L. Development of a technique for continuous perineural blockade of the palmar nerves in the distal equine thoracic limb. Vet Anaesth Analg 2008;35:432–48.
34. Peterbauer C, Larenza PM, Knobloch M, et al. Effects of a low dose infusion of racemic and S-ketamine on the nociceptive withdrawal reflex in standing ponies. Vet Anaesth Analg 2008;35:414–23.
35. Sellon DC, Roberts MC, Blikslager AT, et al. Effects of continuous rate intravenous infusion of butorphanol on physiologic and outcome variables in horses after celiotomy. J Vet Intern Med 2004;18:555–63.
36. Malone E, Ensink J, Turner T, et al. Intravenous continuous infusion of lidocaine for treatment of equine ileus. Vet Surg 2006;35:60–6.

Complications of Unilateral Weight Bearing

Gary M. Baxter, VMD, MS[a],*, Scott Morrison, DVM[b]

KEYWORDS

- Laminitis • Support limb • Distal phalanx • Rotation
- Displacement • Angular limb deformities

SUPPORT LIMB LAMINITIS IN ADULT HORSES

The most common and significant complication of excessive unilateral weight bearing in adult horses is support limb laminitis. This condition can occur in the contralateral limb of any horse with a significant lameness or neurologic deficit in the opposite forelimb or hindlimb. It is unusual for any foot other than the contralateral foot to be affected, suggesting that support limb laminitis is a local pathologic process within the digit that is greatly influenced by the mechanical overload of the limb. This is in contrast to other types of laminitis where a systemic abnormality is believed to contribute to the disease process that most often affects multiple feet.

Pathophysiology

There has been much research performed on laminitis in the past decade but nearly all of it has focused on the more classic forms of laminitis, such as grain overload, the sick horse syndrome (toxemia), and what often is referred to as the fat horse syndrome (metabolic syndrome). There has been little work on support limb laminitis, which potentially has a different pathogenesis than more traditional forms of laminitis. Whether or not all of these various types of laminitis have a unifying pathogenesis currently is unknown, but the many causes seem to make this an unrealistic expectation.

Currently, the pathophysiology of support limb laminitis is not understood. The pathophysiology of the classic forms of acute laminitis has two major schools of thought: hyperperfusion of the digit, which allows destructive enzymes (laminitis-trigger factors) access to the lamella and subsequent damage to these cells,[1-3] and hypoperfusion followed by reperfusion by some chemical mediators or subsequent to arteriovenous shunting leading to laminar ischemia and cellular damage.[3-5] Regardless of which theory is agreed with, the common theme is that an intense inflammatory

[a] Department of Clinical Sciences, James L. Voss Veterinary Teaching Hospital, Colorado State University, 300 West Drake Road, Fort Collins, CO 80523-1620, USA
[b] Rood and Riddle Equine Hospital, 2150 Georgetown Rd, PO Box 12070, Lexington, KY, USA
* Corresponding author.
E-mail address: gbaxter@colostate.edu (G.M. Baxter).

Vet Clin Equine 24 (2009) 621–642
doi:10.1016/j.cveq.2008.10.006
0749-0739/08/$ – see front matter © 2009 Elsevier Inc. All rights reserved.

vetequine.theclinics.com

process occurs within the laminar tissue.[5] Inflammatory mediators, such as matrix metalloproteinases (MMPs), are believed to target the basement membrane of the lamella, causing lysis and separation of the basement membrane from the epidermal cell.[2,5,6] Alternatively, circulating white blood cells may gain access to the laminar tissue through damaged endothelium resulting in lamellar destruction through release of intracellular enzymes.[5] This intense inflammatory response mirrors what is believed to occur with systemic inflammatory response syndrome and multiple organ dysfunction syndrome in people.[5] The end result of these events (separation of laminar epithelial cells from the underlying dermis) likely is to the result of a combination of (1) basement membrane breakdown from MMP release and activation and (2) inflammatory and possibly hypoxic injury to the lamellar basal epithelial cells responsible for adhesion of the cells to the underlying matrix.

Laminitis associated with metabolic syndrome or endocrine abnormalities is believed associated with insulin resistance (IR), which causes hyperinsulinemia and hyperglycemia.[7,8] It also has been shown that ponies with recurrent laminitis episodes are insulin resistant and that increased levels of cortisol can lead to IR.[9] Lamellar cells are highly dependent on glucose, and disruption of glucose use by lamellar cells is believed to contribute to laminitis in these obese horses.[7,10] In addition, glucotoxicity of the endothelium, which is known to occur in people, could result in emigration of white blood cells and cytokines into the laminae initiating a severe inflammatory response.[7] Alternatively, high levels of insulin may contribute directly to laminitis, as shown in a recent study. Ponies given human recombinant insulin for 72 hours to create hyperinsulinemia developed laminitis in all four feet.[11] Control ponies given saline did not develop laminitis. In addition, there seems to be a direct correlation between insulin levels and the severity of laminitis in horses with metabolic syndrome.[7,8]

How does the pathophysiology of other types of laminitis fit into the picture of support limb laminitis in horses? One major difference between other forms of laminitis and support limb laminitis is that there usually is no systemic abnormality (that the authors are aware of) in horses with support limb laminitis. These horses usually are healthy with some musculoskeletal lesion contributing to excessive weight bearing on the opposite limb. Other forms of laminitis have some type of systemic abnormality (grain overload, toxemia, metabolic syndrome, Cushing's disease, glucocorticoid treatment, and so forth) that is manifested locally in the feet. In addition, it is unusual for support limb laminitis to manifest in more than one foot, which is in direct contrast to all other forms of laminitis. A rational conclusion from this is that the mechanical forces acting on the contralateral limb must contribute greatly to the disease progression in support limb laminitis. Venographic studies of the foot have revealed that when the carpus was constantly loaded, perfusion to the dorsal hoof wall was reduced.[12] This suggests that excessive unilateral weight bearing may reduce perfusion to the laminae, potentially contributing to hypoxic injury or oxidative stress to the laminar tissues. In addition, the deep digital flexor (DDF) constantly pulls on the distal phalanx when the limb is loaded. The combination of reduced perfusion and constant loading of the DDF could contribute to separation of the sensitive and insensitive laminae and signs of laminitis. Alternatively, the pain and stress associated with the unilateral lameness could increase the release of endogenous adrenocorticotropin hormone and cortisol. Cortisol has an antagonistic effect on the action of insulin and could lead to IR, hyperglycemia, hyperinsulinemia, and possibly laminitis.[13] The lamellar cells are dependent on glucose, and IR decreases the uptake of glucose into these cells, reduces hemidesmosome numbers, and causes basal cell structure collapse, potentially leading to separation along the dermoepidermal junction.[14] Why, however, does the systemic hyperadrenocorticism and IR affect only a single foot? In addition, there is debate as to whether or not systemic cortisol is a reliable indicator of pain in horses and multiple studies have found that horses with laminitis do not have increased cortisol concentrations (Charlie F. Owen, Gary M. Baxter, unpublished data, 2006).[15] To the author's knowledge (GMB) blood cortisol and insulin concentrations have not been determined in horses with unilateral weight bearing but may warrant investigation in the future.

The architecture of the foot is designed for constant movement, cycles of loading and unloading. Because there is no muscle mass below the carpus, the lower limb is dependent on this cyclic loading to aid perfusion. It is estimated that the foot receives far more blood volume than what is needed for nourishment of the tissues. This excess fluid volume is believed to aid in shock absorption and support of the tissue (turgor pressure).[16–18] The perfusion to the digit previously was believed to be dependent on loading of the frog and digital cushion to help pump blood out of the foot. Studies have shown, however, negative pressures in the digital cushion during the loading phase.[16,19] Therefore, direct loading of the frog and digital cushion may not aid in perfusion in the manner previously believed. The circulation and venous pressure patterns in the moving horse and during stance support the notion of continuous movement as a requirement for healthy circulation to the lower limb.[20] Digital venous pressures increase rapidly after hoof contact (slightly before peak vertical force) most likely as a result of compression of the venous plexi. The pressure then decreases throughout the stance phase and finally rises slightly before foot lift off (same time as rapid flexion of the fetlock joint). During the swing phase of the stride, mean digital venous pressures were lower than resting pressures (resulting from prevention of back flow by valves in the veins and the pumping action of the muscles).[21] The cyclic loading and unloading of the foot is believed to create cyclic compression and decompression of the venous vasculature. As the foot is unloaded, blood fills the vasculature of the foot with the aid of gravity, normal arterial blood flow, recovery of compressed tissue, and the centripetal force during the swing phase. At ground contact, the vasculature and soft tissues are compressed, forcing blood out of the foot through areas of low resistance, such as the collateral cartilages and the porous partial surface of the distal phalanx. The circulatory pattern is believed to aid in shock absorption as external vibrations received by the tissues are transferred by the movement of fluid within a closed space, acting as a hydraulic shock-absorbing mechanism.[16,17,22] Although this mechanism is demonstrated in a moving horse, the normal horse, at stance, also undergoes constant movement. This is known as quasistatic loading.[23] Horses have been observed to shift weight from one forefoot to another as many as 125 ± 55 times per hour.[23] The constant weight shifting allows blood to perfuse the tissues, providing nutrients, hydration, and waste removal. When a horse is forced to stand continuously on one foot, the normal foot biomechanics deprive regions of the foot of circulation resulting in tissue fatigue, damage, and necrosis. Venogram studies show a lack of contrast or vascular filling of the dorsal laminar region when the foot is fully loaded compared with the unloaded model. It is hypothesized that the fully loaded vertical limb in which the DDF tendon is engaged and under tension pulls on its insertion site at the semilunar crest of the distal phalanx and causes rotation of the coffin joint and subtle movement of the distal phalanx away from the hoof wall. This subtle movement stretches the submural tissues and vasculature at the same time the subsolar soft tissues are compressed by the anterior solar surface of the distal phalanx.[24] This scenario probably is a normal movement, which aids in shock absorption and circulation; however, it does temporarily result in perfusion deficits in the dorsal laminae. Trying to maintain perfusion in a constantly static loaded foot remains a challenge and can lead to fatigue of the laminar interface and persistent perfusion deficits, resulting in laminitis and eventually coffin bone displacement or chronic laminitis. The long-term, low-magnitude constant loading of the supporting foot is believed to lead to vascular deficits, tissue damage, and support limb laminitis.

Risk Factors

The risk for developing support limb laminitis is believed related to the duration and severity of lameness on the opposite limb.[24,25] It often is associated with complete fractures, sepsis of a synovial structure, catastrophic breakdown, and other conditions causing significant unilateral lameness. There is no known association between the type of unilateral lameness and the risk for developing contralateral limb laminitis. Horses that are unwilling to bear any weight on a diseased limb for even small periods of time, however, seem more prone to developing support limb laminitis than are horses that can shuffle or hobble around, periodically relieving the added weight bearing on the contralateral limb.[24] Increased body weight is considered a risk factor by the author (GMB) but this was not found to be a significant factor in a case-control study of horses with support limb laminitis.[25] Clinically, the author believes that support limb laminitis occurs more commonly in the forelimbs than the hindlimbs and racehorses are at greater risk than horses of other disciplines. An epidemiologic study of traditional laminitis, however, did not reveal any associations between age, breed, gender, or weight and the occurrence of laminitis.[26] Redden reported that horses with healthy, robust feet are less likely to develop support limb laminitis than are horses with thin soles, low heels, negative palmar angles, hoof wall defects, and other structural abnormalities.[24]

Clinical Signs

Any horse with unilateral weight bearing should be monitored closely for signs of laminitis in the contralateral limb. Most cases of support limb laminitis are insidious in nature and easily can go unnoticed until there is significant structural damage. Clinical signs often develop between 2 and 5 weeks of contralateral limb weight bearing. The first signs usually are an increased digital pulse and then a sudden tendency to unweight the contralateral limb. Lameness may be difficult to assess, however, depending on the original injury, and significant lameness may be masked resulting from the need to bear increased weight on the support limb and an inability to unload the limb. A horse may try to shift its weight from the toe to the heel to relieve pressure and pain from the dorsal aspect or may constantly shift its weight from the support limb to the lame limb. Palpation of the digital pulses and the coronary band and changes in hoof wall temperature should be used to help determine if a horse has support limb laminitis. Baseline digital pulses and characteristics of the coronary band are important to establish so that subtle changes can be interpreted accurately. Palpation of the coronary band is believed a more reliable indicator of distal displacement of the distal phalanx than radiography.[25,27] The soft tissue immediately proximal to the coronary band becomes depressed inside the margin of the hoof capsule when the distal phalanx "sinks" within the hoof.[27] This coronary indentation or depression can be palpated and should be assessed frequently in horses at risk for support limb laminitis. Even though hoof wall surface temperature can fluctuate with the environment and debate exists as to whether or not it increases or decreases in early laminitis, it still should be assessed as in indicator of inflammation in the foot.[2,28] Many of these clinical signs may be subtle and difficult to interpret in the early stage of support limb laminitis. If treatment of the suspected laminitis is delayed until the clinical signs are obvious, however, the disease process often is well advanced. In general, preventative measures for the laminitis should be instituted well before any clinical signs are present.

Types of Movement of the Distal Phalanx

The mechanical collapse of the distal phalanx can occur at any point around the lamellar attachment of the bone to the hoof wall. Clinically, movement of the distal phalanx tends to occur in one of three different patterns: dorsal rotation, symmetric distal displacement, and unilateral distal displacement.[29] Dorsal rotation occurs more commonly than symmetric distal displacement, which is more common than unilateral distal displacement. Dorsal rotation is the classic form of laminitis where the distal phalanx separates from the dorsal hoof capsule and rotates about the distal interphalangeal (DIP) joint. It is best diagnosed with a lateral radiograph of the foot. Symmetric distal displacement, or sinking, occurs when the lamellae mechanically collapse evenly all around their attachment to the hoof wall and the bone drops into the hoof capsule. The solar margin of distal phalanx becomes closer to the ground surface and the distance between the parietal surface of the distal phalanx and the inner hoof capsule increases. Displacement often can be difficult to diagnose on a single lateral radiograph, but the depression at the coronary band often can be palpated digitally.[25,27,29] Unilateral distal displacement (medial or lateral) occurs when mechanical collapse occurs on the medial or lateral aspect of the hoof. Medial displacement is more common and the solar surface of the distal phalanx on the affected side moves distally within the hoof capsule. This type of displacement can be diagnosed only radiographically using a horizontal dorsopalmar/plantar view of the distal phalanx.[29] Although each type of displacement may occur independently, a combination of the three types of displacement often is exhibited in many horses (**Fig. 1**).[29]

Symmetric distal displacement appears to occur more commonly in horses with support limb laminitis than the other types of distal phalanx displacement.[25] Many horses may exhibit mild clinical signs of laminitis, however, and have no abnormalities on radiographs in the early stages of the disease. The lack of radiographic changes does not indicate that a horse does not have support limb laminitis. Any horse with even subtle signs of support limb laminitis should be treated and preventative measures continued. Once movement of the distal phalanx occurs in horses with unilateral

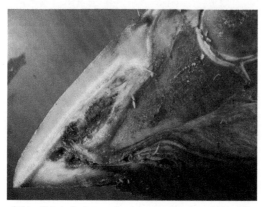

Fig. 1. Cross-section of the distal phalanx of a Quarter Horse gelding that developed support limb laminitis after treatment for a severely comminuted phalangeal fracture. Rotation and distal displacement of the distal phalanx were evident radiographically and at postmortem examination.

lameness, the prognosis for recovery usually is reduced because of the extreme diffi-culty of managing a horse with severe bilateral lameness.

Once laminitis develops, the region of the foot under the most load usually is the first area to become compromised. The normal foot during stance loads the anterior me-dial toe region. This can be seen on pressure sensor mat studies. The center of pres-sure (COP) generally is located just caudal to the apex of the frog and slightly medially. Therefore, most horses at stance load the medial toe region.[23,30,31] When the laminae become compromised, it often is the toe region that shows structural collapse first. When there is reduced weight bearing from severe lameness or the limb lengthened with a brace or cast, the loading pattern of the contralateral limb often is exaggerated. Support limb laminitis cases in the hind limb usually sink laterally and rotate. In an ef-fort to unload the sore hind limb, the contralateral foot often is positioned closer to a horse's midline (base narrow stance) shifting the COP laterally. These cases often show lamellar damage and structural collapse in the anterior and lateral regions of the foot (**Fig. 2**). Cases that have rotation and horizontal plane laminitis can be prob-lematic to treat as addressing the rotational forces can exaggerate strain in the heels/quarters.

Radiographic Diagnosis

Radiography of the digit is a useful method of monitoring horses with support limb laminitis but cannot be used as the definitive diagnostic tool. Radiography also is a rel-atively insensitive tool to document early abnormalities in the laminar region in horses

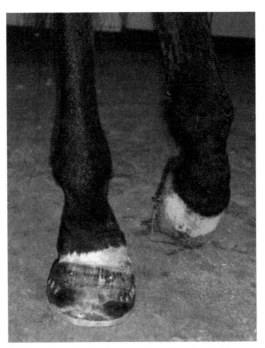

Fig. 2. Thoroughbred filly with right hind–supporting limb laminitis, secondary to a left hock infection. Note the hoof capsule deformity and abnormal wall growth. This foot had severe rotation and lateral sinking of the coffin bone. This foot was rehabilitated with axial sup-port, wall cast, and shoe with a small wedge and rolled toe/rolled shoe branches.

with laminitis but venograms may be helpful in recognition of early vascular deficits and damage (**Fig. 3**). In addition, MRI has been performed on cadaver limbs with chronic laminitis and revealed many additional abnormalities not apparent on radiographs.[32] MRI may be especially applicable in horses with support limb laminitis to detect early and subtle laminar and hoof abnormalities that often are difficult to detect on radiographs. Unfortunately, MRI not always is feasible in many of these horses. To make the best use of radiographs, baseline lateral and dorsopalmar radiographs of the contralateral limb should be obtained. The same radiographic technique and positioning should be performed on subsequent radiographs to permit direct comparisons between the films. Soft tissue thickness between the parietal surface of the

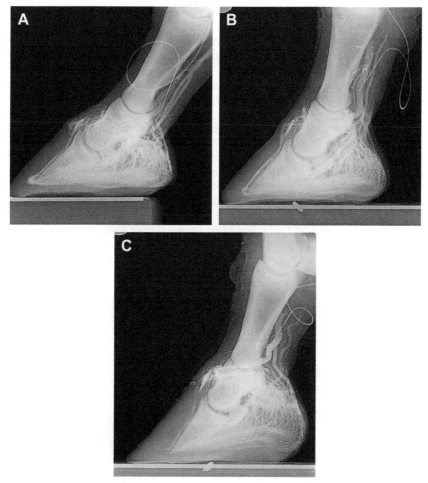

Fig. 3. (*A*) Example of a normal venogram. Note the thick vascular plexus of the sole corium and continuous vascular pattern over the coronary band and down the parietal surface of P3. (*B*) Venogram of a mild case of laminitis. Slight compression of the vasculature of the anterior sole. (*C*) Venogram pattern of a foot with chronic laminitis. The pedal bone has displaced compressing and destroying the vasculature on the sole corium. The vasculature is thinned over the extensor process as a result of stretching and compression from the displacement.

distal phalanx and the inner hoof wall (horn-lamellar zone) should be determined on subsequent lateromedial projections and compared with baseline. In most normal horses this distance is similar at the proximal and distal aspects of the dorsal hoof wall and should be approximately 16 mm (range 11–20 mm) thick.[33,34] This thickness may vary with breed, age, and size of horse,[34] however, emphasizing the need for baseline radiographs for the most accurate interpretation. In a study by Peloso and colleagues,[25] the soft tissue thickness dorsal to the distal phalanx was expressed as a percentage of the palmar cortical length of the distal phalanx (distance from the tip of the distal phalanx to the midpoint of the articulation between the distal phalanx and navicular bone) to adjust for variations in foot size (**Fig. 4**). A contralateral limb with a soft tissue thickness dorsal to the distal phalanx of greater than 29% of the palmar cortical length of the distal phalanx was suggestive of support limb laminitis.[25] In that study, only one of 16 horses with support limb laminitis had evidence of rotation on a lateromedial radiograph.[25]

In addition to the dorsal soft tissue thickness, the distance from the proximal limit of the dorsal hoof wall (as distinguished with a metal marker) to the proximal limit of the extensor process of the distal phalanx (so-called *founder distance*) should be determined and compared with subsequent films to help document symmetric distal displacement of the distal phalanx. This distance was found quite variable in normal horses with a mean distance of 4.1 mm (range −1.8 to 9.7 mm) whereas other investigators have stated that this distance varies from 0 to 15 mm in normal horses (**Fig. 5**).[33,34] Increases in the founder distance suggest that the distal phalanx is displacing down into the hoof capsule (sinking) and may be the only radiographic sign suggestive of laminitis in some horses with support limb laminitis. In a study by Cripps and Eustace, the founder distance was determined to be the most significant radiologic prognostic measurement for acute laminitis cases.[35] Other radiographic signs of distal displacement include cavitation of the coronary band, more visible proximal aspect of the hoof wall (soft tissue line along proximal hoof wall), and a reduced distance between the apex of the distal phalanx and the solar surface.[25,27,29] Unilateral displacement of the distal phalanx can be identified only on a dorsopalmar radiograph

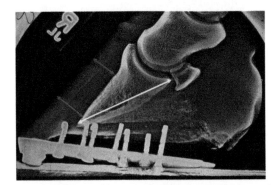

Fig. 4. Lateral radiograph illustrating two methods to document early abnormalities in horses with support limb laminitis. The hoof-lamellar zone (*red arrows*) should be similar in width at the proximal and distal aspects of the dorsal hoof wall and approximately 15 to 18 mm (range 11–20 mm) thick. The soft tissue thickness dorsal to the distal phalanx also should be <30% of the palmar cortical length of the distal phalanx (*yellow arrow*). Subtle abnormalities in the hoof-lamellar zone are better documented by comparisons to baseline radiographs of the same horse rather than relying on standard measurements obtained from healthy horses.

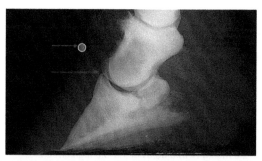

Fig. 5. A lateral radiograph of a horse with distal displacement of the distal phalanx. The distance from the proximal limit of the dorsal hoof wall (metal marker) to the proximal limit of the extensor process of the distal phalanx (*red arrows*) was increased compared with radiographs taken 2 weeks previously. This measurement is referred to as the founder distance or the coronary band-extensor process relation. This distance was found quite variable in normal horses, with a mean distance of 4.1 mm (range −1.8–9.7 mm) whereas other investigators have stated that this distance varies from 0 to 15 mm in normal horses. Comparison of this measurement on subsequent radiographs to baseline radiographs provides the most accurate information.

as an increased distance between the outer hoof wall and the distal phalanx and a reduced distance between the distal phalanx and the sole on the affected side.[29] In addition, the joint space of the DIP joint may be increased on the affected side and narrowed on the unaffected side.[29] Many of these radiographic abnormalities can be subtle, emphasizing the need for good-quality baseline lateral and dorsopalmar radiographs of the contralateral foot in horses with significant unilateral lameness.

Prevention/Treatment

Treatment of horses with support limb laminitis should focus on prevention and should not be delayed until clinical or radiographic signs of laminitis are present. Many horses develop support limb laminitis, however, despite preventative treatment, suggesting that preventative treatments may not be effective. This is not surprising because the pathogenesis of support limb laminitis most likely is different from the more traditional forms of laminitis (and unknown), yet preventative measures may be the same. In general, prevention of support limb laminitis should be directed toward the primary lameness and the contralateral foot. The primary risk factor shown to contribute significantly to support limb laminitis is duration of unilateral lameness.[25] Therefore, anything that can be done to treat the primary cause of the unilateral lameness that enables more normal weight bearing as quickly as possible helps prevent laminitis in the opposite limb. Therapies directed toward the contralateral foot usually are aimed at preventing the development of acute laminitis or minimizing any type of displacement of the distal phalanx.

Systemic medical therapy

Preventative and treatment strategies for horses with support limb laminitis often are similar to those for other types of laminitis and directed toward one of several potential mechanisms. These include reducing inflammation (nonsteroidal anti-inflammatory drugs [NSAIDs], antioxidants, or lidocaine), improving lamellar blood flow (acepromazine, nitroglycerin, isoxsuprine, or pentoxifylline), preventing platelet aggregation/thrombosis (aspirin or heparin), and inhibiting MMPs (doxycycline) (**Box 1**).[36] Whether or not these same mechanisms are important in the development of support limb

---

Box 1
Medical therapy to potentially prevent support limb laminitis

To reduce inflammation

- NSAIDs
  - ○ Phenylbutazone—2.2–4.4 mg/kg IV or orally every 12 hours
  - ○ Flunixin meglumine—0.5–1.1 mg/kg IV every 12 hours
  - ○ Firocoxib—0.1 mg/kg every 24 hours

- Lidocaine—1.3–2.0 mg/kg IV as a bolus or 1.8–3.0 mg/kg/h CRI
- Antioxidants (vitamin E)—10–20 IU/kg orally every 24 hours

To improve lamellar blood flow

- Acepromazine—0.02–0.04 mg/kg IM every 4–6 hours
- Isoxsuprine—0.6–1.2 mg/kg orally every 12 hours
- Nitroglycerin—40–80 mg/horse/day (10–20 mg for each vessel/day)
- Pentoxifylline—5–8 mg/kg orally every 8–12 hours

To prevent platelet aggregation/thrombosis

- Acetylsalicyclic acid (aspirin)—20 mg/kg orally every other day
- Heparin—40–80 IU/kg every 8–12 hours IV or subcutaneously

To inhibit MMP activity

- Doxycycline—1 mg/kg (500 mg) orally every 12 hours

---

laminitis is unknown and in general medical therapy has questionable success in preventing laminitis regardless of the cause. Many combinations of these drugs and procedures are used, however, in horses at risk for support limb laminitis in hopes of delaying or preventing the disease process.

Local foot therapy

Specific objectives aimed at the foot to prevent laminitis or limit displacement of the distal phalanx should include (1) reducing effective bodyweight, (2) recruiting all or part of the sole and frog to bear weight, (3) redistributing weight bearing from the most stressed wall to the least stressed wall, and (4) decreasing the moment arm around the DIP.[37] Most of these principles can be met by removing the existing shoes, shortening and beveling the toe or wall, applying frog support, placing a horse in soft bedding or sand, and encouraging a horse to lie down.[37,38] Effective body weight could be reduced further by casting the foot[39] or slinging a horse.[37] Slinging is the ultimate method to reduce effective body weight and unweight the opposite limb but it requires the expertise to apply and use a sling and closely monitor patients. There also is horse variability as to how well they tolerate the sling. Intermittent slinging for a few hours each day, however, is tolerated by most horses and can be beneficial in preventing contralateral limb laminitis. Unfortunately, this often is labor intensive and not practical in many situations.

Frog supports not only recruit the back part of the foot for weight bearing but also elevate the heel to reduce the pull of the DDF tendon. Heel elevation also can be achieved by applying wedge pads to the bottom of the foot, which is accomplished most easily with a commercial wedge and cuff combination (Redden Modified Ultimate) (**Fig. 6**).[29] Styrofoam padding or commercial wedge pads combined with dental impression material also may be used to provide frog support and heel elevation. In a study by Redden, less than 2.5% of horses with unilateral non–weight-bearing lameness developed laminitis in the contralateral limb when a heel wedge and cuff combination device had been applied to the opposite foot.[24]

Cryotherapy has been shown to reduce the signs of acute laminitis in horses receiving carbohydrate overload.[40,41] Cryotherapy was administered continuously before induction of the model, suggesting that it may be more effective as a preventative measure than treating the condition once clinical signs have developed. The proposed mechanism was vasoconstriction, which prevented laminitis trigger factors induced by the carbohydrate overload from gaining access to the foot. Cryotherapy was not effective, however, unless it included the entire limb up to or past the level of the carpus. It is unknown if similar trigger factors are involved in support limb laminitis and whether or not cryotherapy is beneficial as a preventative measure in horses with unilateral lameness. Cryotherapy also is believed, however, to reduce the metabolism of the laminae, potentially protecting the foot from the adverse effects of increased MMP activity, which should be beneficial with any type of laminitis. Continuous cryotherapy often is impractical to use in many clinical patients, especially those with unilateral lameness. Whether or not intermittent cryotherapy is as effective as continuous treatment in preventing laminitis is unknown.

Pain Management

The severity of pain in horses with laminitis often parallels the severity of the disease process. The clinical assessment of a horse (degree of lameness or pain) can be predictive of survival,[42] suggesting that the degree of pain and the severity of laminar damage often are similar. Therefore, horses with mild discomfort and laminar pain do not need to be treated as aggressively as those horses that are severely painful. The amount of time a horse remains standing often can be used as a guide to determine the level of pain and, therefore, how aggressive to be with analgesia treatment.[43] Management of pain in horses with support limb laminitis often is complicated by the

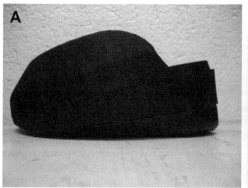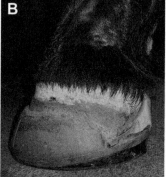

Fig. 6. (*A*) Nanric Ultimate cuff (Nanric, Lawrenceburg, Kentucky). The 18° wedge helps decrease tension of the DDF tendon and improve circulation to the anterior laminae and sole corium. (*B*) Nanric Ultimate cuff adhered to the foot with acrylic. The cuff was placed on the supporting limb along with an elastomer arch support to help prevent laminitis.

primary musculoskeletal problem because that limb often is not back to normal when laminitis develops in the contralateral foot. The horse does not have a good foot to stand on, which often creates considerable anxiety and often is one of the main justifications for euthanasia in these patients.

Mild laminitis pain often is managed with oral NSAIDs alone. Horses with moderate pain usually require additional treatments, such as systemic opioids (morphine IM or fentanyl patches), epidural analgesia (detomidine plus morphine), and sedatives to reduce anxiety (intramuscular [IM] xylazine/detomidine or acepromazine).[43] Morphine can be given at 0.1 mg/kg IM every 4 to 6 hours and then reduced as dictated by patient comfort. Acepromazine (0.02 mg/kg IM or 10 mg/450 kg body weight every 4 to 6 hours) can be used with morphine to prevent the central nervous system excitement that may accompany the use of morphine[43] and potentially improve distal limb perfusion in these horses.[44] Epidurals used for laminitis in the hind feet usually contain detomidine (0.030 mg/kg) and morphine (0.2 mg/kg) and are repeated as necessary.[45] One or two fentanyl patches (10 mg each) may be applied to the foreleg to provide opioid analgesia instead of morphine, but the author (GMB) has found fentanyl of little value in horses with severe laminar pain. Horses with severe pain may require aggressive treatment, including constant rate infusion (CRI) of analgesics, such as lidocaine/ketamine or a solution called pentafusion, which contains a combination of lidocaine/ketamine/morphine/detomidine and acepromazine.[43] The ketamine/lidocaine solution is made by combining 3 g (6 mg/kg) ketamine and 400 mg (0.8–1 mg/kg) lidocaine into 5-L sterile fluids and administered initially at a rate of 500 to 600 mL/h. The authors have not used pentafusion but this combination is reported an effective method to control severe pain in horses with laminitis.[43] The authors report combining lidocaine (3 mg/kg, 1.35 g/450 kg) and ketamine (0.6 mg/kg, 4 g/450 kg) into 1 L of saline, and morphine (0.025 mg/kg, 170 mg/450 kg), detomidine (0.004 mg/kg, 30 mg/450 kg), and acepromazine (0.002 mg/kg, 15 mg/450 kg) into another 1 L of saline and administering both 1-L solutions at a CRI of 70 mL/h. The amount of drug administered can be titrated according to the level of pain of a horse and the response to treatment. Loading doses of lidocaine (1.3 mg/kg intravenously [IV]) and morphine (0.1 mg/kg IV) can be used with either CRI combination to speed the onset of pain relief. Horses receiving these CRI combinations should be monitored closely during the early stage of infusion to adjust the flow rate if ataxia or other complications develop. The duration of use is variable depending on the response to treatment but the flow rate should be reduced and discontinued as quickly as possible because of the risk for overuse of these drugs.

Specific Foot Management

For horses with casts on the injured limb, elevated wooden support blocks on the contralateral limb can be used to counteract the differences in limb length (**Fig. 7**).[46–48] The casted limb usually is longer than the "good" leg, which means that a horse preferentially bears weight on the noncasted limb. Placing an elevated block on the contralateral limb permits a horse to stand squarely preventing overuse of the contralateral limb and development of support limb laminitis. A plastic full flat pad (0.52-in thickness) cut to match the circumference and shape of the foot, is attached to a block of wood (1.5- to 1.75-in thickness) using standard wood deck screws directed distally. Dental impression material is applied to the frog and heels beneath the block and is permitted to exit the back of the foot when the horse stands on the block.[46] This allows even frog, sole, and heel support to the palmar/plantar aspect of the foot. The wooden support block is applied to the hoof with five 1.5-inch wooden deck screws placed proximally to distally on the dorsal hemicircumference of the hoof.

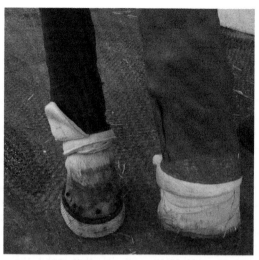

Fig. 7. A wooden block has been applied to the contralateral foot in this horse with a half-limb cast to adjust for the differences in limb length. This permits the horse to bear weight more evenly on both limbs to prevent support limb laminitis caused by overloading of the normal foot.

Screws should not be placed behind the widest part of the foot and the block should be placed in an awake patient to avoid inadvertent placement into the sensitive structures of the hoof.

The goals of providing axial support to the foot in horses with support limb laminitis are to decrease the tensile forces on the anterior laminae and to unload the laminae to some degree by transferring load to the sole, frog, and bars.[49] Axial support of the foot is used as a preventative measure and to treat horses in the acute phase of laminitis. There are several sole/frog support materials available, including impression materials, foam, and rubber pads. Which material used often is based on personal preference of clinicians, but the softer the material the less support and immobilization it provides. Rubber mats cut from gym mats are useful and effective and give horses the ability to mold the material into the configuration they are most comfortable with.[49] These materials usually are fitted to the foot, attempting to unweight the toe and move the weight-bearing surface palmarly/plantarly and are held in position with elastic bandage or duct tape. Decreasing the tensile forces of the anterior laminae is best addressed by reducing the pull of the DDF tendon on the distal phalanx.[49] This is done by elevating the heel, moving the breakover point of the hoof more palmar/plantar (trimming and beveling the toe), or both.[50–54] Heel elevation can be provided with commercial products, such as the Nanric Ultimate cuff, by riveting plastic wedge pads together, or by using a block of wood or styrofoam pads. In most cases, the amount of heel elevation should not exceed 10° as artificial wedges may put additional stress on other regions.[49] In addition, not all horses respond the same and the clinical response of these horses to heel elevation should be monitored closely and the device removed if a horse appears more uncomfortable.

Applying a hoof cast with a heel wedge recently has been shown to unload the dorsal hoof wall but increase the load on the quarters of the hoof in vitro.[39] Whether or not this occurs clinically is unknown but may be another option to provide axial support to the foot in horses at risk for support limb laminitis or as a treatment in horses with acute laminitis. Hoof casts are easy to apply in healthy horses but this may be complicated in horses with an opposite limb musculoskeletal problem because of the inability to pick the foot up. Horses seem to tolerate foot casts well, however, once they are applied even with a half-limb or full-limb cast on the primary injured limb (**Fig. 8**). The authors have not used foot casts as a preventative for support limb laminitis but do not believe they have been that helpful in horses with acute laminitis.

Prevention of supporting limb laminitis can be difficult if a horse is unable to load or walk on an injured limb. If possible, frequent periods of hand walking are ideal. If a horse is left on strict stall rest or unable to walk, the contralateral limb is not sufficiently unloaded until it becomes painful. Unfortunately most cases do not become painful until there already is significant structural damage acquired. Various techniques have been attempted to prevent overloading of the supporting limb, such as slings and water stalls. Devices applied to the foot for support are useful and most practical. Axial support refers to loading of the structures within the perimeter of the hoof wall, such as the frog, bars, and sole, and helps unload the perimeter wall and the lamellar interface.[55] There are many products on the market available for axial support, such as silicone, polyurethane, and elastomers. Some products are moldable, which set up creating an impression; materials that match the consistency of the frog (35–45 durometer) seem to work best and are well tolerated (**Fig. 9**). Other materials, such as rubber and closed cell foams, can be used; these products seem to work best if they are approximately 1- to 1.5-in thick for an average-sized foot and compress 50% under the weight of the horse. Venogram studies have shown cuff shoes with a 10° heel elevation and axial support to enhance dorsal laminae filling with contrast in the fully loaded limb.[24] Thompson and colleagues[52] found that wedging a heel of a cadaver limb by 23° significantly decreased tension on the DDF tendon but increased strain in the quarters, especially medially. Decreasing tension on the DDF tendon improves vascular filling of the anterior lamellar vessels in a loaded limb by

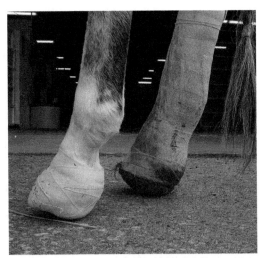

Fig. 8. A fiberglass foot cast with a heel wedge was applied to the right hind foot of this horse after it developed support limb laminitis secondary to a comminuted second phalanx fracture. The cast made the horse more comfortable and willing to bear weight on the foot but did not seem to change the progression of the laminitis. Using foot casts earlier in the course of the disease may be more beneficial.

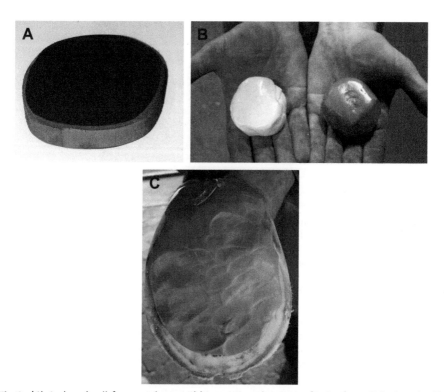

Fig. 9. (*A*) A closed cell foam pad or a rubber mat can be cut to fit the foot. This closed cell foam is 1-inch thick and compresses approximately 50% under the weight of an average size horse. The pad can be bandaged to the foot or placed inside a hoof boot. (*B*) Various products can be used to load the frog and sole. Here is an example of a two-part elastomer, which is mixed and placed on the solar surface. The foot is held up until the elastomer sets up, then bandaged to the foot. (*C*) Foot with impression material compressed into sulcus and throughout sole.

reducing the rotational force and decreasing tension on the anterior laminae. This also is shown with venogram studies to decrease compression on the anterior solar corium by the distal phalanx and enhance perfusion to the anterior solar corium.[24] Although heel elevation helps decrease rotation, it moves the COP caudally, increasing strain on the heels, in particular the medial quarter.[52] It is the author's experience (SM) that prolonged periods of wedging can lead to unilateral distal displacement laminitis (medial or lateral sinking), especially on the low-heeled foot conformation. Therefore, selection of foot support should take into account the foot conformation.[49] The modification of rolling the ground surface of the shoe in the toe and heel regions to create a rocker effect or air wedge is believed by some to create the wedge effect without creating direct compression on the heel region, as does a conventional wedge (**Fig. 10**). This shoe modification has not been evaluated objectively, however.

After the application of foot support, the foot should be examined frequently for subtle changes in the coronary band, which may be the first signs of regional overloading. The first signs of sinking in the quarters or unilateral distal displacement laminitis usually are slowed or ceased wall growth in the quarters followed by a palpable ledge, then coronary band separation. These cases usually do not become painful until there is coronary band separation and impingement by the proximal wall, which usually is

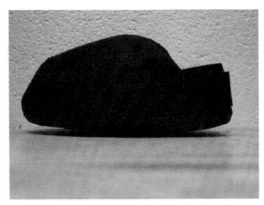

Fig. 10. Modified Nanric Ultimate. The rolled toe and rolled heel increase the mechanics of the wedge. The foot can tip forward creating an increased wedge effect.

approximately 2 months post displacement. Once signs of overloading are detected, preferably at the first sign of decreased wall growth but before a palpable ledge, the pressure can be taken off the coronary band by grooving the proximal hoof wall just below the compromised regions.[56] The groove is made with the edge of a rasp or a 0.25-inch dremmel, parallel to the coronary band and only in the region of compression/ceased wall growth. The entire thickness of the stratum externum and medium is grooved and the groove is performed below the coronary cushion (0.25 to 0.5 in below the hairline) (**Fig. 11**). Strategic and timely subcoronary band grooving can prevent a shear lesion or separation and restore normal wall growth. Once a case is diagnosed as sinking (medial, lateral, or vertical), the author (SM) prefers to remove the wedge, groove the compromised coronary band regions, and apply a foot cast. The foot cast for a sinker should include axial support and ease of breakover in all directions. The author usually places sole support on the solar surface of the foot and casts the foot up to the level just distal to the fetlock. The ground surface of the cast usually is rounded with acrylic or urethane to create a dome, which allows the foot to roll in all directions with little resistance (**Fig. 12**). The foot cast is believed to immobilize or stabilize the entire foot to decrease independent movement of the hoof capsule and

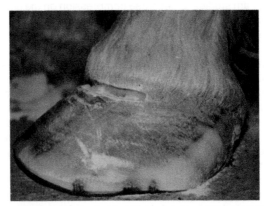

Fig. 11. Subcoronary grooving performed in the toe region of a foot with chronic laminitis. The grooving promotes wall growth in the toe region and relieve shearing/compression of the proximal hoof wall.

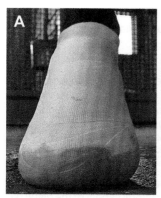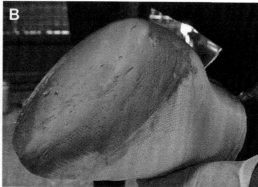

Fig. 12. (A) Fiberglass foot cast used in a foot with early signs of sinking. Elastomer was placed on the sole surface for arch support. (B) The ground surface of the foot cast was coated with acrylic in a mild dome shape, to ease brake over in all directions. The foot cast is believed to decrease independent movement of regions of the hoof wall with the goal of decreasing the propagation of laminar separation and shearing of adjacent laminae.

boney column, with the goal of reducing shearing and twisting of the lamellar interface. Small areas of lamellar damage may propagate to adjacent areas as the hoof capsule moves independently, creating more diffuse areas of separation. Immobilizing the foot with a foot cast, sole support, and rolling the ground surface has been a method the authors used to save many horses that sink.[49] The prognosis for rehabilitating a sinker remains poor, however, once a palpable ledge or separation is evident around the entire coronary band. These cases usually slough the entire wall and are euthanized or go through extensive rehabilitation to regrow the hoof capsule.

Prognosis

Although radiography can be beneficial in monitoring the progression of laminitis, it may not be that helpful in predicting prognosis, especially in horses with acute laminitis. Hunt suggested that the clinical assessment of horses (how lame a horse is) was a more reliable means of determining the final outcome and should be given precedence over radiographic findings.[42] In that study, however, horses that returned to athletic soundness had significantly less distal phalangeal rotation than horses that remained intermittently lame or those that had permanent severe lameness, suggesting that the degree of phalangeal rotation affects the future soundness of horses with chronic laminitis. Many horses that develop severe acute laminitis may not survive long enough to permit rotation or displacement of the distal phalanx and this may explain why there was no significant difference in the amount of phalangeal rotation between the horses that returned to athletic soundness and those that did not survive. In the study by Cripps and Eustace, the type of laminitis as determined by clinical examination (laminitis, acute founder, sinker, or chronic founder) was the most important prognostic parameter, emphasizing the importance of clinical assessment of these horses.[35] Whether or not clinical assessment or the severity of radiographic abnormalities can be used to predict the prognosis in horses with support limb laminitis currently is unknown. What is known, however, is that horses that develop support limb laminitis are more likely to be euthanatized than horses with similar problems that do not develop laminitis.[25] In many of these horses, the lack of a good foot to stand on creates a difficult management situation that may lead to prolonged periods of recumbency, severe pain when standing, and a questionable quality of life.

CONTRALATERAL ANGULAR LIMB DEFORMITIES IN FOALS

Young horses with unilateral lameness problems develop support limb laminitis infrequently compared with adult horses. This most likely is related to smaller body mass and greater likelihood that young horses will lie down. The increased weight bearing on the contralateral limb, however, contributes to physeal growth imbalances leading to angular limb deformities (ALDs). A varus deformity of the carpus is the most common lameness-induced ALD that develops in the contralateral limb and associated most frequently with some type of fracture in the opposite limb. The increased weight bearing is believed to compress or potentially cause microtrauma to the medial aspect of the distal radial physis, leading to slower growth medially. The lateral aspect of the distal radial physis grows normally but the end result is a varus deformity of the carpus resulting from an imbalance in physeal growth. In addition there often is lateral bowing of carpus in many cases presumably from stretching of the ligaments of the limb associated with the increased weight bearing. There is no known prevention for ALD in young horses with unilateral lameness other than minimizing the severity and duration of the primary lameness. Support limb bandaging, limb braces, and corrective shoeing (lateral extensions) may be attempted but often are not effective. Surgical treatment of a contralateral limb carpal varus deformity may be attempted depending on the age it develops but has not been tried by the authors. Many times these foals are older than 6 months when the deformity develops, minimizing the ability to surgically correct the angulation. In addition, the growth potential of medial aspect of the physis often is compromised, further decreasing the ability to manipulate the growth of the distal radial physis.

SUPPORTING LIMB COMPLICATIONS IN FOALS

Since the contralateral limb is overloaded in foals, it is common to see fatigue of the flexor tendons and suspensory ligaments. This is seen more commonly in foals with less developed musculature. If a foal also is on stall rest and has not exercised for a prolonged period of time, muscular atrophy and weakness also can contribute. When the fetlock is noticed to drop or the DIP joint hyperextended (toe flipping up), a heel extension should be placed for support and leverage (**Fig. 13**). Conversely, the lame limb can acquire a contractural flexural deformity as the tendons and ligaments are not loaded normally during a period of rapid bone growth, resulting in an acquired clubfoot (contracture of DIP joint). These cases can be transient and slowly improve as normal weight bearing is achieved or can result in a permanent contracture. Mild cases in younger horses (less than 6 months) often can be treated with toe extensions and shoeing. More severe cases or those that have not responded to toe extensions/shoeing, however, may require an inferior check ligament desmotomy or special shoeing to manage.

Overloading the growth plates in the growing horse can result in ALDs. It seems that varus and valgus deformities commonly are seen in the front limbs (**Fig. 14**A); however, it is more common to see varus deformities in the hind limbs (**Fig. 14**B). This probably is for reasons similar to lateral sinking in adult cases (described previously). A varus deformity of the carpus not uncommonly develops in the contralateral limb, however, secondary to some type of fracture in the opposite limb. The increased weight bearing is believed to compress or potentially cause microtrauma to the medial aspect of the distal radial physis leading to slower growth medially. The lateral aspect of the distal radial physis grows normally but the end result is a varus deformity of the

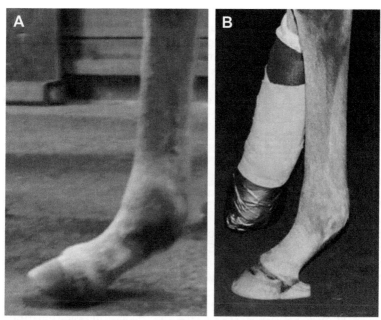

Fig. 13. (*A*) Flexor tendon laxity in a 1-month-old foal. Laxity of the DDF tendon allows hyperextension of the DIP joint and flipping up of the toe. (*B*) Ibex foal shoe with a heel extension to help support the flexor tendons in supporting limb of a foal with a severe left hind coffin bone infection.

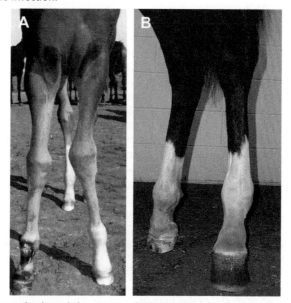

Fig. 14. (*A*) Left carpal valgus deformity in a foal. The right front limb was born with a flexor tendon contracture, which was treated with bandages and splints. During the first few weeks the foal overloaded the left limb causing an angular deformity of the carpus. (*B*) Left hind fetlock varus deformity in a saddlebred weanling. The weanling was born without a coffin bone on the right hind and overloaded the medial aspect of the physis on the left hind distal cannon bone.

carpus resulting from an imbalance in physeal growth. In addition there often is lateral bowing of carpus in many cases, presumably from stretching of the ligaments of the limb associated with the increased weight bearing. There is no known prevention for ALDs in young horses with unilateral lameness other than minimizing the severity and duration of the primary lameness. Foals that develop a varus deformity at the carpus/tarsus or fetlock, however, benefit from a shoe with a lateral support. If a case is developing a valgus deformity, a medial extension may be indicated. Care should be taken to match limb length in foals that are in casts, braces, or special shoes to promote even weight distribution.

REFERENCES

1. Pollitt CC. Basement membrane pathology: a feature of acute equine laminitis. Equine Vet J 1996;28:38–46.
2. Pollitt CC. Equine laminitis. Clin Tech Equine Pract 2004;3:34–44.
3. Moore RM, Eades SC, Stokes AM. Evidence for vascular and enzymatic events in the pathophysiology of acute laminitis: which pathway is responsible for initiation of this process in horses? Equine Vet J 2004;36:204–9.
4. Hood DM. The pathophysiology of developmental and acute laminitis. Vet Clin North Am Equine Pract 1999;15:321–43.
5. Belknap JK. Pathophysiology of acute laminitis. Presented at the 46th BEVA Congress; 2007. p. 201–2.
6. Kyaw-Tanner M, Pollitt CC. Equine laminitis: increased transcription of matrix metalloproteinase-2 (MMP-2) occurs during the developmental phase. Equine Vet J 2004;36:221–5.
7. Johnson PJ, Messer NT, Slight SH. Endocrinopathic laminitis in the horse. Clin Tech Equine pract 2004;3:45–56.
8. Johnson PJ, Messer NT, Ganjam VK. Cushing's syndromes, insulin resistance and endocrinopathic laminitis. Equine Vet J 2004;36:194–8.
9. Bailey SR, Menzies-Gow NJ, Harris PA, et al. Effect of dietary fructans and dexamethasone administration on the insulin response of ponies predisposed to laminitis. J Am Vet Med Assoc 2007;231:1365–73.
10. French KR, Pollitt CC. Equine laminitis: glucose deprivation and MMP activation induce dermo-epidermal separation in vitro. Equine Vet J 2004;36:261–6.
11. Asplin KE, Sillence MN, Pollitt CC, et al. Induction of laminitis by prolonged hyperinsulinaemia in clinically normal ponies. Vet J 2007;174:530–5.
12. Redden RF. A technique for performing digital venography in the standing horse. Equine Vet Educ 2001;3:172–8.
13. Reeves HJ, Lees R, McGowan CM. Measurement of basal serum insulin concentration in the diagnosis of Cushing's disease in ponies. Vet Rec 2001;149:449–52.
14. Pass MA, Pollitt S, Pollitt CC. Decreased glucose metabolism causes separation of hoof lamellae in vitro: a trigger for laminitis? Equine Vet J Suppl 1998;133–8.
15. Galey FD, Whiteley HE, Goetz TE, et al. Black walnut (Juglans nigra) toxicosis: a model for equine laminitis. J Comp Pathol 1991;104:313–26.
16. Bowker RM. The anatomy of the ungula cartilage and digital cushion. Presented at the 12th Annual Bluegrass Laminitis Symposium; 1998. p. 75–88.
17. Bowker RM. Contrasting structure morphologies of "good" and "bad" footed horses. AAEP Proc 2003;49:186–209.
18. Hood DM. The effect of weight bearing on digital perfusion. Presented at the 12th Annual Bluegrass Laminitis Symposium; 1998. p. 94–105.

19. Dyhre-Poulsen P, Smedegaard HH, Roed J, et al. Equine hoof function investigated by pressure transducers inside the hoof and accelerometers mounted on the first phalanx. Equine Vet J 1994;26:362–6.
20. Dyson S, Lakhani K, Wood J. Factors influencing blood flow in the equine digit and their effect on uptake of 99m technetium methylene diphosphonate into bone. Equine Vet J 2001;33:591–8.
21. Ratzlaff MH, Shindell RM, DeBowes RM. Changes in digital venous pressures of horses moving at the walk and trot. Am J Vet Res 1985;46:1545–9.
22. Barrey E. Investigation of the vertical hoof force distribution in the equine forelimb with an instrumented horseboot. Equine Vet J Suppl 1990;35–8.
23. Hood DM. Center of digital load during quai-static loading. Presented at the 12th Annual Bluegrass Laminitis Symposium; 1998. p. 47–62.
24. Redden RF. Preventing laminitis in the contralateral limb of horses with non-weightbearing lameness. Clin Tech Equine Pract 2004;3:57–63.
25. Peloso JG, Cohen ND, Walker MA, et al. Case-control study of risk factors for the development of laminitis in the contralateral limb in Equidae with unilateral lameness. J Am Vet Med Assoc 1996;209:1746–9.
26. Slater MR, Hood DM, Carter GK. Descriptive epidemiological study of equine laminitis. Equine Vet J 1995;27:364–7.
27. Baxter GM. Equine laminitis caused by distal displacement of the distal phalanx: 12 cases (1976–1985). J Am Vet Med Assoc 1986;189:326–9.
28. Hood DM, Wagner IP, Brumbaugh GW. Evaluation of hoof wall surface temperature as an index of digital vascular perfusion during the prodromal and acute phases of carbohydrate-induced laminitis in horses. Am J Vet Res 2001;62:1167–72.
29. Parks AH. Patterns of displacement of the distal phalanx and its sequelae. Presented at the 46th BEVA Congress; 2007. p. 204–5.
30. Judy CE, Galuppo LD, Snyder JR, et al. Evaluation of an in-shoe pressure measurement system in horses. Am J Vet Res 2001;62:23–8.
31. Hood DM. The mechanisms and consequences of structural failure of the foot. Vet Clin North Am Equine Pract 1999;15:437–61.
32. Murray RC, Dyson SJ, Schramme MC, et al. Magnetic resonance imaging of the equine digit with chronic laminitis. Vet Radiol Ultrasound 2003;44:609–17.
33. Redden RF. Hoof capsule distortion: understanding the mechanisms as a basis for rational management. Vet Clin North Am Equine Pract 2003;19:443–62.
34. Cripps PJ, Eustace RA. Radiological measurements from the feet of normal horses with relevance to laminitis. Equine Vet J 1999;31:427–32.
35. Cripps PJ, Eustace RA. Factors involved in the prognosis of equine laminitis in the UK. Equine Vet J 1999;31:433–42.
36. Belknap JK. How to: choose appropriate medical therapy for the acute stage of laminitis. Presented at the 46th BEVA Congress; 2007. p. 206–7.
37. Parks AH. Prevent and/or manage distal phalanx displacement in the acute stages of laminitis. Presented at the 46th BEVA Congress; 2007. p. 206–7.
38. Parks AH, Balch OK, Collier MA. Treatment of acute laminitis. Supportive therapy. Vet Clin North Am Equine Pract 1999;15:363–74.
39. Hansen N, Buchner HH, Haller J, et al. Evaluation using hoof wall strain gauges of a therapeutic shoe and a hoof cast with a heel wedge as potential supportive therapy for horses with laminitis. Vet Surg 2005;34:630–6.
40. van Eps AW, Pollitt CC. Equine laminitis: cryotherapy reduces the severity of the acute lesion. Equine Vet J 2004;36:255–60.
41. Pollitt CC, van Eps AW. Prolonged, continuous distal limb cryotherapy in the horse. Equine Vet J 2004;36:216–20.

42. Hunt RJ. A retrospective evaluation of laminitis in horses. Equine Vet J 1993;25: 61–4.

43. Abrahamsen EJ. How to: effective pain management in the acute stage of laminitis. Presented at the 46th BEVA Congress; 2007. p. 211–2.

44. Leise BS, Fugler LA, Stokes AM, et al. Effects of intramuscular administration of acepromazine on palmar digital blood flow, palmar digital arterial pressure, transverse facial arterial pressure, and packed cell volume in clinically healthy, conscious horses. Vet Surg 2007;36:717–23.

45. Goodrich LR, Nixon AJ, Fubini SL, et al. Epidural morphine and detomidine decreases postoperative hindlimb lameness in horses after bilateral stifle arthroscopy. Vet Surg 2002;31:232–9.

46. Carpenter RS, Wallis TW, Baxter GM. How to apply a half limb cast and elevated support limb shoe in the standing equine patient. American Association Equine Prac 2007;53:403–8.

47. Hendrickson DA, Stokes M, Wittern C. Use of an elevated boot to reduce contralateral support limb complications secondary to cast application. AAEP Proc 1997;43:149–50.

48. Steward ML. How to construct and apply atraumatic therapeutic shoes to treat acute or chronic laminitis in the horse. AAEP Proc 2003;49:337–46.

49. Morrison S. Foot management. Clin Tech Equine Pract 2004;3:71–82.

50. Clayton HM. The effect of an acute hoof wall angulation on the stride kinematics of trotting horses. Equine Vet J Suppl 1990;86–90.

51. Riemersma DJ, van den Bogert AJ, Jansen MO, et al. Influence of shoeing on ground reaction forces and tendon strains in the forelimbs of ponies. Equine Vet J 1996;28:126–32.

52. Thompson KN, Cheung TK, Silverman M. The effect of toe angle on tendon, ligament and hoof wall strains in vitro. J Eq Vet Sci 1993;13.

53. Wilson AM, McGuigan MP, Pardoe C. The biomechanical effect of wedged, eggbar and extension shoes in sound and lame horses. AAEP Proc 2001;47:339–43.

54. Willemen MA, Savelberg HH, Barneveld A. The effect of orthopaedic shoeing on the force exerted by the deep digital flexor tendon on the navicular bone in horses. Equine Vet J 1999;31:25–30.

55. Hood DM, Taylor D, Wagner IP. Effects of ground surface deformability, trimming, and shoeing on quasistatic hoof loading patterns in horses. Am J Vet Res 2001; 62:895–900.

56. Ritmeester AM, Ferguson DW. Coronary grooving promotes dorsal hoof wall growth in horses with chronic laminitis. AAEP Proc 1996;47:212.

Selected Urogenital Surgery Concerns and Complications

Rolf M. Embertson, DVM

KEYWORDS

- Complications • Female urogenital surgery
- Castration • Cryptorchidectomy

This article examines selected urogenital surgeies. The discussion focuses on perioperative concerns and complications. The ideal approach to addressing complications resulting from disease processes or surgery is to avoid them. This requires knowledge of what can go wrong, gained by personal experience and that shared by others. The better one is able to anticipate potential complications, the more likely complications can be avoided. It is hoped that this discussion is beneficial in that regard.

OVARIECTOMY

Ovariectomy is a reasonably common procedure. Different approaches to removal of the ovary have been successfully used. The approach used may be dictated by available equipment, available personnel, economics, and experience of the surgeon. As more and more surgeons become familiar with laparoscopic equipment and procedures, and the surgery times for laparoscopy decrease, fewer conventional procedures will be used to remove ovaries. Currently, the conventional approaches are still widely used and may be better suited for ovariectomy in some situations.

General Concerns

The concerns with the ovariectomy procedure primarily involve access and hemorrhage. There is also some concern regarding wound complications.

Approaches

Conventional approaches to ovariectomy include colpotomy; flank (standing or recumbent); ventral midline; and oblique paramedian. The colpotomy procedure has been used for years. It is done standing, avoiding general anesthesia, and allows access to both ovaries. Potential problems during the approach include laceration of a uterine branch of the vaginal artery, incision, and/or dissection into the rectum or bladder.

Rood and Riddle Equine Hospital, PO Box 12070, Lexington, KY 40580, USA
E-mail address: rembertson@roodandriddle.com

Vet Clin Equine 24 (2009) 643–661
doi:10.1016/j.cveq.2008.10.007
0749-0739/08/$ – see front matter © 2009 Published by Elsevier Inc.

During the surgery it is important not to confuse fecal balls for the ovary. Care should be taken that other adjacent tissues are not caught in the chain ecrasure when this is tightened around the ovarian pedicle. When the ovarian pedicle is crushed and severed, a firm grasp on the ovary is necessary to avoid it being dropped into the abdominal cavity. When the chain ecrasure is released, it is difficult to determine if there is bleeding from the ovarian pedicle. If bleeding occurs, laparoscopic equipment is very useful. Ligation of the ovarian stump can be performed by feel; however, this is a difficult endeavor.

Evisceration through the opening created into the abdomen is a concern postoperatively. Other complications that can occur include peritonitis, colic, abscesses or hematomas at the surgery site, and vaginal adhesions. Closure of the colpotomy incision prevents evisceration. Following closure, however, the author has seen mares show signs of abdominal discomfort. Suturing the vulva closed may prevent bowel from exiting the vagina, but does not preclude the bowel from gaining access to the vagina. Placing the mare in cross ties has been recommended to reduce the risk of evisceration, which increases when the mare lies down. Although the potential complications usually are not encountered, other approaches should be considered in valuable horses.

The standing flank approach avoids general anesthesia. Most but not all mares stand well for this procedure using sedation, regional, and local anesthesia. The abdominal wall is thick in the area of the flank approach making exteriorization of the ovary somewhat difficult. Excess tension on the ovarian pedicle causes discomfort. Care must be taken to place secure ligatures on the ovarian pedicle, because once released back into the abdomen, gaining access again to control hemorrhage is very difficult.

The recumbent flank, ventral midline, and paramedium (parainguinal) approaches require general anesthesia. There are complications associated with general anesthesia and recovery. In most surgical facilities, however, the risks of these complications are very low. Very infrequently, tension on the ovarian pedicle during surgery may decrease the heart rate or affect blood pressure.

The recumbent flank approach yields similar problems to that of the standing flank approach. This is primarily caused by thickness of the body wall preventing easy access to the ovary without significant tension on the ovarian pedicle.

The ventral midline approach places the incision too far from the ovarian pedicle to gain easy access for most ovaries. Tilting the pelvis forward with an additional pad under the pelvis improves this access. If the ovary is quite large, the ovarian pedicle has been stretched, which may make this a more appropriate approach.

The paramedian (parainguinal) approach places the incision directly over the ovary and the ovarian pedicle. The incision is actually closer to the inguinal region than the midline. The approach does require some blunt separation of the thick rectus muscle fibers, which are penetrated perpendicular to the dissection plane by one or two large veins, arteries, and nerves. The vein and artery require ligation if cut or torn. The internal rectus fascia should be penetrated carefully, because, at this level, there is little to no fat between it and the peritoneal lining. Access to the ovary is aided by withholding feed for 24 hours and using the Trendelenburg's position. To minimize the incision length, fluid can be decompressed with a needle from most enlarged ovaries because most are granulosa cell tumors, which have several large follicles. This allows shrinkage of the ovary and easier removal through a smaller incision. Stay sutures or grasping instruments are usually needed to exteriorize the ovary.

This approach usually yields good access to the ovarian pedicle. The ovarian pedicle can be stapled, sutured, or both. Stapling decreases surgery time. Even if stapled, stay sutures, which also act as ligatures, are used on the cranial and caudal aspects of the ovarian pedicle. The stapling device used on the ovarian pedicle still may allow minor bleeding from cut vessels within the pedicle. These are best ligated or oversewn. It is important following removal of the ovary to release some of the tension on the pedicle before release, to determine if bleeding will occur. If both ovaries need removal another approach to the other ovary is necessary.

Postoperative Complications

The postoperative complications include bleeding of the ovarian pedicle, which is rare if the ligatures are carefully placed. Bleeding within the body wall is very uncommon if attention is paid to ligation of the vessels that traverse the musculature. Edema occurs at the surgery site, but is usually mild.

CAESAREAN SECTION

Caesarean section is generally performed as an emergency procedure because of dystocia, but is infrequently done as an elective surgery. The general concerns when faced with a dystocia are obtaining a live foal and a reproductively sound mare. Delivering a live foal by caesarean section from any mare in dystocia requires preparation and teamwork. If the mare is anesthetized and controlled vaginal delivery is attempted, most foals can be delivered within 15 minutes. If one is not successful within that time period, a caesarean section should be performed. Once the abdomen is opened, the uterine horn containing the hind limbs is exteriorized. An incision into the uterus is made from near the apex of the horn to the level of the calcaneal tuber of the fetus (**Fig. 1**). Stay sutures are used at the ends of the incision to stabilize the uterus. Occasionally, the hind legs are not in the horn of the uterus. The incision is then made in the body of the uterus with the uterus still in the abdomen (**Fig. 2**). This allows the contaminated contents of the uterus to spill more easily into the abdomen.

Once the foal is partially delivered, the umbilicus is clamped and transected. The entire foal is delivered and taken to a nearby area for resuscitation. The chorioallantois is separated from the endometrium along the edges of the uterine incision to ensure that the placenta is not inadvertently sutured into the uterotomy incision when closed. Any large vessels bleeding along the cut edge of the uterus should be individually ligated. In addition, a continuous hemostatic suture line over each cut margin of the uterus ensures that attention is also paid to the smaller bleeding vessels. The uterine incision

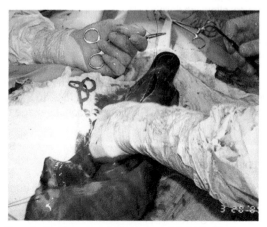

Fig. 1. Incision into the uterine horn containing the distal hindlimb.

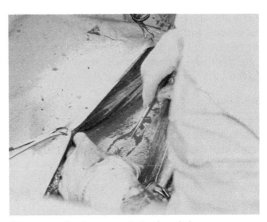

Fig. 2. Incising into the uterine body, uterus is in the abdomen.

is closed in two layers. The suture patterns used depend on the surgeon. An inverting pattern is necessary in the outer layer to provide a serosa-to-serosa seal with no protruding tissue. This helps prevent adhesions. Oxytocin is administered (40 IU, intravenously) following placement of the second layer, to contract the uterus and expel the placenta. This contraction occurs rapidly, and the administration of the oxytocin should wait until closure of the uterus is accomplished. The body wall of the abdomen is closed in routine fashion as for colic surgery. More attention is paid to the strength of the closure, however, because of the length of the incision.

During surgery, the following comments and concerns deserve consideration. Although stay sutures are placed at either end of the proposed uterine incision, delivering the foal often tears the uterus slightly beyond the suture placed toward the uterine body. These sutures help stabilize the uterus during closure, but often the assistant surgeon needs to grasp the uterus using laparotomy sponges to facilitate uterine closure. Spillage of the contaminated uterine contents (fluids, lube, hair, hippomane, and so forth) should be minimized. Laparotomy sponges can be helpful, but may also hinder surgical speed and become loose in the abdomen. Following uterine closure and contraction, the abdomen is lavaged with 15 to 25 L of saline to remove any contaminated fluid and debris. Some surgeons choose to place an abdominal drain during surgery to allow abdominal lavage for a couple days postoperatively. The author has found this unnecessary, provided a thorough abdominal lavage is performed during surgery.

Following recovery from the surgery the concerns are possible infection, bleeding, and the effects of a frequently retained placenta. Oxytocin should be used as needed to help the passing of the placenta, because endometritis and laminitis can develop quickly. To prevent endometritis the uterus is lavaged for 2 to 3 days postoperatively with 5 L of either saline or a 1% povidone-iodine solution. Leakage through the uterine incision should be of minimal concern.

MANAGEMENT OF UTERINE TEARS

The main concern regarding uterine tears is peritonitis. This can occur from tears in the uterine horns or body. A delay in recognition and treatment can be fatal to the mare. Much less common, but of great concern with a uterine body tear, is evisceration, which can also be fatal.

Most uterine tears are foaling injuries, although tears can occur with uterine torsion and hydroallantois. Most uterine tears occur near the tip of the horns and are not associated with dystocia (**Fig. 3**). Tears that occur in the uterine body are usually associated with dystocia. Usually, the tear is diagnosed postpartum during the investigation of the origin of peritonitis. Infrequently, the tear is diagnosed during parturition, usually when eviscerated bowel is noted alongside the foal. Each situation is unique but the quickest way to address evisceration during foaling is to anesthetize the mare, hoist her hind-end, and repel the fetus. This enables the placement of the bowel into the abdomen, delivery of the foal, and subsequent assessment of the extent of the tear. A caesarean section and abdominal exploration may be needed. It may be ideal to close the tear at that point or to suture the vulva closed to prevent evisceration and address the tear in the standing mare following recovery. Postpartum dystocia mares should have a manual vaginal examination performed to check for vaginal, cervical, and uterine tears. This is usually done the day postpartum when the uterus is also lavaged. The tissues are usually edematous making it possible to miss identifying a caudal uterine body tear. Tears at the tips of the uterine horn are rarely palpable vaginally or rectally.

Diagnosis of a leak of uterine contents into the peritoneal cavity is generally not difficult. The typical history is a 1- to 3-day postpartum mare with an increased temperature, increased heart rate, depression, and sometimes abdominal pain. An abdominal fluid sample should be obtained as soon as possible. This generally reveals elevated white blood cell and total protein values. Other diagnostic tests that are beneficial include a rectal examination, which may reveal free gas in the abdomen; a vaginal examination; an ultrasound examination, which shows increased cellular abdominal fluid; and a complete blood count. In the author's opinion, the best resolution for uterine tears is surgical repair.

If a caudally positioned tear is found on manual examination of the uterus, it is best repaired in a standing mare. If a tear is not identified on palpation, exploratory

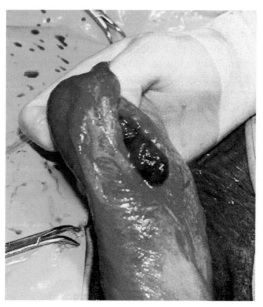

Fig. 3. Uterine horn tear.

celiotomy is indicated. Repair of tears in the caudal uterus generally requires retraction of that area of the uterine wall into the vaginal vault to access for closure. This is accomplished by retraction stay sutures, #2 polyglactin 910 placed at each end of the wound, and inadvertently aided by air and lack of negative pressure within the abdominal cavity. Even so the closure can be tedious and frustrating. Following repair, ideally the mare should be anesthetized, placed in dorsal recumbency, and her abdomen and uterus examined thoroughly through a short caudal midline incision. This also enables a thorough abdominal lavage. An abdominal drain can be placed at the surgeons' discretion. It is possible for repaired uterine body tears to form adhesions to the abdominal floor at the brim of the pelvis.

Repair of a uterine horn tear can be accomplished through a short incision, centered over the umbilicus. The edges of the tear are resected and the defect closed in two layers. The abdomen should then be lavaged with copious amounts of fluid, as previously explained.

REPAIR OF CERVICAL INJURIES

Cervical injuries are essentially the result of too large of an object (foal) passing through too small of an opening (cervix). This can occur from forceful delivery without full dilation of the cervix. It is not necessarily associated with dystocia or fetotomy.

Most cervical injuries result in a full-thickness defect in the cervical wall, of variable length, extending from the external os cranially. Defects in the musculature with intact mucosa can also occur, leaving a thin cervical wall. Most of the muscular defects also extend from the external os cranially; however, some of these are more centrally located with intact cervical muscle cranial and caudal. The site of the defect within the circumference of the cervix is identified by likening the external os to the face of a clock.

Infrequently, more than one defect is present. Sometimes the cervical muscle is so stretched that little intact musculature is palpable and functional. Occasionally, scar tissue is found extending from the external os into the fornix of the vagina, placing tension on the caudal margin of the cervix in the direction of the scar tissue.

The general concern regarding all of these abnormalities is the inability of the cervix to remain competent (ie, form a tight enough seal to prevent an ascending infection, placentitis, and abortion). Some mares with cervical defects can conceive but if the defect prevents a good seal they cannot carry the foal to term because of the ascending infection. Whether or not a cervical defect needs to be repaired is based on the mare's fertility history and the clinician's experience. In general, if a defect extends more than one third of the length of the cervix it should be repaired. Many cervical defects are found after foaling and are repaired before they have a chance adversely to affect fertility. It is often more important in evaluation of the cervix to palpate the cervix and then visualize the cervix through a speculum.

Timing for repair of the cervical defect depends on the surgeon's preference. If the cervix is soft, it is easier to retract within the vaginal vault for surgery. Palpation of the cervix when quite soft makes it difficult, however, to distinguish the different layers easily when the repair is done. Repairing the cervix when it is tight (author's preference) allows more easily identifiable edges of tissue and more accurate apposition of these edges. The cervix can still be retracted well enough within the vaginal vault to perform the surgery.

Preoperative concerns pertain to adequate lighting, adequate access, and surgeon's safety. Even though the mare is sedated and epidural anesthesia induced, mares can still kick the back of the stocks and kick over the padding on the back of the stocks. Adequate lighting is provided by a head lamp worn by the surgeon. Adequate exposure to the cervix is obtained by using Finochietto retractors, modified with long (8-in) blades, which extend beyond the vaginovestibular junction. Stay sutures (#2 polyglactin 910) placed through the wall of the cervix to retract the cervix caudally allow access to the defect for repair. Scar tissue around the cranial vagina may prevent adequate caudal retraction of the cervix. Longer-handled instruments may help overcome this problem. If more than one defect is present in the cervix it is the author's preference to stagger their repair, performing the second surgery 3 to 4 weeks following the first. The tissues swell enough during surgery to make repair of the second site more difficult than needed if done at the same time.

There are several intraoperative concerns. It is important to carefully palpate the defect to determine its extent. The stay sutures placed through the wall of the cervix should be 2 to 3 "hours" away from the edge of the defect. If placed closer to the defect, once the tissue is resected the edge of the defect may retract into the area where the retraction suture is present. With the cervix retracted caudally, Allis tissue forceps are placed on the caudal edge of the mucosa to be resected (**Fig. 4**). These are then used as markers when the mucosal edges are resected. Following removal of this tissue the freshened edges are apposed in three layers using polyglactin 910 (size #1). The first layer closed is the inner-cervical mucosa. This is closed in a continuous horizontal mattress pattern inverting the edges of the mucosa into the cervical lumen. The second layer closed is the cervical muscle. This is the strength layer of the repair and the needle should be placed through adequate amounts of muscle for the repair to hold. The third layer closed is the outer cervical (vaginal) mucosa. This is closed in a continuous pattern catching cervical muscle with each bite. If the tissue layers are not accurately apposed, thinned areas devoid of musculature, or even a full-thickness defect may result. During the repair, the lumen of the cervix is checked frequently for inadvertent penetration of mucosa across the lumen from the defect. If mucosa across the lumen is penetrated this mucosa is digitally torn away from the suture to ensure the lumen is patent. When resecting mucosa along the edge of the defect, very infrequently the abdominal cavity is entered at the very cranial extent of the dissection. This is closed while suturing the layers together and has not proven to be a problem.

It is important to work as efficiently and quickly as possible because the tissues swell with time making the surgery more difficult. Many of the defects are ventral, and the dorsal mucosa may hang down over the area that needs to be visualized. This mucosa may need to be sutured dorsally to allow visualization of the repair.

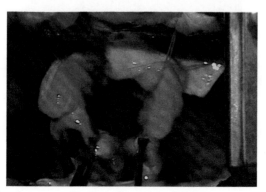

Fig. 4. Cervical defect between Allis tissue forceps. Retraction sutures in place above.

Immediately following the repair and removal of the retraction sutures, the uterus is infused with antibiotics initially to treat the uterine contamination that is often created by the repair.

Postoperatively, minimal complications result from the surgery. Occasionally, the external os that is created is small and tight enough to be of concern. This is generally caused by closure of a large defect. If one is able to insert a finger through the external os the repair should be adequate. Rarely, an adhesion may occlude the lumen of the cervix. In general, pushing the finger through this adhesion and using steroid ointment for several days topically resolves this problem.

It is important to realize that 40% to 50% of the cervical tears that are repaired tear again at subsequent foalings. The cervix tends to tear again at the previous site of repair because the scar tissue is not as elastic as the adjacent tissues.

MANAGEMENT OF RECTOVAGINAL AND PERINEAL INJURIES

The injuries discussed here occur during foaling. Forceful contractions push the foal's foot, feet, or muzzle up through the ceiling of the vagina (vestibule) and into the rectum. If the mare relaxes and the foaling attendants recognize and correct the problem, the result is a rectovaginal (RV) fistula. If not corrected and the mare continues to push, the foal often tears through the remaining tissue creating a third-degree perineal laceration, and creating a cloaca of the rectum and vestibule.

General Concerns

If the tear occurs very cranially in the vagina, the abdomen may be entered, risking evisceration (**Fig. 5**). Fortunately, the tear usually starts around the vaginovestibular junction, which is caudal to the peritoneal reflection. There is temptation and often pressure from the owner and referring veterinarian to close the fresh wound. The wound quickly becomes contaminated, however, and it is difficult to determine which

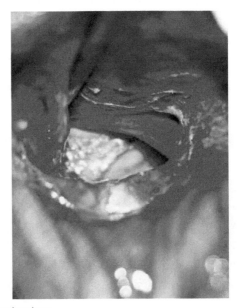

Fig. 5. Vaginal tear postpartum.

shredded tissues are or are not viable. Local hygiene, antibiotics, and nonsteroidal anti-inflammatory medications are indicated initially. It is ideal to wait to repair the tear surgically for 2 to 3 months following the injury. This allows for contraction and healing of the tissues. Some smaller RV fistulas close without surgery. If the injury occurs early in the breeding season it can usually be successfully repaired in 30 days. This allows the mare to be bred approximately 30 days following the repair and perhaps conceive and maintain the pregnancy from that breeding season.

Approaches to Repair

Many different approaches have been successfully used to repair these injuries. There are a few principles inherent to successful repair, regardless of the approach. The tissues must be healed well enough to hold suture under tension. Meticulous closure, especially of the rectal side of the repair, is imperative. This involves using strong sutures placed close together, often just 5 to 6 mm apart. Enough tissue layers should be used to provide strength to the repair. Also important is preventing postoperative impaction of the rectum by maintaining soft feces and reducing postoperative pain with nonsteroidal anti-inflammatory medication. Straining to defecate with a full rectum may lead to dehiscence of the repair. The result of trying different techniques for repair of RV fistulas and third-degree perineal lacerations has led to the techniques the author currently uses.

Preoperative Concerns

The primary preoperative concerns regarding repair of these defects are having healthy tissue to hold the sutures and a reduced volume of soft feces in the gastrointestinal tract during the repair. It is recommended that the horse not eat for 18 to 24 hours preoperatively. The horse should have soft feces on arrival to the hospital. This is best accomplished by allowing green grass pasture and administering mineral oil if needed.

Rectovaginal Fistula Repair

RV fistulas are easier and more reliably repaired than third-degree perineal lacerations. The author does not advise converting a RV fistula into a third-degree perineal laceration for repair, unless there is only a narrow strip of tissue at the anal sphincter creating the fistula.

Following epidural anesthesia and evacuation of the rectum, the perineal region is prepared for surgery. Local anesthesia is used subcutaneously in this area, because sometimes the epidural anesthesia does not desensitize the cutaneous perineum. A horizontal perineal approach is made to gain access to the fistula. An incision is made midway between the anal sphincter and the dorsal commissure of the vulva and dissection is continued cranially. A couple of moderate-sized arteries, which may require ligation, are often encountered in the initial dissection through the musculature. The dissection is continued cranially with scissors and a plane of dissection is reached where the tissues separate fairly easily. The strength layer of the repair is the rectal floor. An effort is made for this to be the thicker layer during the dissection. The perineal tissue on the dorsal side of the incision is distracted dorsally by assistants using Allis tissue forceps. With the surgeon's hand in the vagina and a finger in the fistula, dissection is continued between the rectum and the vagina around both sides of the fistula. The caudal wall of the fistula is incised where the junction between the rectal and vaginal mucosa is anticipated. This junction can then be visualized and the incision is continued around the wall of the fistula separating the rectal floor from the vaginal ceiling. Dissection is then continued another 3 to 4 cm cranial to the fistula. This creates two sheets of tissue: the rectal floor and the vaginal ceiling, each with a hole. The rent in the rectal floor is closed from cranial to caudal using #1 polyglactin 910 in an interrupted Lembert-type pattern. This is started in the center of the defect and extended to the left and the right alternately. The suture inverts the edges of the rectal floor slightly into the rectum, but does not penetrate the mucosa. Sutures are placed in a similar fashion 5 to 6 mm apart until the cranial and caudal margins of the rectal floor are tightly apposed. Closure of the rectal floor from cranial to caudal reduces tension on the sutures when the mare strains to defecate. Defecation likely places more tension perpendicular to the long axis of the rectum than parallel to the long axis. During defecation the tension acts more to extend the suture line rather than pull apart the suture line. The hole in the vaginal ceiling is then closed with #1 polygalactin 910 in a continuous Lembert pattern from side to side. Tension on the vaginal ceiling, perpendicular to the long axis of the vagina, is much less than that occurring within the rectum.

Following closure of the holes in the rectal floor and the vaginal ceiling, the space between the rectum and the vagina created by dissection is closed. This is done with #1 polyglactin 910 in several interrupted purse string sutures. The subcutaneous tissue and the skin are routinely closed.

Third-Degree Perineal Lacerations

These are repaired in three layers: (1) the vaginal ceiling, (2) the rectal floor, and (3) the space between (**Fig. 6**). It can be difficult to determine what tissues should be reapposed and how. The surgical approach should be planned before making an incision. An incision is made along the junction of the rectal and vaginal mucosa and around the entire defect. When the cutaneous perineum is reached, the incision is continued along the scar between it and the vaginal mucosa. Flaps of tissue are created by deeper dissection along this edge, leaving some tissue that will hold suture attached to the mucosa. Dissection is extended cranially between the rectal floor and the vaginal ceiling to allow for the suture line to start cranial to the incised edge. It is important as the tissues are apposed to keep reassessing where the tissues should fit together. The rectal floor is partially closed first in the same manner as was done for the RV fistula closure, except the rectal floor is closed from side to side. Then the vaginal ceiling is created by suturing the edges together in a continuous vertical mattress pattern for approximately 5 to 6 cm. The space between the rectal floor and the vaginal ceiling

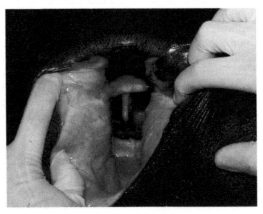

Fig. 6. Third-degree perineal laceration.

is then closed using #1 polyglactin 910 in interrupted purse string sutures. The closure is continued out to the cutaneous perineum in this manner, creating a thicker perineal body as the repair continues caudally. The cutaneous perineum is usually closed in a continuous vertical mattress pattern suture. Often, it is not possible accurately to appose the anal sphincter and this is usually not necessary.

Postoperative Concerns

The primary concern is development of a leak and partial dehiscence. This is prevented by placing the sutures close together and with secure knots. It is very important to keep the feces soft in the immediate postoperative period (grass, mineral oil) and keep the mare comfortable so that she defecates and does not develop a rectal impaction. If a large quantity of feces accumulates within the rectum and the mare appears uncomfortable, the feces should be evacuated.

Assuming the repair heals, tissue strength should be sufficient for natural breeding after 30 days postoperatively. They generally need to go through a heat cycle to resolve the contaminated uterus that often develops.

These mares generally do not develop an RV fistula or third-degree perineal laceration during subsequent foaling. It is advisable, however, for the foaling to be attended.

TREATMENT OF URINE POOLING

Urine pooling usually results from the reproductive tract angling downward cranially. This angling of the reproductive tract develops in most broodmares to some degree with advancing age. As the mare urinates some of the urine runs cranially and downhill into the cranial vagina. This is especially true if the urine hits the sutured area of the dorsal vulva and splashes back cranially toward the vagina. Infrequently, foaling trauma tears the transverse fold, which then predisposes to urine pooling. Urine pooling can also be seen in recent postpartum mares. As the tissues regain tone the urine pooling can resolve.

The general concerns regarding urine pooling are the effects on the cervix and endometrium, irritating these structures and creating infertility. The concerns with surgical repair primarily involve intraoperative tension on the relatively friable tissues that are used to create an extension of the urethra. This may result in leaking of urine through the surgical site.

Urine pooling in the cranial vagina can usually be resolved by extending the urethra caudally to the caudal brim of the pelvis. A tube is created from the mucosa on the floor of the vagina, more properly termed "vestibule" in this region. The original urethral extension technique made a U-shaped incision around the ventral left and right walls of the vagina and then split the transverse fold into dorsal and ventral flaps. Starting at the transverse fold, the left side was sutured to the right side with the ventral edges inverted into the new urethra and the dorsal edges inverted into the vaginal floor. There was often excessive tension on the mucosal edges in the broader, flatter cranial aspect of the vagina leading to leaks in the extended urethra. The technique was modified to reduce tension in the cranial aspect of the urethral extension. Following the U-shaped incision, the transverse fold was pulled caudally and sutured to the left and right sides of the vaginal floor. Beyond the caudal extent of the transverse fold, the left and right sides were then sutured together to the very caudal extent of the urethral extension. This creates a Y-shaped suture line. One technique uses a partial thickness of mucosa, suturing the ventral edges of the incised tissue together following some dissection of this tissue away from the wall of the vagina. The other technique uses full-thickness tissue, suturing the ventral edges together, then the dorsal edges together. Leaks in the modified urethral extension techniques do still occur, but at a lower incidence. The author uses the latter technique, a full-thickness, two-layer closure using 2-0 polyglactin 910.

If the mare has urine scalding or urine crystals present on the skin just ventral to her vulva, she may have a problem with urethral sphincter tone. The sphincter is damaged in some mares following foaling, which results in the constant dribbling of urine and often the pooling of urine in the cranial vagina. The urethral extension should resolve the urine pooling in the cranial vagina but does not resolve the dribbling of urine caused by the incompetent urethral sphincter.

Preoperative Concerns

Safety is of concern while working on the back end of the mare. The other preoperative concerns include adequate lighting, best addressed by the use of a headlamp, and adequate exposure and access, solved by the use of Balfour retractors and long-handled instruments.

Procedure

Following epidural anesthesia and placement of the Balfour retractors, which are tied to the base of the tail, the tissues are further anesthetized with topical lidocaine. Creating the horizontal cut in the transverse fold requires tension on the tissue edge. This incision is facilitated by stretching the middle section across the cranial vagina using Allis tissue forceps and long-handled thumb forceps. Once this incision is started it is continued to the junction of the transverse fold and the vaginal wall on both the left and the right sides. The incision is then extended along the left and right sides of the ventral aspect of the vaginal walls in a similar fashion caudally to the caudal brim of the pelvis. The initial incision along the floor of the vagina should be made just through the mucosa, and then separated using blunt dissection with scissors. Blunt dissection creates less bleeding than a deeper incision. The reason for the dissection is to create a large flap of tissue to suture. The transverse fold is pulled caudally as far as possible with the Allis tissue forceps. Traction on this tissue should not be so excessive as to tear a hole in the transverse fold. The area at most risk for leaking is at the start of the caudal leg of the Y-shaped suture line, where the left and right suture lines converge and the single midline suture line begins. To reduce tension and seal on this area further, a simple continuous suture line is placed over the dorsal edges that have been inverted into the floor of the vagina. If there still seems to be considerable tension, tension-relieving incisions on each side of the incision may be beneficial. The incision can be partially protected by use of a balloon-tip Foley catheter placed into the bladder and left in place for 3 to 4 days. This keeps the bladder decompressed preventing trauma to the suture line from the forceful urination. A condom with a hole cut in the tip is taped over the end of the catheter to prevent aspiration of air into the bladder.

It is important that the caudal aspect of the incisions made into the left and right sides of the vaginal floor are far enough apart to have enough mucosa to create a tunnel large enough to accommodate the surgeon's index finger.

The mare should not be bred for approximately 30 days postoperatively. At 30 days, the urethral extension should be examined for leaks and, if found, repaired. The site of most leaks is obvious because there is a hole present in the floor of the vagina over the extended urethra (**Fig. 7**). If the site of the leak is not obvious, yet urine is still gaining access to the cranial vagina, the urethral extension can be distended with saline to look for the site of the leak. This is done by placing a balloon-tip Foley catheter in

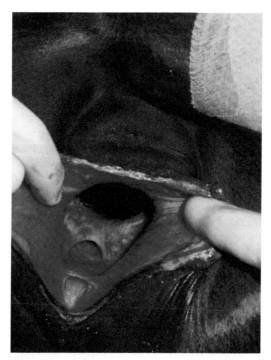

Fig. 7. Urethral extension, large defect.

the caudal opening, manually occluding the urethral sphincter area, and infusing saline under pressure into the extended urethra.

Leaks are usually successfully repaired by incising the roof of the urethral extension cranially to the defect. The mucosal edge of the defect is then incised in a horizontal plane, which continues around each side to the cut edge of the roof of the urethral extension. This creates dorsal and ventral edges of tissue. The open area is then closed in two layers using 3-0 polyglactin 910 in a continuous horizontal mattress pattern. The ventral edges are inverted into the new urethra and the dorsal edges inverted into the vestibule. Occasionally, the urethral extension is damaged during subsequent foaling and requires repair.

CASTRATION

There are several approaches and surgical techniques that have been used successfully to remove testicles positioned in the scrotum. The techniques used are based on what the veterinarian originally was taught, with modifications based on experiences, financial concerns, the experiences and desires of the owner or agent, the demeanor of the horse, and the equipment and facilities available, among other reasons. Castrations can be performed with the horse standing or recumbent using an open or closed technique. An "open" castration refers to when the parietal layer of the vaginal tunic is opened and the testicle, epididymus, and the contents of the vaginal tunic are emasculated. Little to no vaginal tunic is resected. A "closed" castration refers to when the vaginal tunic is either not opened or just partially opened and some of the vaginal tunic is removed with the testicle. Castrations are usually performed through a surgical site that is left open to heal by second intention. Primary closure of the surgery site can also be used, but requires strict adherence to aseptic technique. The different surgical techniques are well described in the additional reading texts listed.

This discussion is directed toward how to avoid potential complications and approaches to treatment if encountered. More complications develop following castration than any other surgical procedure routinely performed. The potential complications are somewhat similar between techniques; however, some procedures minimize the risks of various complications. The primary complications of concern include hemorrhage, swelling, infection, and evisceration, with a few other complications possible. The risks of encountering these complications can be minimized by the veterinarian having a good understanding of the anatomy of the structures involved and knowledge of what complications can occur and why.

Hemorrhage

There are many small vessels that may be cut or torn during dissection to expose the testicles. These may create a small amount of bleeding postoperatively and are generally of little concern, except to the owner. This bleeding can be avoided or minimized by using blunt dissection as much as possible during the procedure. Hemorrhage from the testicular artery or pampiniform plexus can be significant. This is best avoided by leaving the emasculator in place long enough to ensure the vessels are crushed (2–3 minutes). Double ligation of these structures provides the best prevention of bleeding. It is very important that the ligatures are tight and the knots secure. Bleeding from the vessels in the cremaster muscle can create concern. This can be avoided by crushing the muscle with the emasculator separately, if the entire spermatic cord is large, or ligating the cremaster muscle with or without the spermatic cord. Bleeding from the larger vessels in the inguinal region is unusual and can be avoided by careful dissection.

If there is a steady stream of blood from the castration wound 30 to 60 minutes postoperatively, or the site continues a steady drip for several hours postoperatively, the hemorrhage should be addressed. This is also true of a primary closure site where significant swelling is noted within a couple hours of surgery. Packing the surgical site with roll gauze may stop mild bleeding; however, it generally does not stop significant hemorrhage. The pressure from continued bleeding separates tissues in the inguinal region, creating a large hematoma adjacent to the pack. The most direct, effective, and fastest way to resolve the bleeding is to anesthetize the horse, explore the surgery site, and ligate the offending vessel. If an obvious source of hemorrhage is not found, double ligate the spermatic cord and cremaster because these are the likely source of origin of the bleed. In addition, tightly accordion several gauze rolls (tied to each other) into the space that was created in the inguinal area. Suture the opening closed, also going through the gauze, leaving long tags for easy access when the pack is removed (**Fig. 8**).

Evisceration

The vaginal tunic is an out-pouching of the abdominal peritoneum. The internal inguinal ring is the entrance to this diverticulum. If the internal inguinal ring is large enough, small intestine can fit through this ring and migrate down the vaginal tunic. Fortunately this occurs infrequently. In the intact horse, this is called an indirect inguinal hernia. In the recently castrated horse, this allows evisceration. Even though the vaginal tunic is crushed and sealed in the closed castration, this seal can be easily opened by the pressure of the small intestine.

To prevent evisceration through the vaginal tunic, it must be occluded, which is easily done by ligation. By extending one's index finger through a hole created in the

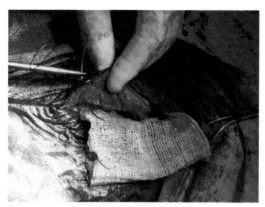

Fig. 8. Scrotal surgery site. Suturing gauze packing into the incision.

parietal layer of the vaginal tunic, the internal inguinal ring can be palpated. It has been suggested that if the internal inguinal ring is less than two fingers wide (3–3.5 cm), ligation is unnecessary. The author has found that unreliable and ligates the vaginal tunic (#2 polyglactin 910) to prevent evisceration.

Evisceration following castration usually occurs within several hours postoperatively. If this occurs, the horse should be anesthetized, the exposed intestine lavaged, placed back into the scrotum, and the scrotal incision closed. The horse should then be transported to a surgical facility for definitive repair. On arrival, the horse is again anesthetized and the abdomen and scrotal region prepared for surgery. A short incision is made at the umbilicus to allow palpation of the abdominal side of the internal inguinal ring. The intestines are again lavaged, and pulled back into the abdomen. The bowel should be exteriorized again and closely examined for adherent debris and viability. Resection and anastomosis may be necessary. The abdomen is lavaged; some of the fluid may exit the vaginal tunic. The vaginal tunic is then closed. The abdomen is closed in routine fashion and the scrotal and inguinal area is packed with roll gauze as described previously. The prognosis is related to the amount of bowel eviscerated and the duration and degree of exposure and strangulation.

Swelling

This is the most common complication encountered for castrations, where the surgery site was left open to heal by second intention. The primary causes of postoperative swelling include surgical trauma, hemorrhage, infection, lack of drainage, and postoperative management.

Surgical technique plays a role in the development of postoperative edema. Knowing exactly what is planned and proceeding quickly through surgery minimizes trauma to the tissue and postoperative swelling. Minimize bleeding, as mentioned previously; blood adds fluid to the tissues and obscures visualization of the surgery site. The incision left open must be large enough to allow adequate drainage. Often, the skin between the two incisions is removed to leave one large opening.

Postoperative management can help lessen the amount of swelling that develops. Exercise causes movement of these tissues, which encourages ventral drainage and probably lymphatic drainage. Nonsteroidal anti-inflammatory drugs should also help reduce swelling.

Infection

All castration sites not primarily closed become contaminated and many develop a low-grade infection, leading to more swelling. Good drainage lessens the amount of serum that accumulates in the dissected spaces and lessens the risk of persistent infection. Perioperative antibiotics should also help lessen the risk of infection.

Persistent infection may develop within the spermatic cord, which is referred to as a "scirrhous cord." This condition may be predisposed by leaving the entire, or much of the, vaginal tunic during the castration. Early recognition and treatment with antibiotics and drainage may resolve the infection, but surgical excision is often necessary. These horses usually present to a surgical hospital weeks after the castration with a palpably thickened spermatic cords. There is usually drainage from an opening at the previous castration site. An elliptic incision is made around the opening and dissection is continued around the thickened spermatic cord, isolating it from the surrounding tissue. The proximal extent of the infected cord is determined by a change from the thickened cord to the more normal cord. The spermatic cord is either emasculated or ligated and transected at that site (**Fig. 9**). The surgery site is left open to heal by second intention.

Miscellaneous

Other complications of castration are rarely encountered, with a few listed here. Septic peritonitis may occur from extension of a severe infection within the spermatic cord. A hydrocele may form within the end of the healed vaginal tunic. Penile trauma by the emasculator has been encountered.

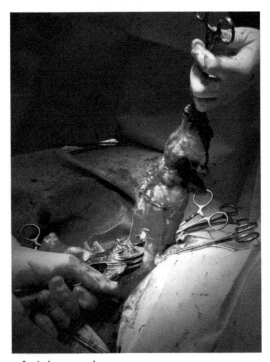

Fig. 9. Emasculation of scirrhous cord.

Primary Closure

Primary closure of the castration site usually avoids the complications that can occur following castration. The castration is performed as a clean surgical procedure. The skin is closed, avoiding the influence of contamination and the spaces created by dissection are closed, avoiding serum accumulation. The contents of the vaginal tunic are ligated, preventing it as a source of hemorrhage. The vaginal tunic itself is ligated, preventing bowel herniation. The author uses this technique almost exclusively because of the low risk of complications and minimal to no aftercare for the owner. A small amount of edema may develop at the surgery site and migrate down to the sheath. The only significant complication experienced using this technique has been hemorrhage in a couple cases. If this occurs, a large hematoma develops in the scrotum and inguinal region. The castration site is opened and the source of the hemorrhage is identified and ligated. The surgical site is then left open to heal by second intention.

Following castration with primary closure, horses are walked for 5 to 7 days, and then started back into training.

CRYPTORCHIDECTOMY

This section discusses the complications and concerns regarding the surgical procedures for removal of a retained or cryptorchid testicle. The assumption is made that a cryptorchid testicle is present based on known history, physical examination, or other diagnostic tests.

There are a few different approaches or procedures that have been used successfully to remove cryptorchid testicles. These include the inguinal, parainguinal, suprapubic paramedian, and standing flank conventional approaches and the standing flank and dorsally recumbent laparoscopic approaches. The approach used should be based primarily on minimizing the risks of complications, but also on the surgeon's experience, and economic factors. It is difficult to recommend the use of the conventional flank and suprapubic paramedian approaches in North America, with the availability of referral hospitals and trained surgeons. Currently, the inguinal and laparoscopic procedures are the most commonly used. The laparoscopic approaches are discussed elsewhere in this issue.

The complications and concerns regarding cryptorchidectomy are similar to those for castration. The primary concerns are swelling, infection, evisceration, hemorrhage, and sometimes most importantly the inability to find the retained testicle.

Finding the Retained Testicle

This can occasionally be difficult. During the preoperative standing examination, an inguinal testicle is usually partially palpable. An abdominal testicle is often not identified on rectal examination. An ultrasound examination may or may not be helpful. If the testicle is not identified, it is ideal to prepare for dorsally recumbent laparoscopic surgery, if the equipment is available, and starving the horse for 12 to 18 hours does not present a scheduling problem. With the horse anesthetized and positioned in dorsal recumbency, it is rare to not be able to feel an inguinal testicle. If present, an inguinal approach is indicated. Importantly, the retained testicle still looks like a testicle, not the tail of the epididymus. If the testicle is not palpable and is present in the abdomen, the inguinal approach may still be a faster way to find and remove the testicle. The laparoscopic approach, however, is a more reliable way to find and remove the testicle.

Hemorrhage

Generally, hemorrhage, is not a large concern. Inguinal testicles and related structures are smaller than if found in the scrotum. Isolation of an inguinal testicle using an inguinal approach allows most to be removed in similar fashion as for scrotal testicles. During closure, the large inguinal vessels should be avoided.

Infection

Performing the surgery as a clean procedure and using perioperative antibiotics, the risk of infection is low. If the site becomes infected, it should be treated like other infected surgery sites.

Swelling

The surgery site often develops some edema. This is usually mild and is related to the amount of soft tissue trauma created during surgery. Hemorrhage and infection also create swelling at the surgery site.

Evisceration

This becomes a risk if the internal inguinal ring is significantly enlarged or another opening is created into the abdomen and the surgery site is not closed. Some surgeons still use an inguinal pack to occlude the opening created. The pack is removed in 24 to 48 hours when the soft tissues have swollen enough to close the opening into the abdomen. Occasionally, the opening is not yet closed or the pack has adhered to intestine, enabling evisceration when the pack is removed. If this occurs, it is addressed in a similar fashion as that described previously.

Inguinal Approach to the Cryptorchid Testicle

This is the most direct approach to the inguinal cryptorchid testicle, with little risk of complications. For removal of the abdominal testicle, this approach may also use less of the surgeon's time than laparoscopy. A 6- to 7-cm incision is made over the external inguinal ring through the skin and subcutaneous tissue. Blunt dissection is then continued through the fat, fascia, and blood vessels to the external inguinal ring. This minimizes any bleeding that may occur. Often the distal end of the vaginal tunic containing the tail of the epididymus is found during this dissection. If not, the area is examined for the inguinal extension of the gubernaculum testis. This is usually present as a thin, diffuse band of fibrous tissue. Clean dissection, patience, adequate lighting, and a narrow malleable retractor aid in finding this structure. Tension placed on this tissue everts the end of the vaginal tunic, to which it is attached, into the inguinal canal. The vaginal tunic is grasped with Ochsner forceps and incised. The epididymus is exposed, grasped, and tensed. The internal inguinal ring needs to be digitally enlarged to allow exteriorization of a small deformable testicle, exteriorized by placing traction on the epididymus. The testicle is resected using ligatures for hemostasis. The surgery site is closed by apposing the tissue in the inguinal region with several interrupted sutures, then the subcutaneous tissue and skin. The author has not found it necessary to close the external inguinal ring.

If the inguinal extension of the gubernaculums testis cannot be found, which is unusual, a parainguinal approach or laparoscopy is used to find and remove the testicle. The parainguinal approach involves separating the loose fascia from the body wall, medial to the external inguinal ring. An incision is made long enough to allow two fingers into the abdomen to feel for and exteriorize the testicle. If needed, the incision can be lengthened to allow a hand into the abdomen. Following resection of the testicle, this incision can be closed, and then the rest of the inguinal approach is closed. Following removal of a cryptorchid testicle, using the inguinal approach, horses are hand-walked for 5 to 7 days, and then started back into training.

FURTHER READINGS

Auer JA, Stick JA, editors. Equine surgery. 3rd edition. St. Louis (MO): Saunders Elsevier; 2006.

Samper JC, Pycock JF, McKinnon AO, editors. Current therapy in equine reproduction. St. Louis (MO): Saunders Elsevier; 2007.

Wolfe DF, Moll HD, editors. Large animal urogenital surgery. Baltimore (MD): Williams and Wilkins; 1999.

Complications of Equine Wound Management and Dermatologic Surgery

R. Reid Hanson, DVM

KEYWORDS

- Equine • Wounds • Complications
- Management • Dermatologic surgery

Complications of wounds and cosmetic surgery although frequent can be accurately managed with a combination of timely surgical and medical intervention to ensure the best possible outcome. The lack of soft tissue protection and a large quantity of susceptible synovial, tendon, ligament, and neurovascular structures make early and meticulous evaluation of limb wounds critical. Chronic wounds should be considered infected and may become afflicted with sarcoid, *Pythium* spp, *Habronema* spp, or *Draschia* spp, and rarely neoplasia. Methicillin-resistant *Staphylococcus aureus* (MRSA) infections can consequently be difficult to treat and are associated with increased morbidity, mortality, and treatment costs. Skin grafting is usually used following a period of open wound management and after healthy granulation tissue formation. Penetrating wounds of the abdomen or thorax have a guarded prognosis resulting from the ensuing potential for infection and pneumothorax. Gunshot wounds limited to the skeletal muscles have a good prognosis, whereas injuries that involve vital organs decrease survivability.

COMPLICATIONS OF REPAIR
Osseous Sequestration

The distal limbs of horses are extremely susceptible to damage of the periosteum and underlying bone because of the lack of soft tissue protection. Because the periosteum provides the blood supply to the outer one third of the cortical bone, disruption of the periosteum leads to ischemia of the bone with eventual bone death secondary to these alterations in blood flow. This ischemic locale is very susceptible to bacterial colonization and proliferation originating from the inciting trauma. Blunt trauma with no external entry wound may result in sequestrum formation indicating that bacterial

Department of Clinical Sciences, College of Veterinary Medicine, Auburn University, JT Vaughan Hall, 1500 Wire Road, Auburn, AL 36849, USA
E-mail address: hansorr@auburn.edu

Vet Clin Equine 24 (2009) 663–696
doi:10.1016/j.cveq.2008.10.005
0749-0739/08/$ – see front matter © 2009 Elsevier Inc. All rights reserved.

vetequine.theclinics.com

inoculation may also occur by way of the bloodstream. This type of injury is more commonly present with trauma to the metacarpal or metatarsal bones.[1]

The body may be able to resorb the sequestrum or expel it from the draining tract depending on the size of the devitalized bone fragment. Larger fragments usually persist and lead to more extensive clinical disease. The sequestrum can become a chronic nidus thereby delaying the healing process. Because of the lack of vascularization, the immune response at the site is inadequate, leading to a chronic infection that persists in the face of a normal immune system.[2,3] The lack of a relative reliable blood flow impedes the migration of osteoclasts to the site hindering the natural resorption of bone. These two events collectively result in a chronic inflammatory focus that the body cannot or only slowly resolves.[1]

The most common sites for sequestrum formation are those with a relative lack of soft tissue covering, such as the phalanges, metacarpal or metatarsal bones, calcaneous, distal radius, medial tibia, and skull (**Fig. 1**). The affected site most commonly involves some degree of soft tissue swelling and usually has a coexisting draining fistulous tract. There is usually not a significant lameness, but some deep palpation over the sequestered bone generally produces a painful response.[1,4]

Sequestra formation may not be readily noticeable on survey radiographs until 3 to 4 weeks after the inciting injury has occurred.[5,6] Correct radiographic orientation and contrast radiography may be useful to the location and extent of a sequestrum. Ultrasound evaluation may also benefit in further localizing a fistulous tract and bone fragment.[7] The chronic fistulous tract is identified as an anechoic fluid or gas-filled tract surrounded by an echogenic fibrous scar tissue. The sequestrum is identified as a highly echogenic bone fragment surrounded by an anechoic pocket of fluid.

Complete resection and removal of the fistulous tract, involucrum, and sequestrum is best performed with the horse under general anesthesia. Preoperative bacterial

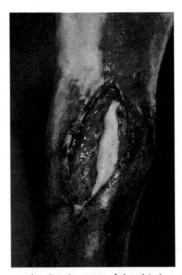

Fig.1. Sequestrum formation on the distal aspect of the third metacarpus in a chronic wound that is healing by third intention. There is relative lack of soft tissue covering in this area, which predisposes the underlying bone to more trauma. Disruption of the periosteum leads to ischemia of the bone with eventual bone death secondary to these alterations in blood flow.

culture of the tract or the sequestrum itself is not considered essential because surgical removal of all necrotic debris is the procedure of choice. The tract should be dissected carefully from the adjacent soft tissue until the sequestrum is reached. All nonviable debris and bone should be removed. The surrounding bone should be curetted until the underlying healthy bone bleeds. Excessive bony proliferation may be removed with an osteotome or chisel to contour the bone. Excessive contouring of long bones may result in the development of fissure lines in the cortex that could lead to significant fracture of the bone when the horse is recovering from anesthesia. Healthy adjacent periosteum should be preserved if possible to minimize excessive bone remodeling. If a clean and complete resection of the involucrum and the surrounding necrotic debris adjacent to the involucrum is achieved, primary closure of the skin defect is preferred. With sequestra involving the distal limbs, it is important to be conservative in the amount of tissue removed. If complete resection of the contaminated tract is not possible, open drainage and second-intention healing signify the best choice.[1]

A nonadherent permeable or semiocclusive dressing to keep the bone moist and allow for granulation tissue formation should be applied to wounds left to heal by second-intention healing. A protective bandage is applied over this primary covering and changed as often as needed based on the quantity of the exudate. Skin grafts may be used to speed healing in large wounds once the defect has filled in with granulation tissue. This is especially important in wounds of the dorsal third metacarpal or metatarsal bone.

Most horses that develop sequestra have a good prognosis once the local infected nidus is removed. Return to full function after complete resolution of clinical signs is possible in most cases. Secondary trauma to the soft tissue, tendon, or bone sustained during the initial injury is the most likely factor leading to permanent problems in those horses that do not return to full function.[2]

Exposed Bone

Exposed or denuded bone is a common complication of wounds of the distal aspect of the limb.[8] Exposed cortical bone in which the periosteum has been removed is prone to desiccation of the superficial layers of the cortex, which may result in infectious superficial osteitis and sequestrum formation.[9] Exposed bone within a wound can delay wound healing directly if the bone becomes infected, or indirectly because its rigid structure can delay the formation of granulation tissue and wound contraction.[10]

Distal limb avulsion wounds with exposed bone increase in wound size for 14 to 21 days. Wound expansion predominantly is caused by the distraction forces applied across the wound during the inflammatory and debridement stages of wound healing, and the lack of a granulation tissue bed in the center of the wound to neutralize the tensile forces exerted on the wound margins from the surrounding skin. Wounds with a small amount of exposed bone, or wounds without exposed bone, expand for a shorter period because less time is required for granulation tissue to seal the wound. Larger wounds with exposed bone take longer to form a granulation bed and subsequently wound contraction is postponed.[10]

Periosteal insults from blunt trauma, tendon or joint capsule strain, surgical manipulation, or laceration or degloving injuries may result in extensive periosteal exostosis.[11-13] Injuries involving bones in horses stimulate more periosteal new bone growth than similar wounds in other species and ponies.[11,12] More extensive periosteal reaction in young compared with adult horses has been attributed to a more active osteoblastic activity of the periosteum in young horses.[13] The extensive periosteal new bone growth seen in adult horses is poorly understood. Deferred collagen lysis compared with other species may be a contributing factor.[11] The more extensive periosteal new bone formation in horses compared with ponies is alleged to be the result of a slower onset and longer duration of the periosteal response and prolonged extensive limb swelling in horses, as compared with ponies.[12]

Despite the common occurrence of exposed bone associated with trauma to the distal aspect of the limb, there has been little investigation into methods of stimulating coverage of granulation tissue over exposed bone in horses. Granulation tissue development is a very important role in second-intention healing because it provides a barrier to infection and mechanical trauma for the underlying tissues. Healthy granulation tissue is resistant to infection and provides a moist surface for epithelialization. The delay in wound healing caused by exposed bone has prompted the search for different methods to promote granulation tissue coverage of bone in other species.

Head trauma, thermal injury, and surgical oncology often results in exposed bone of the cranium in humans.[9,14] In these cases the outer cortex of the uncovered portion of the cranium is fenestrated with drill holes, burrs, or lasers to expose the medullary cavity from which granulation tissue grows to cover the exposed bone.[9,15–17] Similarly, exposed cortices of long bones in humans have been fenestrated with drill holes to promote granulation tissue formation.[12] It has been suggested that the drill holes promote healing by allowing osteogenic factors from the medullary cavity access to the wound, or by the enhancement of healing of bone and soft tissue by a nonspecific response known as "the regional acceleratory phenomenon."[18] Cortical fenestration combined with drugs that promote topical granulation tissue may accelerate granulation tissue coverage compared with control wounds, but further investigation is needed.

Cortical fenestration of 1.6-mm drill holes in the cortex of the second metacarpal bone in experimentally created wounds in dogs resulted in clot formation over the bone that promoted granulation tissue formation and may have protected the bone's outer layers from desiccation.[19] The effects of cortical fenestration with 3.2-mm drill holes were evaluated in experimentally created wounds of the distal aspect of the limb of horses.[20] Cortical fenestrated wounds became covered with granulation tissue earlier than control wounds, and fenestration had no significant effect on sequestrum formation. The granulation tissue growing directly from the bone surface also contributed to granulation tissue formation (**Fig. 2**). If the wounds are not large (<6 × 6 cm) it may be difficult to realize a significant contribution from the granulation tissue growing from the cortical fenestration sites alone. Cortical fenestration may also be advantageous if it is used with other methods of promoting granulation tissue.[20] Splinting of the limb is usually not necessary for the recovery from general anesthesia unless there are associated traumatic injuries to the limb that suggest instability.

Degloving Injuries

Degloving or avulsion injuries are not uncommon in equine practice, and their management can be challenging because of prolonged treatment, cost, and sometimes unknown outcome.[20–22] The body that becomes entrapped in hazards or a limb that becomes intertwined in fencing can quickly sustain tissue damage. The most common sites for this type of trauma are the hemithorax, dorsal aspect of the metacarpus or metatarsus, and the cranial aspect of the tarsus.[22] Vascular, soft tissue, and bone damage is directly proportional to the length of time and effort the horse uses to free itself. Some injuries that seem to be superficial and innocuous on the surface may involve vital structures surrounding the wound or later develop cutaneous and internal abscesses or ulcerative cellulitis. Local wound care should be an integral part of the initial treatment.[23] Severity and duration and location of the laceration determines

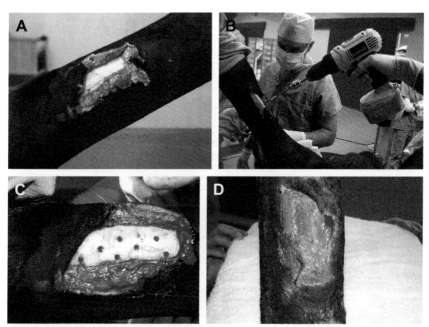

Fig. 2. (*A*) Degloving injury (9 × 5 cm) of the dorsal metatarsus with exposed bone proximal to the fetlock. Exposed bone within a wound can delay wound healing directly if the bone becomes infected, or indirectly because its rigid structure can delay the formation of granulation tissue and wound contraction. (*B*) Cortical fenestration of the dorsal metacarpus with a 4-mm drill penetrating into the medullary canal. (*C*) Cortical fenestrated area after drilling. The granulation tissue growing directly from the cortical fenestration sites to serve as an extra source for granulation tissue production. (*D*) Granulation tissue production and complete coverage of the wound 12 days after cortical fenestration. A significant contribution of the granulation tissue from the cortical fenestration sites is especially noticeable in wounds larger than 6 × 6 cm.

the best approach to the treatment of degloving injuries because healing of wounds involving the distal limb is often delayed when compared with other areas of the body, further complicating the healing process.

Primary repair of the wound is the preferred treatment for wounds that involve detachment of skin with maintenance of an intact blood supply (**Fig. 3**). Complications, such as sequestrum formation, are lessened and healing is improved when the exposed bone and tendons are covered with skin and soft tissue in the immediate posttrauma period. Closing as much of the wound as possible improves the cosmetic and functional outcome and lessens the amount of healing having to occur by second intention.

Delayed closure of a degloving injury is preferred when there is significant contamination, swelling, and trauma of the wound without loss of skin. Initial treatment for the first 2 to 3 days after injury includes debridement and lavage of the wound followed by wet to dry bandages to facilitate further debridement. Pressure bandaging is indicated to remove edema associated with the injury. Debridement of the wound edges and appropriately applied tension sutures facilitate closure of the wound because skin retraction is a complication of delayed closure.

Second-intention healing is indicated for degloving injuries in which there is a considerable loss of skin immediately at the time of injury or in which a closed degloving

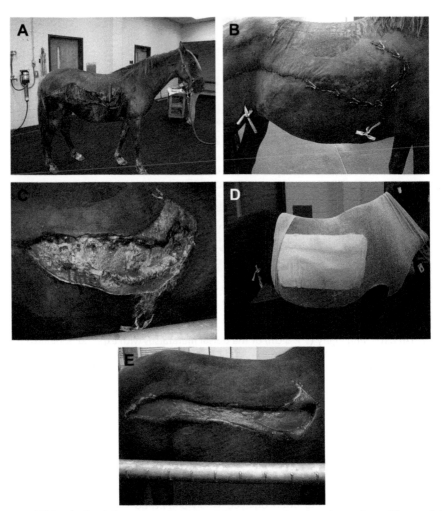

Fig. 3. (A) Degloving injury to the right hemithorax secondary to a laceration with a metal post. There is extensive undermining of the skin along the dorsal and ventral caudal aspects of the wound. (B) Primary repair of laceration. Debridement of the wound edges, walking sutures, and appropriately applied tension sutures facilitate closure. (C) The laceration repair dehisced 6 days after primary repair. The wound is debrided, cleansed, and honey is applied topically to facilitate third-intention wound healing. (D) A secondary topical pad and reusable body meshing is used to facilitate wound cleansing. (E) Laceration 25 days after initial injury. Contraction, epithelialization, and granulation tissue formation is progressing well.

injury has developed avascular necrosis of the skin with subsequent sloughage. The wound is sharply debrided until only healthy tissue remains. A hydrogel Carradress dressing (Carrington, Irving, Texas) is applied to the region of the wound that remains open. These dressings are able to contribute moisture to dehydrated tissue, augment autolytic debridement, and absorb some moisture from an exudating wound. The dressing is applied to the wound bed followed by application of a conformable absorptive dressing (Kerlix, Kendall, Mansfield, Massachusetts). A firm cotton bandage is used to provide warmth and support and to minimize excessive movement of the limb and associated wound area. Depending on the size and location of the wound, skin grafting may be indicated to facilitate complete healing. Grafting should be delayed to permit maximum wound contraction, which depending on the location and size of the wound may be 4 to 8 weeks after injury.

Dorsal knuckling of the fetlock and an inability to extend the digit is a common complication of distal limb wounds that is usually associated with the loss of the extensor tendon of the distal limb.[24] Supporting the dorsal aspect of the limb to counteract the pull of the flexor tendons on the palmar or plantar aspect of the limb is the premise for management of extensor tendon disruption. The wound and extensor tendon laceration is managed by second-intention healing without suturing the extensor tendon.[22,25] A rigid polyvinyl chloride splint is applied to the dorsal or palmar or plantar aspect of the distal limb after wound bandaging. The bandage and splint, which maintains the limb in extension and prevents dorsal knuckling of the fetlock, are retained until normal limb function returns, which may vary from 7 days to 6 weeks.[1]

Wound Infection and Dehiscence

Wound infection and dehiscence occur in both surgically or trauma-induced wounds. Tissue integrity and perfusion, wound repair processes, and bacterial challenge and host responses heavily influence infection. A very important determinant of wound infection is the bacterial inosculation dose. An inoculum size of 10^5 organisms per gram of tissue is a bacterial challenge below which soft tissue wounds may heal without infection. Samples from infected wounds should be taken on a sterile swab from deep within the infected site or tract after cleansing of the wound with dilute povidone-iodine or chlorhexidine scrub, followed by a thorough lavage with sterile isotonic fluid or by harvesting fresh exudate on a sterile swab. Debridement of wounds should be performed on cleaned wounds before the administration of systemic antimicrobials. Necrotic, devitalized, or macerated tissue and organic debris should be removed. Copious lavage should be performed with dilute solutions, such as 0.1% povidone-iodine or 0.05% chlorhexidine solution, which maintain antiseptic properties and minimize tissue toxicity. Pressures of greater than 8 psi and up to 70 psi dislodge adherent bacteria without forcing them deeper into tissue. A 60-mL syringe with a 14-gauge needle can generate 8 psi and a Water Pik (Water Pik, Fort Collins, Colorado) can generate up to 70 psi.

There is no replacement for a representative culture and sensitivity of a wound. It is helpful, however, to have an idea of the organism to expect when faced with a need for therapy in the absence of culture results. Common isolates from equine wounds include *Streptococcus* spp most predominantly followed by coagulase-positive and coagulase- negative *Staphylococcus* spp in addition to Enterobacteriaceae, *Pseudomonas* spp, and anaerobes. Gentamicin and penicillin or cephalothin is a good treatment choice. Aminoglycosides have a concentration-dependent bactericidal action and a good concentration-dependent postantibiotic affect that remains for several hours after the dose is administered and bacteria continue to take up the drug through a combination of passive and oxygen-dependent facilitated processes. Antimicrobial susceptibility of *Pseudomonas* spp is unpredictable and therapy should be based on culture and sensitivity. Local wound care with silver sulfadiazine is effective in most confirmed pseudomonas skin infections. Systemic antibiotics are generally administered for 7 to 10 days in combination with local wound debridement and care.[21]

Regional Limb Perfusion

Regional intravenous infusion achieves high concentrations of antibiotic by diffusion from the vascular space into the traumatized and infected synovial membranes.

Survival rates of horses treated with systemically injected antibiotics in conjunction with regional intravenous antibiotic infusion is greatly increased. Higher concentrations of antibiotic are detected sooner in joints after regional intravenous compared with regional intraosseous antibiotic infusion.

To perform standing regional intravenous perfusion, the horse is sedated. A high four-point block is performed using mepivacaine when the synovial structure to be treated is located at or below the fetlock. Anesthesia of the ulnar and median nerves, or tibial and peroneal nerves, is performed when the area to be treated is located at the level of the carpal or tarsal joints, respectively.

An Esmarch's bandage or a pneumatic tourniquet is applied proximal to the affected synovial structure to occlude the venous system. Usually, the bandage or tourniquet is applied to the mid-metacarpus or metatarsus, but in cases of infection of the carpal or tarsal structures, the bandage or the tourniquet is applied to the distal aspect of the radius or the mid tibial region. The Esmarch's bandage is maintained in place after antibiotic infusion for a period of 30 to 40 minutes and then released.

The antibiotic, generally an aminoglycoside or cephalosporin (amikacin, 1 g diluted in 20–30 mL of saline solution; gentamicin, 1 g diluted in 20–30 mL of saline solution; cephotaxim [Claforan], 1–2 g diluted in 20–30 mL of sterile water) is injected into one of the local superficial veins when the Esmarch's bandage is in place. The palmar-plantar medial and lateral veins are used when the infusion is performed at the level of the fetlock. The cephalic and saphenous veins are used when the tissues intended to be perfused are localized at the levels of the carpal and the tarsal joints. The skin over the vein is surgically prepared using an antiseptic technique. The vein is catheterized using a 22-gauge, 2.5-cm catheter with an infusion plug. A 23-gauge butterfly catheter with an incorporated extension set also works well for this purpose.

The volume of infusion varies between 20 and 30 mL, but smaller volumes can be used for treating foals. Different recommendations for the rate of infusion are reported. The rate of infusion can be as fast as 60 mL/min or 2 mL/min for a total delivery time of 30 minutes for a 30-mL volume. For standing treatment, a fast rate of administration is more convenient and seems to offer satisfactory results. Once the catheter is withdrawn several gauze sponges are applied over the venipuncture site and the site is wrapped with an elastic bandage to avoid a hematoma formation.

Foreign Bodies

Most horses with foreign bodies present with a nonhealing persistent draining tract. This wound is recognized only after prolonged medical treatments have been unsuccessful in resolving a local infection.[22] Most foreign bodies are not evident radiographically unless, however, a gas line is evident secondary to a bacterial infection. Plastic and wood have the same radiodensity as soft tissue and are not visible radiographically. Ultrasound, contrast radiographs, or probing the wound with a surgical instrument may aid in the identification of these foreign bodies.[1,7,22]

Thermal Injuries

Burns are uncommon in horses, with most resulting from barn fires (**Fig. 4**). Thermal injuries may also result from contact with hot solutions; electrocution; lightening strike; friction as in rope burns; abrasions; radiation therapy; and chemicals, such as improperly used topical drugs or maliciously applied caustic agents.[26,27]

Most burns are superficial, easily managed, inexpensive to treat, and heal in a short time. Serious burns, however, have serious complications that can result in rapid, severe burn shock or hypovolemia with associated cardiovascular changes. Smoke inhalation and corneal ulceration also are of great concern.[26,27] Management of severe

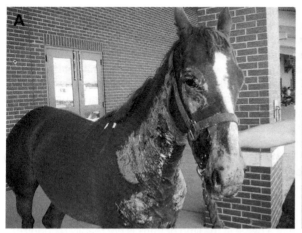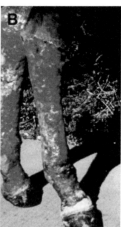

Fig. 4. (*A*) Superficial to deep second-degree burn of the muzzle, periocular region, neck, and chest. These wounds may heal spontaneously in approximately 30 days if further dermal ischemia does not develop, which may lead to full-thickness necrosis. The eye needs to be evaluated daily for evidence of trauma or inflammation. (*B*) Third-degree burn of the distal hind limbs 3 weeks after initial injury. Third-degree burns are characterized by loss of epidermal and dermal components including the adnexa. Healing is by means of contraction and epithelialization from the wound margin or acceptance of an autograft.

and extensive burns is difficult, expensive, and time consuming. The large surface area of the burn dramatically increases the potential for loss of fluids, electrolytes, and calories. Burns covering up to 50% or more of the body are usually fatal, although the depth of the burn also influences mortality. Massive wound infection is almost impossible to prevent because of the difficulty of maintaining a sterile wound environment. Long-term care is required to prevent continued trauma, because burn wounds are often pruritic and self-mutilation is common. Burned horses are frequently disfigured, preventing them from returning to full function. Before treatment, the patient must be carefully examined, with particular attention paid to cardiovascular function, pulmonary status, ocular lesions, and the extent and severity of the burns.[26,28–30]

Although specific guidelines do not exist for burns of horses, euthanasia should be recommended for deep partial-thickness to full-thickness burns involving 30% to 50% of the total body surface area.[29,30] The availability of adequate treatment facilities, cost of treatment, and pain experienced by the horse during long-term care should be considered when deciding treatment. Euthanasia is often an acceptable alternative because convalescence may take up to 2 years.[31] Cost of treatment and prognosis should be thoroughly discussed with the owner.[26,27,32,33]

Excessive Skin Tension

Skin sutured with excessive tension is likely to have complications of healing because of local ischemia with pressure necrosis of the surrounding skin and the pull through of sutures at the skin edge with subsequent wound disruption. Undermining the surrounding skin, relief incisions, and appropriately applied tension sutures are the most common methods that can be used to lessen tension along the skin margins.

The surrounding skin can be undermined up to 4 cm from the wound edge without associated complications.[1,34] Relief incisions can be closed after the primary incision is closed or left to heal by second intention.

To not interrupt the blood supply to the primary suture line, tension sutures are positioned well away from the wound margin. Once the tension suture is in place, the primary incision line is sutured to close the wound edges. Tension suture patterns include vertical mattress, horizontal mattress, far-far-near-near, and far-near-near-far patterns. Vertical mattress sutures with or without skin support to prevent laceration of the wound edges, such as polyethylene or rubber tubing, are useful in reducing tension on the primary suture line. This tension suture support method is used in areas that cannot be bandaged well, such as the upper limb, body, and neck region. It is contraindicated to use tension suture supports under a limb cast or heavy bandage because these supports may cause tissue necrosis and suture line failure. Tension sutures are not effective after 7 to 10 days and should be removed in a staggered fashion with one half removed initially followed by the remaining sutures later.[1]

Nerve Damage

Nerve damage or transection of a nerve in the limb or trunk is not readily recognized at the initial time of the injury. Many lower limb lacerations in the pastern, fetlock, and heel bulb areas with significant injury almost certainly have concurrent transection of the palmar or plantar digital nerve that is not recognized during the examination of the injury. Unilateral transection of the palmar or plantar nerves associated with a traumatic laceration seems to regrow after transection to reinnervate the affected area and cause minimal clinical problems in horses.[4]

Neuroma formation after nerve transection, although rare, can occur and may cause lameness, together with focal pain directly over the wound and nerve site. The lameness improves after local anesthetic is placed at the site of the neuroma. Surgical removal of the neuroma and associated nerve is the treatment of choice to which most horses respond favorably.

Potential sites for wound-associated nerve transection other than the limb include the lateral aspect of the proximal radius and elbow where the radial nerve lies fairly superficial and the shoulder region in which lacerations and blunt trauma may contribute to suprascapular nerve injury (**Fig. 5**). Nerve injury to either location, however, is uncommon.

Injuries to smaller nerve branches most likely occur with all types of traumatic wounds but seem to have minimal impact on wound healing. Occasionally, focal areas of wounds may be hypersensitive to touch and other stimuli, which may indicate previous damage to nerve branches and potential small neuroma formation. This hypersensitivity tends to resolve as the wound is covered with healthy granulation tissue.[1]

Major Blood Vessels

Pastern lacerations are the most common location for wounds to involve a major blood vessel, such as the palmar digital vein or artery. Significant blood loss can occur if the hemorrhage is not controlled soon after injury by temporarily clamping the vessel or applying pressure over the wound with a bandage in the standing horse (**Fig. 6**). Anastomosis of the vessels is usually not possible because the severed ends usually retract into the wound. Large vessel lacerations, which may involve the saphenous vein along the medial aspect of the tarsus, the cephalic vein along the medial aspect of the distal radius, and the greater metatarsal artery along the lateral aspect of the metatarsus, are best treated by ligation of the severed ends if they can be identified. Fortunately, collateral circulation usually develops readily.[1]

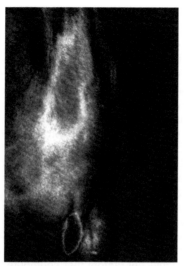

Fig. 5. Sweeney of the left shoulder. Prominence of the scapular spine is present secondary to atrophy of the suprascapular musculature resulting from blunt trauma of the suprascapular nerve.

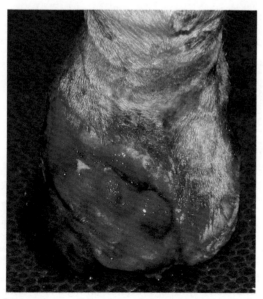

Fig. 6. Laceration of the palmar axial surface of the right fore limb. Temporarily clamping the palmar digital artery or vein or applying pressure over the wound with a bandage in the standing horse can avert significant blood loss. The severed vessels are usually severely damaged, which prevents anastomosis. Collateral circulation of the affected vessels develops rapidly in 2 to 4 weeks.

Movement

The extent of movement of the skin relative to the underlying bed of granulation tissue is usually much higher in the limb regions than in the trunk. This is possibly exacerbated by the relative lack of skin elasticity and the obvious proximity of the limb skin to structures with a high degree of motion, such as joints and tendons. Trunk wounds have a better available reparative blood supply than those of the distal limb.

An injury to the distal limb metacarpal or metatarsal region of a horse that involves the flexor tendons or their sheaths requires healing by the ingress of blood vessels from adjacent structures. As healing attempts to progress, however, repeated tendon contraction and limb movement moves the injury away from the site of the skin wound leaving the damaged tissues with no effective mechanism for healing.

Rigid limb casting of a distal limb wound is very effective in facilitating wound contraction and epithelialization if the tissues are initially sharply debrided and lavaged (**Fig. 7**). The mechanisms for this may be more complex than merely controlling movement. Although movement of the limb and wound is limited, added surrounding pressure applied to the wound may also facilitate the healing process. Warmth, restriction of movement, and the presence of a moist healing environment in conjunction with a cast are probably significant factors that contribute to wound healing. Which aspects of the exudate are desirable and enhancing of wound healing and which are inhibitory is not known in the horse. Heat, pain, swelling, or lameness created by the cast indicate attentive re-evaluation of the wound and the consideration of cast removal or cast change.[1]

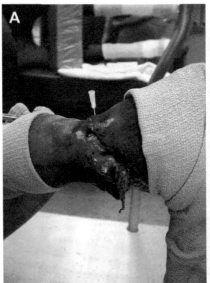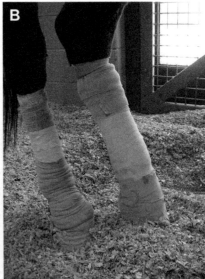

Fig. 7. Laceration of the left hind plantar pastern region. (*A*) Initial debridement of the wound and lavage of affected synovial structures. (*B*) Rigid limb casting is very effective in promoting wound contraction and epithelialization. Warmth, restriction of movement, and the presence of a moist healing environment in conjunction with a cast are significant factors that contribute to wound healing. Heat, pain, swelling, or lameness created by the cast indicate attentive re-evaluation of the wound and the consideration of cast removal or cast change.

Self-Mutilation

Significant self-mutilation of wounds through rubbing, biting, and pawing can occur if the horse is not adequately restrained or medicated. Usually, the most intense pruritic episodes occur in the first weeks of wound healing during the inflammatory phase of repair and during eschar sloughing but can be a later complication associated with burn wounds.[27,35] To prevent extreme self-mutilation, the horse should be cross tied or sedated at this time and use of a neck collar may be considered. Delayed healing, poor epithelialization, and complications of second-intention healing may limit return of the animal to their previous use.

Exuberant Granulation Tissue

Surgical resection is a simple and effective method to control exuberant granulation tissue. The procedure is performed with the horse standing, because granulation tissue is not innervated. Strips of granulation tissue can be shaved from the wound bed in a distal to proximal direction to produce a flat surface level with or slightly (approximately 2 mm) below the surrounding wound edges. The epithelial margin should be preserved to allow continued healing. A pressure bandage is usually necessary to control hemorrhage after excision. In lower limb wounds of horses this technique has been successful in enhancing second-intention healing that was delayed because of protruding granulation tissue. This technique is preferred for the removal of exuberant granulation tissue over other methods, such as application of caustic drugs, because it is easy to perform; provides tissue for histologic evaluation, if needed; and preserves the epithelial margin for continued healing. As with any alternate technique, healing by contraction and epithelialization must subsequently be supported by maintaining the limb in a firm support bandage and limiting excessive motion of the wound or excessive granulation recurs. Corticosteroids may be applied topically to curb the early formation of exuberant granulation tissue, hence facilitating epithelialization and wound repair. The ability of some corticosteroids to suppress the formation of exuberant granulation tissue in the early phases of healing may be related to their ability selectively to decrease the release of profibrotic transforming growth factor-β from monocytes and macrophages, inhibiting lysosomal activity and fibroblastic proliferation. Corticosteroids are generally applied at the earliest signs of formation of exuberant granulation tissue with one or two applications being all that is needed to achieve the desired effect. Continued applications are not recommended, because this may exert negative effects on wound contraction, epithelialization, and angiogenesis. Corticosteroids should not be applied to an infected wound because they inhibit the inflammatory response required to eliminate microorganisms.

Application of a cast to a lower limb wound is indicated in cases in which it is difficult to control exuberant granulation tissue. Wounds over joints or tendons may require immobilization because continued movement disrupts healing. Frequently, the hock or carpus is involved in these types of compound injuries. When the limb is mechanically stable, the wound should be bandaged for a few days before applying a cast, to allow superior wound debridement and permit dissipation of edema, which ensures a better-fitting cast. Casts minimize the formation of exuberant granulation tissue by reducing motion. Casts should be maintained no longer than necessary over lower limb wounds for reasons similar to those mentioned for bandages and to minimize the development of cast sores. Generally, casts over wounds should be changed every 3 to 10 days, but this depends on the nature and location of the wound and the temperament of the horse. Skin grafts can be used after cast removal to facilitate wound coverage. A splint bandage is continued during this period.

COMPLICATIONS OF CONTAMINATED WOUNDS
Methicillin-Resistant Staphylococcus Aureus Infection

There have been increasing reports of MRSA infection and colonization in horses and other domestic animals.[36–39] MRSA is resistant to all β-lactam antimicrobials and frequently to a wide range of additional antimicrobial classes because of the presence of an altered penicillin-binding protein. Infections can consequently be difficult to treat and are associated with increased morbidity, mortality, and treatment costs, compared with infections caused by methicillin-susceptible S aureus strains.[40–42]

Identification of MRSA infection and colonization in horses in veterinary hospitals and in the community, and reports of transmission of MRSA between humans and animals, have raised concern about the role of animals in MRSA infection in humans and the potential for animals to become a reservoir of MRSA.[36,38,39,43] In one recent veterinary hospital study the incidence rate of nosocomial MRSA infection was at the rate of 1.8 per 1000 admissions, with an incidence density of 0.88 per 1000 patient days. Administrations of ceftiofur or aminoglycosides during hospitalization were the two risk factors associated with nosocomial MRSA colonization. In another veterinary hospital study horses that had received at least 72 hours of penicillin treatment had a 5.8-times higher chance (odds) of harboring penicillin-resistant staphylococci than horses that were not admitted to the clinic and did not receive penicillin treatment. Control horses with a 72-hour stay at the clinic but no penicillin treatment still had a 2.4-times higher chance (odds) of harboring penicillin-resistant strains. This work demonstrated that horses entering the hospital harbor staphylococci-containing antibiotic-resistance genes. Shortly after hospitalization, horses acquired a specific multidrug-resistant skin flora that was presumably selected for and maintained in the hospital by the use of penicillin. These authors proposed that antibiotics should be limited to the treatment of infection and not used for infection prevention and that such prudent use could help prevent selection for multidrug-resistant strains, such as MRSA strains in animals.[44] MRSA screening of horses admitted to a veterinary hospital was useful for identification of community-associated and nosocomial colonization and infection, and for monitoring of infection control practices.[45,46]

MRSA infections are generally classified as hospital or community acquired and as superficial colonization of a wound without signs of infection, superficial soft tissue infection or cellulitis, complex skin and skin-structure infection, or osteomyelitis. Superficial wounds may be treated without the use of oral or IV antibiotics. Regular cleansing of the wound with 4% chlorhexidine gluconate and soft tissue debridement is effective at reducing the colony-forming bacteria load. Topical application of honey or silver-coated dressings has been shown to be effective. Careful monitoring of the wound is imperative to ensure adequate response to treatment.[47–49]

Ventral midline celiotomy closures are prone to MRSA infection (**Fig. 8**). Clinical signs usually present 5 to 10 days after surgery with a purulent exudate escaping from the subcutaneous tissue. Opening of the skin closure accompanied by local superficial debridement with the application of 4% chlorhexidine, topical honey, or silver-coated dressings has been an effective treatment. Although intranasal mupirocin can prevent endogenous acquired MRSA infections in an ICU and is effective in overall decolonizing of nasal carriers, mupirocin is less effective in decolonizing extranasal sites, such as wounds.[50,51] Doxycycline in combination with rifampin has been shown to have a synergistic activity against MRSA activity in people.

Local antimicrobial treatment, consisting of implantation of vancomycin-impregnated polymethyl methacrylate beads, has also been performed to increase the concentration of antimicrobials in the local environment and decrease adverse systemic

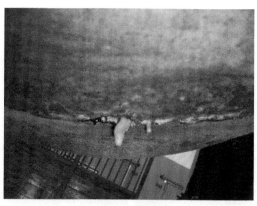

Fig. 8. Ventral midline celiotomy closure. Purulent discharge is present 7 days after closure. Opening the subcutaneous closure completely, debridement of the affected tissue, and daily cleansing of the tissues resulted in complete healing of the wound by third intention.

effects.[52–54] Vancomycin has been documented to elute from polymethyl methacrylate in vitro.[44] The vancomycin-impregnated polymethyl methacrylate beads are changed frequently, because there is concern that daily wound lavage increases the elution rate of vancomycin from the polymethyl methacrylate and reduces the local vancomycin concentration by dilution.[10]

Abdominal Wounds

Most injuries that involve the abdominal wall are best treated with wound exploration, abdominocentesis, ultrasound, and rectal examination to document whether a wound breaches the peritoneal cavity. Injuries to the deep inguinal area are especially prone to penetrating injuries of the abdominal wall (**Fig. 9**). Septic peritonitis and potential bowel eventration are serious complications if left unattended.[22] Most injuries penetrating the abdominal cavities are best treated with the horse under general anesthesia to permit thorough wound exploration, debridement, abdominal lavage, and primary closure.[1]

Large wounds that involve an open abdominal cavity are emergency conditions. Emergency first aid treatment usually requires immediate closure of the wound to prevent bowel from exiting the wound. Provisionally bandaging, suturing, or clamping the wound until exploration and repair of the wound can be used. With severe abdominal contamination abdominal drainage using large-bore catheters egressing the ventral abdomen should be performed for repeated abdominal lavage of the abdomen for several days after surgery (**Fig. 10**). Large abdominal wall defects that cannot be closed primarily at surgery should be bandaged and left to heal by second intention. Many of these defects close completely. Abdominal wall herniation is usually secondary sequelae. A synthetic mesh implant may also be used to facilitate closure 2 to 3 months after injury.[55]

Thoracic Wounds

Injuries of the chest are common and rarely result in penetrating the thorax, and are usually the result of the horse running over or into a fixed natural object, such as tree, fence post, or other substantial stationary object. These wounds should be thoroughly explored for the presence of foreign bodies or secondary rib fractures. Intercostal perineural local anesthesia facilitates a more thorough exploration and assists in the control of pain that often accompanies these injuries.[6] Thorough wound

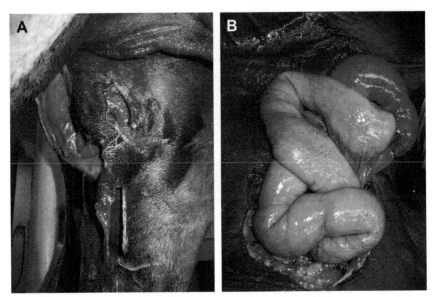

Fig. 9. Deep inguinal injury of the LH limb. (*A*) Multiple deep lacerations and contusions to the medial thigh and abdominal wall. (*B*) Prolapse of small intestine 2 days postinjury through the initial wound. Thorough wound exploration, debridement, abdominal lavage, and primary closure of the wound was done immediately after injury under general anesthesia.

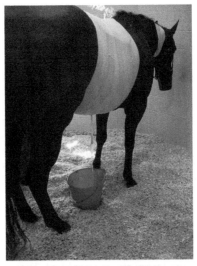

Fig. 10. Eggressing lavage fluid from an abdominal lavage catheter. A penetrating abdominal wall injury was left undetected for 12 days postinjury. A large-bore catheter exiting the ventral abdomen should be inserted for repeated abdominal lavage of the abdomen for several days after surgery.

debridement and lavage should be performed, followed by removal of rib fragments, foreign bodies, and other debris that may be present within the depths of the wound. It is imperative that the wound be closed primarily or covered with an airtight dressing and left to heal by second intention. Primary muscle flaps of the longissimus and external abdominal oblique muscles, diaphragmatic advancement flaps, or prosthetic meshes can be used to facilitate closure of the wound over the lateral thorax.[52,56] General anesthesia may be used if pneumothorax is not present; however, it is not recommended because of further undefined respiratory and cardiovascular risks.[1]

Horses with large axillary wounds should be closely observed for the development of subcutaneous emphysema and impending pneumothorax, however, which may develop secondarily to axillary wounds that do not initially penetrate the chest (**Fig. 11**). The wounds of this area often expand deep into the axilla along the thoracic wall and tend to aspirate air into the wound and deeper structures.[56] To inhibit air from moving into the tissues the wound may be packed with sterile gauze and the skin over the defect temporarily closed using stent bandages. The packing should be removed every 24 to 48 hours and the wound repacked until healthy granulation tissue has developed to occlude the defect. To reduce the potential for subcutaneous emphysema the horse should be confined to a stall or cross tied to minimize movement of the limb.[1]

Emergency triage is necessary in some cases when pneumothorax is the result of interruption to the thoracic wall. If there is any evidence of respiratory distress, including flaring of the nostrils or short rapid breaths, the wound should be covered with an airtight dressing (saran wrap) to prevent further incursion of air into the thorax.

Pneumothorax may be detected by ultrasound, thoracocentesis, and radiography. Diagnostic thoracocentesis may be performed by placing a 3.5-teat cannula or 14-gauge catheter high into the thirteenth intercostal space adjacent to the caudal margin of the rib into the thoracic cavity and attaching a fluid extension line with sterile fluid (2–3 mL). If the fluid foams out of the extension, pneumothorax is confirmed; if the fluid is aspirated into the thoracic cavity it is not likely that pneumothorax is present. If pneumothorax is present a three-way stop cock is attached to the extension line and then to a 60-mL syringe or active suction pump. The air is removed by active suction

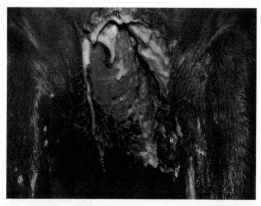

Fig. 11. Deep ventral chest and axillary wound. This wound went into the axilla along the thoracic wall penetrating the chest. To inhibit air from moving into the tissues the wound was sharply debrided, packed with sterile gauze and the skin was temporarily closed. This procedure was performed with the horse standing to avoid complications of pneumothorax with general anesthesia. The packing was changed every 48 hours until healthy granulation tissue developed to occlude the defect.

with precautions to prevent the introduction of more air through the original wound (**Fig. 12**). Radiography is useful to determine if air is present within the thoracic cavity and reveal the presence of a collapsed lung, secondary rib fractures, or foreign bodies. In horses experiencing severe respiratory distress intranasal oxygen may be beneficial.

Horses with acute and especially chronic chest wounds should be closely evaluated for secondary pleuritis by means of radiography, ultrasound, and fluid analysis obtained by thoracocentesis. Pleuritis secondary to thoracic trauma is uncommon if the thoracic wounds are suitably treated. The caveat is that penetration of the thoracic cavity may not be readily apparent and accurate treatment with broad-spectrum antibiotics and surgical debridement of the wound is delayed. Thoracoscopy is indicated to identify associated injuries and foreign bodies in horses with severe or complicating injuries.[1]

Gun Shot

Traumatic wounds caused by acts of violence are an increasingly important cause of injuries to horses.[57,58] Wounds limited to the skeletal muscles have a good prognosis, whereas injuries that involve vital organs decreased survivability. Ten horses with injuries caused by gunshots or stab wounds by spears or knives were treated. The depths of many soft tissue injuries were initially underestimated. Seven of 10 horses survived requiring surgical and medical treatments.[58] In another study 22 horses were evaluated for injuries caused by firearms. Most had been shot with 0.22-caliber rimfire cartridge bullets or lead shotgun pellets, although other weapons included BB pellets, a 0.35-caliber rimfire cartridge bullet, and airgun pellets. In eight of these horses the injury was confined to the skin or skeletal muscles, seven of which returned to their previous use. In 14 horses, additional injuries included the sinus, pharynx, mandible, tooth, aorta, eye, tibia, gastrointestinal tract, joint, and trachea. Of the 11 horses with injuries to deep or vital structures other than the eye, three died, five were euthanatized, and three survived.[57]

Debridement of the wound and delayed primary closure 4 to 5 days after injury are the preferred treatment for gunshot injuries. Treatment by minimal debridement, lavage, and the establishment of drainage allows for excellent results when only skin and skeletal muscle were involved. The benefit of using antimicrobial agents remains equivocal, but may be indicated if the wound is heavily contaminated or vital

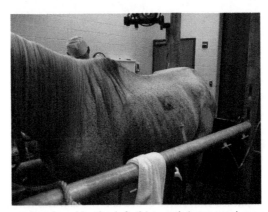

Fig. 12. Thoracoscopy tube placed in the left thirteenth intercostal space. This horse developed pneumothorax secondary to a right thoracic injury. Air was removed by active suction with precautions to prevent the introduction of more air through the original wound.

structures are in close proximity to the site of injury. Small-caliber ammunition may have sufficient velocity to enter the abdomen, respiratory tract, or skull. In such situations more aggressive treatment aimed at repairing damaged vital structures may be indicated.[57]

Pythiosis

Infections in horses caused by *Pythium insidiosum* are most commonly restricted to the cutaneous and subcutaneous tissues in horses that have prolonged contact in lakes, ponds, and swampy areas.[59–61] There may be single or multiple nonhealing, rapidly enlarging, tumor-like, ulcerative, nodular masses with multiple draining tracts and serosanguineous discharge.[60] These lesions are usually on the limbs and ventral abdomen but can occur anywhere on the body including tendons, ligaments, and bone in chronic cases (**Fig. 13**). The lesions are usually intensely pruritic and horses may mutilate the wounds if not closely monitored.[60,61] There may be mild to marked lymphadenopathy. Skin lesions often contain "kunkers," yellowish gritty coral-like bodies ranging from 0.5 to 1.5 cm in diameter. Kunkers are composed of necrotic eosinophils, *Pythium* sp hyphae, and necrotic vessels.[60,61] Cutaneous pythiosis, although seemingly straightforward, is often misdiagnosed as cutaneous habronemiasis, sarcoids, or excessive granulation tissue, which are characterized by similar gross lesions.[60–62]

Because of possible recurrence, it has been recommended that surgical excision be followed by systemic administration of antifungal drugs.[60,61] Antifungal therapy may not be effective, however, because of the lack of ergosterol (the target molecule of antifungal drugs) in the plasma membranes of oomycetes. This probably explains why antifungal chemotherapy alone has shown very little success in treating phycomycosis.[62] Topical application of "Phycofixer" consisting of ketoconazole, rifampin, dimethyl sulfoxide, and hydrochloride (University of Florida, Gainesville, and Franck's

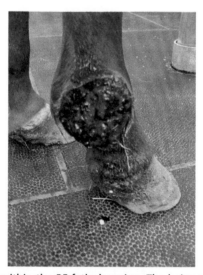

Fig. 13. Pythiosis present within the RF fetlock region. The lesion was markedly pruritic resulting in the horse mutilating the lesion. Pythiosis is often misdiagnosed as cutaneous habronemiasis, sarcoids, or excessive granulation tissue, which is characterized by similar gross lesions.

Compounding Pharmacy, Ocala, Florida) beneath an absorbent bandage has met with good success in wounds that cannot be surgically debrided.

Recently, immunotherapy using a newly formulated vaccine has been successful in treating cutaneous pythiosis in horses and dogs.[62] This vaccine has been shown to be effective for both acute and chronic cutaneous pythiosis in the horse.[61,62]

For most phycomycosis infections the prognosis is guarded to poor regardless of the advances in treatment. The reason is that many horses have multiple bone lesions at the time of initial presentation.[60,61] The rate of recurrence after attempted surgical excision has also been a major factor in the failure of treatment.

Myiasis

Chronic open wounds can become contaminated with habronemiasis, a common cause of ulcerative cutaneous granulomas in horses. Habronemiasis is a result of infection with larvae of the nematodes *Habronema muscae*, *Habronema majus*, and *Draschia megastoma*.[63] Infection of a wound with these larvae induces proliferative, exuberant granulation tissue caused by a presumptive hypersensitive reaction to dead or dying larvae.[64,65] Lesions of chronic wounds are most commonly seen on the limbs and any area of traumatized skin.[63,64,66,67]

The onset of habronemiasis is often characterized by the rapid growth of papules or failure of a wound to heal with the development of exuberant granulation tissue. Lesions may be solitary or multiple and are characterized by ulceration, exudation, intermittent hemorrhage, exuberant granulation, and pruritus (**Fig. 14**). Wounds often contain small yellow granules commonly called "sulfur granules" representing necrotic, caseous, or calcified material surrounding nematode larvae.[64,68]

The disease is most common during the spring and summer when fly populations are active, and lesions often regress during the winter. The diagnosis is often made exclusively on the basis of history, compatible clinical signs, the location of lesions, and the presence

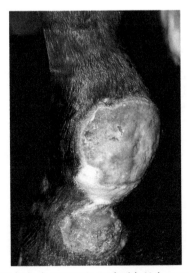

Fig. 14. Chronic wound of RF fetlock contaminated with *Habronema* spp larva. The two large lesions are characterized by ulceration, exudation, intermittent hemorrhage, and exuberant granulation tissue. Small yellow granules (sulfur granules) are present in the wound representing necrotic, caseous, or calcified material surrounding nematode larvae.

of yellowish granules. Biopsy is the method of choice for confirming the diagnosis, which reveals nodular to diffuse eosinophilic dermatitis. Multiple foci of coagulative necrosis with or without degenerating nematode larvae in the center are characteristic of this disease.[64] Habronemiasis must be differentiated from proliferative granulation tissue, sarcoids, pythiosis, squamous cell carcinoma, and other neoplasms.[63–67]

A combination of local and systemic treatment aimed at reducing the size of the lesions, reducing associated inflammation, and preventing reinfestation is most effective.[63–67] Massive lesions and wounds refractory to medical treatment may be removed surgically or at least debulked before topical and systemic treatment. Corticosteroids are used to reduce inflammatory hypersensitivity reactions, and for smaller lesions, topical or intralesional application is favored. Topical preparations that contain anti-inflammatory, larvicidal, antimicrobial, penetrating, and protective ingredients are commonly used.[63–67] Ivermectin has been reported to be effective in the treatment of habronemiasis in horses, because it kills infective larvae and adult worms in the stomach.[69]

COMPLICATIONS OF NEOPLASIA
Squamous Cell Carcinoma

A variety of tumors have been reported in association with chronic wounds. Neoplasia secondary to trauma or thermal injury is not uncommon in humans, and can develop acutely but more often latently, several years after the injury.[70] Squamous cell carcinoma has a prevalence rate of almost 2% in human burn wounds.[70] Although scar malignancy in animals is less frequently diagnosed than in humans, various causes, including chronic irritation, as in the case of the chemicals applied to a wound, may potentially lead to development of squamous cell carcinoma.[70] Squamous cell carcinoma and fibrosarcoma have been identified in association with scars resulting from burns in the horse (**Fig. 15**). Squamous cell carcinoma has been associated with cutaneous scars in a llama and a horse.[71,72] Other complications include habronemiasis, keloid-like fibroblastic proliferations, sarcoids, and other burn-induced neoplasia.[31]

The clinical management of squamous cell carcinoma can include surgical excision, cryosurgery, electrosurgery, intralesional chemotherapy with such agents as cisplatin or 5-fluorouracil cream, immunotherapy, hyperthermia, and radiotherapy.[72,73] Cryotherapy controls squamous cell carcinoma of the skin but is not optimal for recurrent

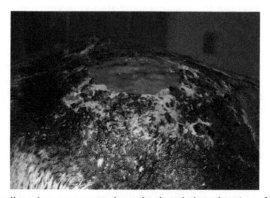

Fig. 15. Squamous cell carcinoma present along the dorsal gluteal region of a horse, which developed secondarily after deep second-degree burn to the area. (*Courtesy of* J. Schumacher, DVM, MS, DACVS, Knoxville, TN.)

squamous cell carcinoma or larger tumors.[74] Intralesional injection with cisplatin in oil or topical or intralesional administration of 5-fluorouracil is effective. Hypertrophic scars, which commonly develop following deep second-degree burns, generally remodel in a cosmetic manner without surgery within 1 to 2 years. Because scarred skin is hairless and often depigmented, solar exposure should be limited. Chronic non-healing areas should be excised and autografted to prevent neoplastic transformation. Return of squamous cell carcinoma associated with incomplete removal of the lesion is not uncommon, which subsequently requires chronic retreatment.

Interstitial brachytherapy with iridium-192 sources has several advantages compared with other possible treatments.[74] Although management is intensive and more costly than other treatments, it is very effective in eliminating the lesion and causes little tissue defect. Delayed healing, poor epithelialization, and complications of second-intention healing may limit return of the animal to previous uses.

Sarcoid

Sarcoid is a benign tumor of fibrous tissue of horses, donkeys, and mules. Sarcoids are the most frequently diagnosed tumor in horses, with sarcoid transformation an increasingly important cause of wound healing failure. Surveys have estimated the prevalence of sarcoid at 20% of all equine neoplasms and 36% of all skin tumors.[75–79]

Sarcoids are presumably caused by bovine papilloma virus type 1 and 2 infection, although retrovirus etiologies have been suggested.[75–79] The mode of virus transmission and presence of latent infections are not clearly understood. Peripheral blood mononuclear cells may serve as host cells for bovine papilloma virus type 1 and 2 DNA and contribute to virus latency.[80] Sarcoids are recognized as having six different clinical manifestations (occult, verrucose, nodular, fibroblastic, mixed, and malignant-malevolent) and can occur at any cutaneous site.[34,81–83] These lesions are characterized by proliferation of neoplastic fibroblasts and thickening or ulceration of the skin.

Horses with sarcoids at other sites seem to be particularly prone to sarcoid transformation, as are those that have close contact with other horses having sarcoids.[34,79] Transformation is also more likely in uncovered wounds in summer months when flies are abundant.[81] Body, trunk, or facial wounds that contain sarcoid cells usually develop verrucose sarcoids, whereas limb wounds develop fibroblastic sarcoids that are easily confused with exuberant granulation tissue.[34,81,82] Some wounds partially heal, whereas others fail to heal at all even if the overall extent of sarcoid involvement is small. Wounds on horses with sarcoids at other sites should be treated particularly carefully, with attention not to cross-contaminate the wounds, no matter how small and insignificant the wound.

Fibroblastic sarcoids strongly resemble exuberant granulation tissue or staphylococcal pyogranuloma, especially when it progresses at the site of a wound, and especially in limb wounds.[34,81,82] Traumatic skin injuries that fail to heal may contain considerable sarcoid components in the wound margins, and the sarcoid tissues can be interdispersed with granulation tissue. Sporadic infiltration of sarcoid tissue at a granulation wound site is very difficult to identify and can be easily missed on biopsy. Careful deep biopsy and a skilled pathologist are essential. The presence of sarcoid transformation in a wound site adds critically to the therapeutic challenges.[82] Early diagnosis and treatment is the most effective course for resolution because most sarcoids involving wounds are prone to getting worse with time and develop into larger more invasive lesions.

Surgically debulking a wound with sarcoid tissue is the most effective treatment for lesions involving wounds. Surgical removal is complicated by the regrowth of the sarcoid at the surgical site and complications of complete wound healing because of lack of a suitable means for wound closure or the subsequent interference with normal function. The rate of regrowth of the equine sarcoid following surgical excision is closely dependent on the extent of the tumor and the degree to which the surgeon can define its limits. Small, well-defined tumors carry the best prognosis for surgical removal, whereas extensive areas of poorly defined verrucose and mixed sarcoid may result in rapid regrowth of a more aggressive sarcoid type. The earliest regrowth of sarcoids occurs within days of incomplete excision and is usually accompanied by rapid wound dehiscence and subsequent failure to heal.[83] Viral latency may be one explanation for the high rate of recurrence following surgical excision of sarcoids. In one study bovine papillomaviral DNA was detected in essentially all sarcoids examined. There seems to be a regional variation in the prevalence of viral types with sarcoid tumors. Viral DNA in normal skin samples from horses with sarcoids suggests the possibility of a latent vial phase.[84]

Cryotherapy and immune-mediated therapy have mixed results when used to eliminate sarcoid tissue in wounds. Cryotherapy is generally used as an adjunct therapy after surgical debulking of the wound and in areas where complete excision of the sarcoid is not possible. Repeat treatments are often needed and complicate the healing of the wound. Poor cosmesis related to regrowth of white hair and scarring is one of the most common "cosmetic" complications associated with cryotherapy.

Radiation therapy using interstitial brachytherapy with iridium-192 sources has been used for the treatment of equine sarcoids affecting the eyelid, lower limb, and joints with good results of greater than 90% efficacy (**Fig. 16**). These procedures are relatively simple to use when the clinician and radiation oncologist can work as a team to maximize the efficacy of the treatment. Although expensive and management intensive, more clients are willing to pay the expense to achieve the excellent results associated with this approach.[4]

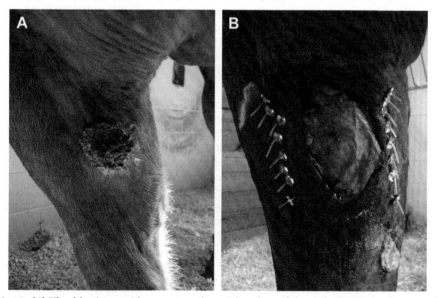

Fig.16. (*A*) Fibroblastic sarcoid present on the axial surface of the right forelimb. The sarcoid developed secondarily from a wound to the same area. Other sarcoids were previously present on the body. (*B*) The wound was surgically debrided and interstitial brachytherapy with iridium-192 in plastic straws was applied within the wound.

COMPLICATIONS OF SKIN GRAFTS

Skin grafting decreases healing time and is one of the best techniques for covering a wound that has been chronically affected by exuberant granulation tissue. Skin grafting of lower limb wounds should be considered to cover the granulating wound bed if contraction has ceased and the wound bed is large.[8,85] Frequently, however, wounds in horses are treated for several weeks before skin grafting is initiated. At this point granulation tissue is mature, fibrous, and has less of a blood supply than newly formed granulation tissue. Other complications of graft acceptance and healing are wound infection and sequestra formation.

Chronic inflammation, inherently present during second-intention healing of wounds on the distal portion of limbs of horses, may be at least as important as infection because it reduces the quality of the granulation bed and results in the production of a moderate amount of purulent exudate, both of which negatively influence acceptance of grafts.[12] As a result, the ability of a wound bed to accept a graft is lessened. It is imperative that chronic granulating wounds be debrided to a level below the skin surface down to a level of healthy granulation tissue before graft application.[8,86–88]

To increase the success of graft acceptance wound bacteria must be minimized. β-Hemolytic *Streptococcus* spp, *Proteus* spp, and *Pseudomonas* spp are capable of producing destructive proteolytic enzymes and excessive purulent discharge that breakdown fibrinous attachments between the graft and recipient bed.[89,90] Topical antiseptics have better efficacy than antibiotics in reducing bacterial wound load because the latter increase the risk of patient sensitization and the development of resistant organisms especially when used routinely over prolonged periods in uninfected wounds.[88,90] Infected wounds, however, should be treated with broad-spectrum antibiotics while awaiting culture results. The bone underlying the wound should be radiographed for evidence of sequestra and excessive pericortical dystrophic mineralization. Large wounds often develop healthy granulating tissue around the perimeter before a sequestrum completely defines itself.

Donor site is influenced by the method of grafting, color and texture of the donor hair, cosmesis of the donor site, and ease of obtaining skin. Common sites for obtaining donor skin include pectoral, dorsal neck region, perineum, ventral midline, ventral lateral abdomen, and sternal region caudal to the girth area.[8,91]

Pinch Grafts

Pinch grafts are distinct pieces of skin (3 mm in diameter) produced by excising an elevated cone of skin. Graft acceptance is as high as 75% using pinch grafts partially because of the fact that the pockets of granulation tissue hold the graft in contact with the wound. Complications include necrosis of the graft, slower wound healing, improper orientation of hair, and thin skin coverage of the wound.

Necrotic spots along the top of the granulation pockets normally occur during healing, after which the graft epithelializes circumferentially. Because pinch grafts are small, complete epithelialization of the wound often takes more than 70 days.[91] Improper orientation of hair growth is a complication of pinch graft application despite repeated efforts properly to align the hair to match that of the recipient area. A cobblestone appearance with thin subcutaneous tissue is sequelae of pinch graft applications that may not be cosmetically acceptable for show horses.

Punch Grafts

Punch grafts are circular pieces of skin that are directly removed from the locally anesthetized donor site or by obtaining biopsies from an excised piece of donor skin.

Common complications of punch graft failure are incomplete removal of the underlying subcutaneous tissue from the graft, recipient site hemorrhage, and motion.

Because punch grafts are full thickness they must have the subcutaneous tissue and fascia removed from the dermis with a surgical blade before implanting, because these layers prevent revascularization and subsequent graft failure. Placing grafts in saline-soaked sponge gauze for a short period of time minimizes graft desiccation while recipient beds are created. Accumulation of blood and serum beneath the graft displaces the grafts from the recipient site. Hemorrhage can be avoided by ensuring that it is controlled before grafting. Displacement of the grafts can also be minimized by using a biopsy punch a size smaller than used to obtain donor graft to ensure a snug fit in the recipient bed. Displacement of the graft by motion can be minimized by securing the wound under a heavy bandage (**Fig. 17**). Displacement of grafted tissue at wrap changes can be reduced by soaking the primary bandage before removal. Casting is not indicated for punch graft techniques because punch grafts are not indicated for grafting over moveable areas of the body.

Tunnel Grafts

Tunnel grafts are useful for healing of wounds that are hard to immobilize or bandage as on the dorsal surface of the hock or fetlock. Graft survival rates of 80% have been reported with excellent cosmetic results.[92] Complications of tunnel grafting include the placement of tunnel grafts too close to one another, failure of the graft to become exposed, and accidental removal of the tunnel graft when removing the overlying granulation tissue.

This technique requires harvesting of full-thickness or spit-thickness strips of skin 2 to 5 mm wide and slightly longer than the length of the wound's edges. These grafts are placed in granulation tissue that has been allowed to develop 4 to 8 mm above skin level. These tunnels can be created using a cutting needle, flattened K-wire with a trocar point, or malleable alligator forceps. The graft is then tunneled approximately 6 mm below the surface of the granulation tissue at the recipient site ensuring that the

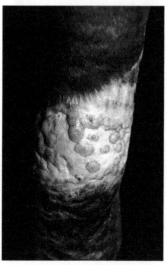

Fig. 17. Punch biopsy grafts in place on the dorsum of the fetlock. Several grafts failed to take because of hemorrhage, displacing grafts at wrap changes, and movement at the grafting site.

epidermal side of the graft faces the surface of the wound. Tunnel grafts should not be placed closer than 2 cm apart to prevent excessive necrosis of granulation tissue.[92] The cut ends of the skin strips are sutured to the skin on either side of the granulation bed. A tourniquet may be useful to control hemorrhage and improve visualization of the strips for procedures that involve grafting on a limb. If placed the correct depth, the granulation tissue overlying the graft should slough in 7 to 10 days.[93] If this does not occur, it should be excised at this time. Adjacent granulation tissue that is raised should be excised at this time. Most tunnel graft failures are attributable to accidental removal of the graft during removal of the overlying granulation tissue or failure of the graft to become exposed. Exposure of the graft if necessary may be facilitated by placing malleable probes or wires through the tunnels to cut through the overlying granulation tissue.[92]

FULL-THICKNESS SHEET GRAFT

Full-thickness or split-thickness grafts can be applied as a sheet or expanded before transplantation. The full-thickness sheet graft is the most cosmetic type of free sheet graft because it contains all the properties of the surrounding skin, provides maximum piliation, and can withstand pressure and friction. Full-thickness grafts are not as readily accepted because there are less exposed blood vessels available for imbibition of plasma and for inosculation (**Fig. 18**).

No specialized equipment is needed for harvesting, and the procedure can often be performed in the standing sedated horse using local anesthesia.[91] Donor sites of full-thickness grafts should be sutured. The graft should be cut slightly larger than the recipient bed to allow for shrinkage after the graft is excised because of recoil of elastic fibers in the deep dermal layers of the graft. The full-thickness graft should be sutured to the donor site with some tension to prevent occlusion of the dermal vessels that may occur if the graft is allowed fully to contract.

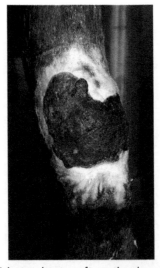

Fig. 18. An unmeshed full-thickness sheet graft on the dorsal surface of the fetlock. Full-thickness sheet grafts often require more nourishment than can be supplied by the granulating recipient wound. As a result, full-thickness grafts are usually reserved for fresh uncontaminated wounds.

A high oxygen gradient between the wound and the graft is essential for neovascularization of the graft and graft acceptance. Full-thickness grafts treated with hyperbaric oxygen therapy developed less granulation tissue, edema, and neovascularization, but more inflammation. The superficial portion of these full-thickness grafts was also less viable than the superficial portion of those not treated with hyperbaric oxygen therapy.[94]

Full-thickness sheet grafts are often considered compromised because they often require more nourishment than can be supplied by the granulating recipient wound. As a result, full-thickness grafts are usually reserved for fresh uncontaminated wounds. The upper layers of a full-thickness graft are more likely to slough because full-thickness grafts require more nourishment and have fewer exposed vessels for this purpose. Because of the lack of abundant donor skin in the horse, the graft often must be meshed and expanded to achieve coverage of the wound larger than the donor area.

Split-Thickness Grafts

Split-thickness grafts are more readily accepted than full-thickness grafts, and may be used to cover granulation beds that are less than ideal.[95] Because blood vessels branch as they become more superficial in the dermis, more vessels are cut and exposed with split-thickness grafts. The greater the number of exposed vessels the better the absorption of nutrients is from the granulation bed. A split-thickness sheet graft is more cosmetic than a pinch or punch graft because the thickness of the graft and orientation of the hair are uniform and coverage by the graft is more complete.

A mechanical dermatome or a free-hand knife (Watson Skin Graft Knife, Down's Surgical, Sheffield, England) is used to split the dermis. The latter is preferred because it is easy and economical to use. General anesthesia is necessary to obtain the graft; split-thickness donor sites are very painful to the horse, because many nerve endings are exposed. Grafts less than 0.5-mm thickness in the horse lack strength, durability, and have sparse or no hair follicles or exocrine glands, which results in less sebaceous secretion. Grafts harvested between 0.63 and 0.75 mm have good coverage of hair and greater durability than do thinner grafts.[96,97] Unlike full-thickness grafts, suturing of the donor site is not required and primary graft contraction is minimal because a portion of the dermis remains intact and heals with a scarred appearance.[97]

The grafts can be applied to the wound after the horse has recovered from general anesthesia. This reduces anesthesia time and the possibility of damage to the graft during the recovery process. The graft can then be affixed to the wound with the horse standing without using local anesthesia by overlapping and gluing the graft with cyanoacrylate to the skin surrounding the wound. To increase graft success in an area that is difficult to immobilize, such as the fetlock or hock, the graft can be further secured by suturing the graft to its recipient bed with simple interrupted absorbable sutures (**Fig. 19**). Meshing grafts greatly enhances graft acceptance by preventing mechanical disruption of the graft from its vascular supply by exudate. Fenestration of the graft also enables topically applied antimicrobial agents to contact the graft bed and allow for the escape of fluid produced by the wound.[95,97]

Although proper graft bed preparation and grafting techniques are important for successful graft application, successful graft acceptance depends greatly on attention to postoperative care. During the initial 4 to 10 days the graft may become edematous and pale. These changes are from a loss of blood supply caused by vessel constriction and the expulsion of erythrocytes while the graft is nourished by passive imbibing nutrients onto its open vessels from the granulating bed by way of plasmatic imbibition. By day 10 the graft typically has a complete union to the graft bed. The epidermis might necrose and slough in some regions of the graft. Generally, only the

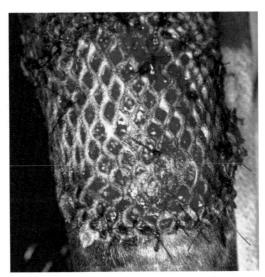

Fig.19. Meshed split-thickness graft on the dorsal metatarsus. Suturing the graft to its recipient bed with simple interrupted sutures minimizes displacement of the grafts and mechanical disruption from the graft bed.

superficial areas of the graft have been lost and small areas of dermis surrounded by granulation tissue are present. The epidermis regenerates from migration of epithelial cells present in the remaining sebaceous glands, sweat glands, and hair follicles (**Fig. 20**).

Periodic bandage changes allow for a clean environment and recognition of graft failure. For many horses frequent bandage changes aid in comfort. Soaking the inner

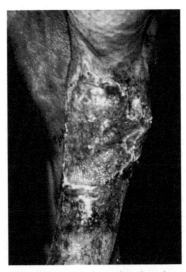

Fig. 20. Meshed split-thickness graft applied to the dorsal tarsus 7 days previously. The epidermis has sloughed and necrosed in some places where the graft is pale, which can be mistakenly interpreted as a graft failure. The epidermis regenerates from the migration of epithelial cells present.

bandage with sterile saline for 5 minutes and then carefully removing the bandage prevents destruction of many grafts. The presence of purulent material on the initial bandage change does not have a detrimental effect on acceptance of individual grafts. Silver sulfadiazine in a 1% water-miscible cream is effective against most gram-positive and gram-negative organisms and may enhance wound epithelialization. Additional immobilization gained with a cast is usually unnecessary to facilitate acceptance of grafts after 10 to 14 days. Immobilization may, however, lessen edema and decrease the possibility of self-mutilation.[8,96,97] Persistence in regrafting on horses that self-mutilate wounds has resulted in satisfactory wound healing in most cases.

SUMMARY

Complications of wounds and cosmetic surgery although frequent can be accurately managed with a combination of timely surgical and medical intervention to ensure the best possible outcome. The lack of soft tissue protection and a large quantity of susceptible synovial, tendon, ligament, and neurovascular structures make early and meticulous evaluation of limb wounds critical. Radiographs of traumatized areas should be performed in all cases of distal limb wounds. Devitalized bone subject to sequestrum formation may not be evident initially. Ultrasonography provides information about the details of soft tissue structures and radiolucent foreign material.

Chronic wounds should be considered infected and may become afflicted with sarcoid, *Pythium* spp, *Habronema* spp, or *Draschia* spp and rarely squamous cell carcinoma. Identification of pathologic tissue from a biopsy sample of the wound confirms the diagnosis. MRSA infections can consequently be difficult to treat and are associated with increased morbidity, mortality, and treatment costs, compared with infections caused by methicillin-susceptible *S aureus* strains. Penetrating wounds of the abdomen or thorax have a guarded prognosis resulting from the ensuing potential for infection and pneumothorax. Gunshot wounds limited to the skeletal muscles have a good prognosis, whereas injuries that involve vital organs decrease survivability.

Skin grafting is usually used following a period of open wound management and after healthy granulation tissue formation. Skin graft may be applied to fresh wounds that are vascular enough rapidly to produce granulation tissue. Failure to adhere to these basic principles in wound care results in poor graft survival.

REFERENCES

1. Hendrix SM, Baxter GM. Management of complicated wounds. Vet Clin North Am Equine Pract 2005;21(1):217–30.
2. Clem MF, Debowes RM, Yovich JV, et al. Osseous sequestration in horses, a review of 68 cases. Vet Surg 1988;11:2–5.
3. Clem MF, Debowes RM, Yovich JV, et al. Osseous sequestration in horses. Compend Contin Educ Pract Vet 1987;9:1219–24.
4. Moens Y, Vershooten F, DeMoor A, et al. Bone sequestration as a consequence of limb wounds in the horse. Vet Radiol 1980;21:40–4.
5. Gift LJ, DeBowes RM. Wounds associated with osseous sequestration and penetrating foreign bodies. Vet Clin North Am Equine Pract 1989;5(3):659–708.
6. Booth LC, Feeney DA. Superficial osteitis and sequestrum formation as a result of skin avulsion in the horse. Vet Surg 1982;11:2–8.
7. Cartee RE, Rumpg PF. Ultrasonic detection of fistulous tracts and foreign objects in muscles of horse. J Am Vet Med Assoc 1984;184:1127–32.

8. Stashak TS. Wound management and reconstructive surgery of problems associated with the distal limbs. In: Equine wound management. Philadelphia: Lea & Febiger; 1991. p. 163–217.

9. Latenser J, Snow SN, Mohs FE, et al. Power drills to fenestrate exposed bone to stimulate wound healing. J Dermatol Surg Oncol 1991;17:265–70.

10. Hurwitz DJ. Osseous interference of soft tissue healing. Surg Clin North Am 1984; 64:699–704.

11. Silver IA. Basic physiology of wound healing in the horse. Equine Vet J 1982;14: 7–15.

12. Wilmink JA, Stolk PW, VanWeeren PR, et al. Differences in second-intention wound healing between horses and ponies: macroscopic aspects. Equine Vet J 1999;31:53–60.

13. Caron JP, Barber SM, Doige CE, et al. The radiographic and histologic appearance of controlled surgical manipulation of the equine periosteum. Vet Surg 1987;16:13–20.

14. Bradley DM, Swaim SF, Stuart SW. An animal model for research on wound healing over exposed bone. Vet Comp Orthop Traumatol 1998;11:131–5.

15. Bailin PL, Wheeland RG. Carbon dioxide (CO2) laser perforation of exposed cranial bone to stimulate granulation tissue. Plast Reconstr Surg 1985;75:898–902.

16. Cabbage EB, Korock SW, Malik PA. Skin grafting denuded skull. Ann Plast Surg 1982;8:318–21.

17. Brown PW. The fate of exposed bone. Am J Surg 1979;137:464–9.

18. Specht TE, Colahan PT. Osteostixis for incomplete cortical fracture of the third metacarpal bone: results in 11 horses. Vet Surg 1990;19:34–40.

19. Lee AH, Swaim SF, Newton JC, et al. Wound healing over denuded bone. J Am Anim Hosp Assoc 1987;23:75–84.

20. Johnson RJ. The effects of cortical fenestration on second intention healing of wounds over exposed bone of the distal aspect of the limb of horses. Masters Thesis, Auburn University July 11, 2000.

21. Adam EN, Southwood LL. Surgical and traumatic wound infections, cellulitis, and myositis in horses. Vet Clin North Am Equine Pract 2006;12:335–61.

22. Baxter GM. Wound management. In: White NA, Moore JN, editors. Current techniques in equine surgery and lameness. 2nd edition. Philadelphia: WB Saunders; 1998. p. 72–80.

23. Farstvedt EG, Hendrickson DA, Dickenson CE, et al. Treatment of suppurative facial cellulitis and panniculitis caused by *Corynebacterium pseudotuberculosis* in two horses. J Am Vet Med Assoc 2004;224:1139–42.

24. Belknap JK, Baxter GM, Nickels FA. Extensor tendon laceration in horses: 50 cases (1982–1988). J Am Vet Med Assoc 1993;203(3):428–31.

25. Bertone AL. Tendon lacerations. Vet Clin North Am Equine Pract 1995;11(2): 293–314.

26. Fubini SL. Burns. In: Robinson NE, editor. Current therapy in equine medicine 2. Philadelphia: WB Saunders; 1987. p. 639–41.

27. Fox SM. Management of a large thermal burn in a horse. Comp Cont Educ Pract Vet 1988;10:88–95.

28. Hanson RR. Management of burn injury in the horse. Vet Clin North Am Equine Pract 2005;21:105–23.

29. Johnston DE. Burns: electrical, chemical and cold injuries. In: Slatter D, editor. Textbook of small animal surgery. Philadelphia: WB Saunders; 1985. p. 516–33.

30. Fox SM, Goring RI, Probst CW. Management of thermal burn injuries, Part II. Compend Cont Educ Pract Vet 1986;8:439–44.

31. Schumacher J, Watkins JP, Wilson JP, et al. Burn induced neoplasia in two horses. Equine Vet J 1986;18:410–3.

32. Baxter GM. Management of burns. In: Colahan PT, Mayhew IG, Merritt AM, editors. Equine medicine and surgery. 5th edition. St. Louis (MO): Mosby; 1999. p. 1843–7.

33. Warden GD. Outpatient care of thermal injuries. Surg Clin North Am 1987;67: 147–57.

34. Bailey JV, Jacobs KA. The mesh expansion method of suturing wounds on the legs of horses. Vet Surg 1983;12(2):78–82.

35. Geiser D, Walker RD. Management of large animal thermal injuries. Compend Cont Educ Pract Vet 1985;7:S69–78.

36. Cefai C, Ashurst S, Owens C. Human carriage of methicillin-resistant *Staphylococcus aureus* linked with pet dog. Lancet 1994;344:539–40.

37. Loeffler AK, Boag J, Sung JA, et al. Prevalence of methicillin-resistant *Staphylococcus aureus* among staff and pets in a small animal referral hospital in the UK. J Antimicrob Chemother 2005;56:692–7.

38. Weese JS, Archambault M, Willey BM, et al. Methicillin-resistant *Staphylococcus aureus* in horses and horse personnel, 2000–2002. Emerg Infect Dis 2005;11: 430–5.

39. Weese JS, Rousseau J, Traub-Dargatz JL, et al. Community-associated methicillin-resistant *Staphylococcus aureus* in horses and humans who work with horses. J Am Vet Med Assoc 2005;226:580–3.

40. Blot SI, Vandewoude KH, Hoste EA, et al. Outcome and attributable mortality in critically ill patients with bacteremia involving methicillin-susceptible and methicillin-resistant *Staphylococcus aureus*. Arch Intern Med 2002;162: 2229–35.

41. Engemann JJ, Carmeli Y, Cosgrove SE, et al. Adverse clinical and economic outcomes attributable to methicillin resistance among patients with *Staphylococcus aureus* surgical site infection. Clin Infect Dis 2003;36:592–8.

42. Melzer M, Eykyn SJ, Graunsden WR, et al. Is methicillin-resistant *Staphylococcus aureus* more virulent than methicillin-susceptible *S. aureus*? A comparative cohort study of British patients with nosocomial infection and bacteremia. Clin Infect Dis 2003;37:1453–60.

43. Manian FA. Asymptomatic nasal carriage of mupirocin-resistant, methicillin-resistant *Staphylococcus aureus* (MRSA) in a pet dog associated with MRSA infection in household contacts. Clin Infect Dis 2003;36:e26–8.

44. Greene N, Holtom PD, Warren CA, et al. In vitro elution of tobramycin and vancomycin polymethyl-methacrylate beads and spaces from simplex and palacos. Am J Orthop 1998;27:201–5.

45. Weese JS, Lefebvre SL. Risk factors for methicillin-resistant *Staphylococcus aureus* colonization in horses admitted to a veterinary teaching hospital. Can Vet J 2007;48(9):921–6.

46. Trostle SS, Peavy CL, King DS, et al. Treatment of methicillin-resistant *Staphylococcus epidermidis* infection following repair of an ulnar fracture and humeroradial joint luxation in a horse. J Am Vet Med Assoc 2001;218:554–9.

47. Schnellmann C, Gerber V, Rossano A, et al. Presence of new mec(A) and mph(C) variants conferring antibiotic resistance in *Staphylococcus* spp isolated from the skin of horses before and after clinic admission. J Clin Microbiol 2006;44(12): 4444–54.

48. Visavada BG, Honneysett J, Danford MH. Manuka honey dressing: an effective treatment for chronic wound infections. Br J Oral Maxillofac Surg 2008;46:55–6.

49. Wright JB, Lam K, Burrell RE. Wound management in an era of increasing bacterial antibiotic resistance: a role for topical silver treatment. Am J Infect Control 1998;26(6):572–7.
50. Wertheim HFL, Verveer J, Boelens HAM, et al. Effect of mupirocin treatment on nasal, pharyngeal, and perineal carriage of Staphylococcus aureus in healthy adults. Antimicrob Agents Chemother 2005;49:1465–7.
51. Muller A, Talon D, Potier A, et al. Use of intranasal mupirocin to prevent methicillin-resistant Staphylococcus aureus infection in intensive care units. Crit Care 2005;9(3):R246–50.
52. Santschi LM. Diagnosis and management of surgical site infection and antimicrobial prophylaxis. In: Auer JA, Stick JA, editors. Equine surgery. 2nd edition. Philadelphia: WB Saunders; 1999. p. 55–60.
53. Holcombe SJ, Schneider RK, Bramlage LR, et al. Use of antibiotic-impregnated polymethyl methacrylate in horses with open or infected fractures or joints: 19 cases (1987–1995). J Am Vet Med Assoc 1997;211:889–93.
54. Swalec Tobias KM, Schneider RK, Besser TE. The use of anitmicrobial-impregnated polymethyl methacrylate. J Am Vet Med Assoc 1996;208:841–5.
55. Kawcak CE, Stashak TS. Predisposing factors, diagnosis and management of large abdominal wall defects in horses and cattle. J Am Vet Med Assoc 1995; 206(5):607–11.
56. Holcombe SJ, Laverty S. Thoracic trauma. In: Auer JA, Stick JA, editors. Equine surgery. 2nd edition. Philadelphia: WB Saunders; 1999. p. 382–5.
57. Vatistas NJ, Meagher DM, Gillis CL, et al. Gunshot injuries in horses: 22 cases (1971–1993). J Am Vet Med Assoc 1995;207:1198–200.
58. Bartmann CP, Wohlsein P. Injuries caused by outside violence with forensic importance in horses. DTSCH Tierarztl Wochenschr 2002;109:112–5.
59. Poole HM, Brashier MK. Equine cutaneous pythiosis. Compend Contin Educ Pract Vet 2003;25:229–36.
60. Reis JL, Queiroz de Carvallo C, Nogueira RH, et al. Disseminated pythiosis in three horses. J Vet Microbiol 2003;96:289–95.
61. Worster AA, Lillich JD, Cox JH, et al. Pythiosis with bone lesions in a pregnant mare. J Am Vet Med Assoc 2000;216:1795–8.
62. Hensel P, Greene CE, Medleau L, et al. Immunotherapy for treatment of multicentric cutaneous pythiosis in a dog. J Am Vet Med Assoc 2003;223:215–8.
63. Vasey JR. Equine cutaneous habronemiasis. Compend Contin Educ Pract Vet 1981;8:290–8.
64. Scott DW. Habronemiasis. In: Large animal dermatology. Philadelphia: WB Saunders; 1988. p. 251–5.
65. Von Tscharner C, Kunkle G, Yager J. Nodular diseases. Vet Demmatol 2000;11: 179–86.
66. White SD, Evans AG. Parasitic skin diseases. In: Smith PB, editor. Large animal internal medicine. St Louis (MO): CV Mosby; 2002. p. 1221–2.
67. Moriello KA, DeBoer DJ, Semrad SD. Diseases of skin. In: Reed SM, Bayly WM, editors. Equine internal medicine. Philadelphia: WB Saunders; 1988. p. 536.
68. Rees CA, Craig TM. Cutaneous habronemiasis. In: Robinson NE, editor. Current therapy in equine medicine 5. St. Louis (MO): WB Saunders; 2003. p. 195–200.
69. Herd RP, Donham JC. Efficacy of ivermectin against cutaneous Draschia and Habronema infection (summer sores) in horses. Am J Vet Res 1981;42:1953–5.
70. Novick M, Gard DA, Hardy SB, et al. Burn scar carcinoma: a review and analysis of 46 cases. J Trauma 1977;17:809–17.

71. Baird AN, Frelier PF. Squamous cell carcinoma originating from an epithelial scar in a horse. J Am Vet Med Assoc 1990;196:1999–2000.
72. Rogers K, Barrington GM, Parish SM. Squamous cell carcinoma originating from a cutaneous scar in a llama. Can Vet J 1997;38:643–4.
73. Paterson S. Treatment of superficial ulcerative squamous cell carcinoma in three horses with topical 5-fluorouracil. Vet Rec 1997;141:626–8.
74. Theon AP, Pascoe JR. Iridium-192 brachytherapy for equine periocular tumors: treatments results and prognostic factors in 115 horses. Equine Vet J 1995;27: 117–21.
75. England JJ, Watson RE, Larson K. Virus like particles in an equine sarcoid cell line. Am J Vet Res 1973;34:1601–3.
76. Cheevers WP, Faemi-Ninie S, Anderson LW. Spontaneous expression of an endogenous retrovirus by the equine sarcoid derived Mc-1 cell line. Am J Vet Res 1986;47:50–2.
77. Baldwin RW. Mechanism of immunity in cancer. Pathobio Ann 1981;11:155–75.
78. Nasir L, Reid SWJ. Bovine papillomaviral gene expression equine sarcoids. Virus Res 1999;61:171–5.
79. Reid SWJ, Smith KT, Jarrett WFH. Detection, cloning, and characterization of papillomaviral DNA present in sarcoid tumors of *Equus asinus*. Vet Rec 1994; 135:430–2.
80. Brandt S, Haralambus R, Schoster A, et al. Peripheral blood mononuclear cells represent a reservoir of bovine papillomavirus DNA in sarcoid-affected equines. J Gen Virol 2008;89(Pt 6):1390–5.
81. Wilmink JM, Van Weeren PR. Treatment of exuberant granulation tissue. Clin Tech Equine Pract 2004;3(2):141–7.
82. Knottenbelt DC. A suggested clinical classification for the equine sarcoid. Clin Tech Equine Pract 2005;4(4):278–95.
83. Knottenbelt DC, Edwards SER, Daniel EA. The diagnosis and treatment of equine sarcoid. In Pract 1995;17:123–9.
84. Carr EA, Theon AP, Madewell BR, et al. Bovine papillomavirus DNA in neoplastic and non-neoplastic tissues obtained from horses with and without sarcoids in the western United States. Am J Vet Res 2001;62(5): 741–4.
85. Meagher DM, Adams OR. Split thickness autologous skin transplantation in horses. J Am Vet Med Assoc 1971;159:55–60.
86. Booth L. Equine wound reconstruction using free skin grafting. Calif Vet 1991;45: 13–6.
87. French DA, Fretz PB. Treatment of equine leg wounds using skin grafts: thirty-five cases, 1975–1988. Can Vet J 1990;31:761–5.
88. Teh BT. Why do skin grafts fail? Plast Reconstr Surg 1979;63:323–32.
89. Hanson RR. Management of avulsion wounds with exposed bone. Clinical Tech Equine Pract 2004;3(2):188–203.
90. Robeson MC, Edstrom LE, Krizek TJ. The efficacy of systemic antibiotics in the treatment of granulating wounds. J Surg Res 1974;16:299–306.
91. Schumacher J, Hanselka DV. Skin grafting of the horse. Vet Clin North Am Equine Pract 1989;5:591–614.
92. Carson-Dunkerly SA, Hanson RR. Equine skin grafting principles and field applications. Comp Contin Educ Pract Veterin 1997;19:872–82.
93. Caron JP. Skin grafting. In: Auer JA, Stick JA, editors. Equine surgery. 2nd edition. Philadelphia: WB Saunders; 1999. p. 152–66.

94. Holder TEC, Schumacher J, Donnell RL, et al. Effects of hyperbaric oxygen on full-thickness meshed sheet skin grafts applied to fresh and granulating wounds in horses. Am J Vet Res 2008;69:144–7.

95. Tobin GR. The compromised bed technique: an improved method for skin grafting problem wounds. Surg Clin North Am 1985;64:653–8.

96. Booth LC. Split thickness autogenous skin transplantation in the horse. J Am Vet Med Assoc 1982;180:754–7.

97. Hanselka DV. Use of autogenous mesh grafts in equine wound management. J Am Vet Med Assoc 1974;164:35–41.

Complications of Ophthalmic Surgery in the Horse

Dennis E. Brooks, DVM, PhD

KEYWORDS

- Horse • Conjunctival graft • Penetrating keratoplasty
- Complications • Surgery • Ophthalmic

COMPLICATIONS OF OPHTHALMIC SURGERY

Advances in the understanding of ophthalmic diseases of the horse and improved microsurgical technologies now allow for more complicated ophthalmic surgical procedures to be successfully performed on the equine eyelids, cornea, lens, and vitreous and for the successful treatment of equine glaucoma. A discussion of the common complications of selected ophthalmic surgical procedures in the horse can perhaps reduce their occurrence and minimize the degree of ocular dysfunction per occurrence.

EYELIDS
Traumatic Eyelid Lacerations

Indications
Lacerations of the eyelids should be repaired promptly to inhibit formation of cicatricial eyelid deformities, prevent a reduction in eyelid blinking function, and reduce the chance of infections and exposure-induced damage to the cornea.[1] Corneal ulcerations, globe perforation, uveitis, periorbital fractures, and orbital cellulitis or abscessation can accompany eyelid lacerations.

Technique of eyelid laceration repair
Surgery to repair a small eyelid laceration may be performed with sedation and local anesthesia alone, whereas severe lacerations that need sophisticated blepharoplastic repair require the animal to be under general anesthesia.[1,2] The eyelids have a rich vascular supply and generally do not require removal of tissue of questionable viability. Even desiccated avulsed eyelids are capable of revascularization after surgical repair.[1,2] For this reason, and because of the concern for exposure keratitis, it is imperative that eyelid tissue tags and pedicles not be amputated and, instead, replaced to as near normal an anatomic position as possible.

Department of Large Animal Clinical Sciences, College of Veterinary Medicine, University of Florida, 2015 SW 16 Avenue, Gainesville, FL 32608, USA
E-mail address: dbrooks@ufl.edu

Vet Clin Equine 24 (2009) 697–734
doi:10.1016/j.cveq.2008.08.001
0749-0739/08/$ – see front matter
vetequine.theclinics.com
© 2009 Elsevier Inc. All rights reserved.

It is wise to consider culturing a traumatic eyelid wound of any long-standing duration before suturing the defect. Thorough flushing of the affected area with saline and a dilute povidone-iodine (2%) solution should be performed to clean the area. The first step taken in the surgical repair is to appose the lid margin accurately.[1,2] A figure-of-eight suture is placed on the eyelid margin, which allows for knot placement away from the cornea. The remainder of the defect is closed in two layers: a deep layer in the palpebral conjunctiva with 4-0 to 6-0 absorbable suture material in a simple interrupted or simple continuous pattern starting at the eyelid margin and a superficial layer through the skin with 4-0 to 5-0 nonabsorbable suture material in a simple interrupted pattern. Sutures are usually left in place for 7 to 10 days.

Administration of topical and systemic antibiotics, systemic anti-inflammatory drugs, and tetanus toxoid are important for postoperative medical care. Protection of the cornea is absolutely imperative if the lids are swollen or compromised in such a way that the cornea is perpetually exposed. Some eyes may need a temporary tarsorrhaphy.

Complications

Some dehiscence of the eyelid margin nearly always occurs after surgery (**Figs. 1–7**). This margin breakdown can cause varying amounts of lid misalignment with resulting entropion or ectropion. Gaping of the conjunctival side of the incision because of poor suture placement can slow healing and allow suture(s) to rub on the cornea, resulting

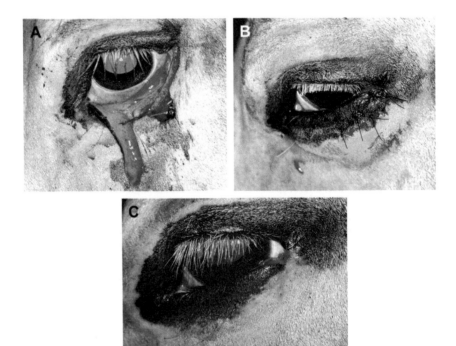

Fig. 1. (*A*) Extensive lower lid laceration is repaired by means of a standard two-layer closure. (*B*) Lid swelling in eyelid laceration repair is common immediately after surgery. (*C*) There is slight dehiscence of the lid margin in the eye 3 weeks after surgery. No further repair was necessary.

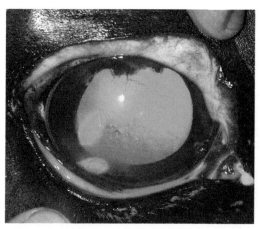

Fig. 2. Removal of the torn upper lid resulted in nonhealing corneal ulcers. Grid keratotomy and medical therapy resolved the ulcers in the short term, but this horse is still at risk for further ulcers.

in painful corneal ulcers. These sutures would need to be replaced or removed. Skin sutures can also become infected.

Intralesional injection of topical anesthetics would cause a performance animal to test positive during a postperformance drug test. Communication with trainers and owners is imperative, but lid pedicle amputation, especially of the upper eyelid, should never be recommended.

Lacerations of the eyelids near the medial canthus may involve the nasolacrimal apparatus and affect tear drainage. The integrity of the duct should be tested by close examination and the passage of fluorescein sodium dye through the nasolacrimal duct.[1–4]

Entropion

Indications
Entropion is the inward rolling of the eyelid margin to allow contact of eyelid hairs with the cornea.[1,2] Clinical signs include excessive tearing and blepharospasm in addition to variable amounts of keratitis and conjunctivitis. Entropion is most often seen in foals and may be anatomic from too much eyelid skin; secondary to enophthalmos from

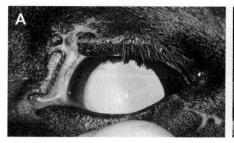
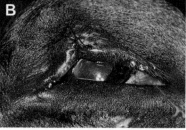

Fig. 3. (*A*) Entropion/ectropion and a corneal ulcer resulted because of scar tissue formation after trauma to the upper eyelid. (*B*) Scar tissue was broken down, and the lid margin was realigned and sutured in the eye.

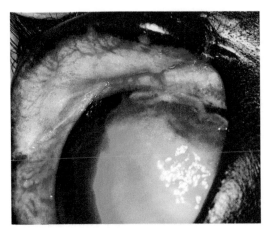

Fig. 4. Suture in the subconjunctival layer in this eye was exposed to cause an ulcer. The suture was removed.

ocular pain; or associated with dehydration, malnutrition, or atrophy of orbital fat from the cachexia present in debilitating systemic diseases. Because the growing foal has a dynamic facial conformation, permanent surgical correction is not recommended until maturity is reached.

Entropion is rarely anatomic in adult horses and is generally associated with spasms of the orbicularis oculi muscle as a result of chronic irreversible ocular pain, or it may be cicatricial as a result of previous eyelid trauma. Topical anesthetics and a local nerve block facilitate differentiation between any existing primary anatomic component of the entropion and any secondary entropic contribution of spasm.

Temporary entropion surgery in foals

Ocular lubricants, and sometimes temporary eversion of the offending eyelid with vertical mattress sutures or staples, are helpful for treating entropion in foals. In rare

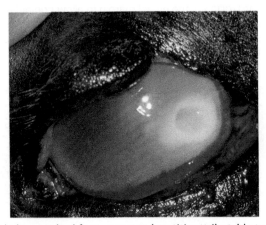

Fig. 5. Large fungal ulcer resulted from exposure keratitis attributable to failure to close an upper eyelid laceration properly. The ulcer appeared after general anesthesia for colic surgery. A conjunctival transplant graft was later used to aid in healing of the ulcer.

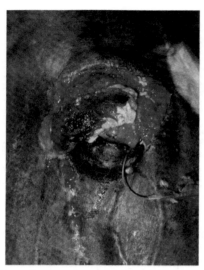

Fig. 6. Skin graft is sloughing after complete avulsion of the upper lid and bony portions of the supraorbital process. Further attempts to form an upper lid also failed; the eye was enucleated, and blepharoplasties were used to cover the cutaneous defect.

cases, eyelid eversion can reduce the strength and ability of the tarsal plate to hold the lid margin in position if the sutures or staples are not removed in 10 to 14 days. Chronic lid margin flaccidity, entropion, and blepharospasm in the adult horse are the result if the sutures or staples are not removed in the foal (**Fig. 8**).

Entropion surgical technique (modified Hotz-Celsus procedure)

The goal of surgical correction of entropion should be slight undercorrection.[1,2] The modified Hotz-Celsus procedure is particularly useful for dealing with most entropion conditions in the adult horse.[2] The procedure is simple and involves removing a crescent-shaped piece of skin and orbicularis muscle. The initial incision is made with a number 15 scalpel blade 2 mm from the eyelid margin; its length depends on the

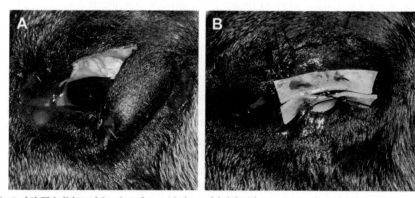

Fig. 7. (*A*) This lid avulsion is at least 10 days old. (*B*) Lid was sutured, and a temporary tarsorrhaphy was placed to reduce lid movement and tension on the incision during the healing phase.

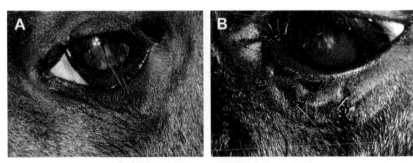

Fig. 8. (A) Entropion in a yearling caused by temporary lid tacking for entropion when it was a foal. There was no muscular tone to hold the lower eyelid off the cornea. (B) Hotz-Celsus entropion procedure was used to repair the condition.

amount of eyelid margin that is entropic. A second elliptic incision made parallel to the first joins the two ends of the first incision. The width of the piece of tissue to be excised should have been previously determined while examining the nonsedated horse. After the skin is incised to the depth of the orbicularis oculi muscle, the skin and a portion of this muscle are undermined and excised with scissors. The defect is then closed using 4-0 to 6-0 nonabsorbable suture material in a simple interrupted pattern. The suture ends adjacent to the cornea are trimmed short to avoid irritation of the cornea. The sutures are left in place for 10 to 14 days.

Complications

Eyelid swelling is common after surgery. If the excised piece of tissue is too narrow, undercorrection of the entropion results, whereas removal of too wide a piece of skin results in ectropion. Ectropion and exposure keratitis with ulcers can result from overcorrection of the entropion. Suture ends can rub on the cornea to cause ulcers and should be removed. Sutures can become infected to cause cutaneous abscesses.

Laser as an Alternative Surgical Technique for Eyelid Tumor Removal

Care must be used in removing superficial or deep eyelid margin or third eyelid (TE) tumors with carbon dioxide (CO_2) or other lasers, because any heat generated can adversely affect the cornea. Melting ulcers are a serious complication in such cases (**Fig. 9**).

NICTITANS
Nictitans or Third-Eyelid Flaps

Indications

The TE, nictitans, or nictitating membrane lies in the ventral-medial orbit of horses, where it produces some of the tears and also acts like a windshield wiper to distribute the precorneal tear film. It consists of a "T"-shaped piece of hyaline cartilage and a large seromucoid gland surrounding the base of the cartilage.[1,2]

TE flaps provide physical support to a weakened cornea, reduce contamination of the surface of injured corneas, and minimize tear evaporation from the exposed corneas of exophthalmic globes. Nictitating membrane flaps do not provide plasma-derived antiproteases to melting ulcers and are not a source of collagen to replace missing corneal tissue. They are indicated in superficial nonhealing and noninfected corneal ulcers, in ulcers caused by facial nerve paralysis, and also to reinforce

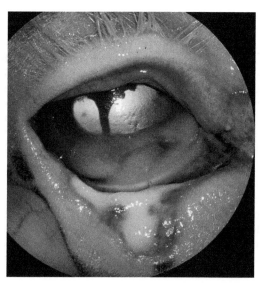

Fig. 9. Heat from a laser used to treat a TE tumor was excessive and induced corneal melting with a complicating *Pseudomonas* infection that slowly responded to topical and systemic antibiotics.

a conjunctival graft.[5] TE flaps are contraindicated for melting corneal ulcers in horses because they do not provide a blood supply or fibrovascular tissues to the ulcer. In addition, they may make it impossible to observe the progression of the disease visually, impede the penetration of topical medications to the cornea, and cause the retention of inflammatory exudates adjacent to the corneal lesion.[5,6]

Technique for third-eyelid flap
General anesthesia is recommended for performing a TE flap. Formation of a TE flap with attachment to the upper eyelid is performed by placing two to four horizontal mattress sutures through stents high in the upper eyelid and dorsal fornix of the desired location. Direct the needle (4-0 suture) through the anterior face of the TE approximately 3 mm from the leading edge and then again through the fornix to the skin adjacent to the first bite. These sutures should pass through the cartilage but not be full thickness in the TE. The flap can be released in 7 to 10 days.[5]

Complications
Cartilage of the TE can be deformed to cause corneal irritation and can necessitate TE removal. Sutures can rub on the cornea and cause an ulcer if placed too low in the fornix. The skin can be ulcerated from the sutures if stents are not used. The globe can rupture behind the flap if not carefully monitored.

Surgical Technique for Removal of the Third Eyelid

Indications
Surgical removal of the TE is strictly reserved for malignant neoplasia of the TE or a nictitans so severely traumatized that it interferes with nictitans and globe function.

Technique
It is possible to remove the entire nictitans with heavy sedation and sensory nerve blocks in most standing horses. The dorsal margin of the TE is gently grasped with

small hemostats or toothed forceps, and the TE is pulled up and outward. A curved hemostat is positioned and clamped below the mass halfway across the base of the TE at the most ventral region of the TE. This minimizes postoperative hemorrhage. A second curved hemostat is positioned and clamped opposite the first hemostat, such that the base of the TE is completely clamped. A number 15 blade is used to cut the TE and neoplastic tissue along the hemostats. The hemostats are left clamped for 2 to 3 minutes after TE removal. The conjunctival area at the base of the TE can be carefully sutured with 5-0 Vicryl but is generally not sutured and is left to granulate. Hemorrhage after surgery is slight in this author's experience but can be controlled with pressure and light cautery. Topical antibiotics are indicated for 5 to 7 days after surgery.

Complications

Complications, although rare, include orbital fat prolapse, slight hemorrhage, keratoconjunctivitis sicca (KCS), or superficial keratitis. TE cartilage incompletely excised can irritate the cornea to cause entropion, conjunctivitis, and infection. The absence of a TE can alter nasal lid conformation, such that environmental debris accumulates and causes persistent inflammation of the nasal conjunctiva and eyelids.

CORNEA
Corneal Lacerations

Indications

Full-thickness corneal lacerations with or without iris prolapse require surgical correction. If the laceration involves the limbus, the adjacent sclera under the conjunctiva should be carefully examined.

Technique

The aim of the repair is to restore corneal integrity and achieve a watertight seal. A prolapsed iris should be amputated, and any hemorrhage should be controlled with pressure or careful and gentle iris cautery. Simple interrupted sutures (7-0 to 8-0 suture) are placed to close the laceration, and the anterior chamber is reformed with lactated Ringer's solution (LRS). The sutures should be perpendicular to the laceration, enter and leave the cornea 1 mm from the wound margin, and be placed two thirds of the thickness of the corneal stroma. Superficial sutures result in incision gaping, and sutures that penetrate the cornea result in microleaks of aqueous humor. Suture tension should be appositional rather than compressive, because some corneal edema is present. The lacerations may be covered with a conjunctival pedicle graft if corneal melting is present. A small syringe with a 25- or 27-gauge needle can be used to reform the anterior chamber with sterile LRS.

Complications

Dehiscence, aqueous humor microleaks, anterior and posterior synechia, corneal infection, infectious endophthalmitis, uveitis, cataract, blindness, and phthisis can occur after the surgical repair of a corneal laceration. Reforming the anterior chamber with sterile water can result in corneal edema (**Fig. 10**). Microleaks must be repaired or persistent uveitis and blindness can result. Leaks around sutures necessitate removal and replacement of the suture. Incisional microleaks require placement of more sutures or repositioning of existing sutures. A leak through a perforation of the tissue can be managed by tissue glue, conjunctival or amniotic grafting, or corneal transplantation. Synechia can realistically only be dealt with pharmacologically. Combined 1% atropine and 2.5% phenylephrine applied topically can aid in breakdown of adhesions.

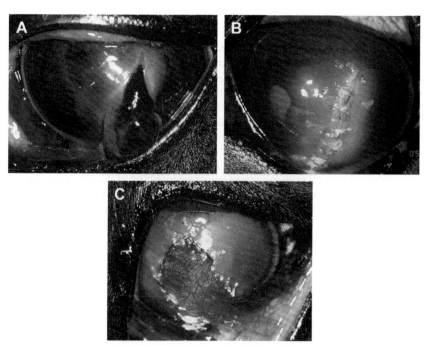

Fig. 10. (*A*) Large traumatic corneal laceration with iris prolapse is present. (*B*) Anterior chamber is shallow, the hyphema is resorbing, and the intraocular pressure is still slightly low after suturing of the incision 1 week after surgery of the eye. (*C*) Conjunctival pedicle graft covers the leaking incision 1 week later in the eye.

Tissue plasminogen activator (TPA) can be injected into the anterior chamber to remove large fibrin adhesions.

Melting Ulcers and Keratectomy, Conjunctival Grafts, and Amniotic Membrane Grafts

Indications
Melting ulcers in horses are sight threatening because they can rapidly lead to globe rupture. This aggressive form of ulcerative keratitis is associated with high levels of tear film proteolytic activity. Neutralizing and normalizing proteolytic activity in the tear film is an important objective of the medical and surgical treatment of melting corneal ulcers in horses.[2,7,8] Melting ulcers that are nonresponsive to medical therapy, ulcers deeper than one half of the thickness of the cornea, and full-thickness corneal perforations with iris prolapse require surgical therapy.[2,5,7] In these cases, superficial keratectomy or direct surgical debridement in conjunction with conjunctival, corneal, or amniotic membrane (AM) transplant grafts is required.

Keratectomy

Indications
A keratectomy involves removal of the corneal epithelium and a portion of the stroma. Keratectomy speeds healing of melting ulcers by removing necrotic and infected tissue, encouraging vascularization, minimizing scarring, and decreasing the stimulus for anterior uveitis.[5,7] It may also be done to prepare the cornea for a conjunctival or amniotic graft.

Technique

Superficial layers of necrotic tissue in melting ulcers can be cut and removed with topical anesthesia, a cellulose sponge or cotton swab, and corneal or tenotomy scissors held parallel to the corneal surface.[5] A microsurgical blade can also be used to debride the epithelial layers before placement of a conjunctival or AM transplant graft.

Keratectomy for removal of deeper layers of degenerate cornea requires general anesthesia. A corneal incision is made to outline the lesion to be removed with a corneal trephine, a diamond knife, or a microsurgical blade. The depth of the incision in the stroma should be adequate to remove the lesion completely. The edge of the tissue to be removed is grasped by forceps, and a corneal dissector is introduced and held parallel to the cornea. The dissector is tangentially used to separate the corneal lamella without penetrating deeper than the original cutting plane. The cornea is then separated until the opposite incision line is reached.[5–7] Depending on the amount of the stromal defect, a conjunctival or amnion graft may then be placed.

Complications

The complications of superficial and deep keratectomy include infection, stromal granulation tissue formation, and globe perforation.[2,5–7] Topical cyclosporine A (CsA) can be used topically after healing of the cornea to reduce granulation tissue formation.

Conjunctival Transplant Grafts

Indications

The conjunctiva is a mucous membrane that begins at the eyelid margin, lines the insides of the eyelids, and then reflects at the fornix to extend over the sclera to end at the limbus. It is composed of nonkeratinized, stratified, squamous epithelium with goblet cells and an underlying fibrous Tenon's capsule. The bulbar conjunctiva is freely movable except near the limbus, whereas the palpebral conjunctiva is not movable.[5]

Conjunctival transplant grafts or flaps are frequently used in equine ophthalmology for the clinical treatment of melting corneal ulcers, deep stromal ulcers and descemetoceles, and perforated corneal ulcers with iris prolapse. Melting ulcers should always be stabilized with medical therapy before the surgical placement of the graft to provide a healthier cornea for suturing and to prevent proteinase digestion of any absorbable sutures that may hold the conjunctival graft in place.[2,3,5,9]

Conjunctival transplant autografts consist of a highly viable epithelium and a stroma with significant antibacterial, antifungal, antiproteinase, and anticollagenase effects. Plasma-derived antibodies and macroglobulin are placed in direct contact with the corneal ulcer bed. The fibrovascular or deeper layer of the conjunctival transplant graft offers fibroblasts and collagen with which to begin rebuilding the corneal stroma.[2,5,7] Although not as strong as corneal tissue, conjunctival transplant grafts do provide some physical support to the weakened cornea.[5]

There are different types of conjunctival transplant grafts based on the source of the mucosa (bulbar or palpebral) and the type of graft (total or 360°, bridge or bipedicle, hood or 180°, and the pedicle conjunctival graft). A 360° conjunctival transplant graft is used for large corneal lesions, but it covers the entire cornea, which makes vision impossible; it prevents monitoring of lesion progression; and it often leaves large blinding corneal scars.[2,5,7] The 360° conjunctival transplant graft is thus no longer recommended. Hood transplant flaps cover half of the cornea and are also associated with large scars. The bridge or bipedicle transplant flap is indicated for large melting ulcers in the central, dorsal paracentral, and lateral paracentral corneal regions. The pedicle or rotational transplant grafts from the dorsal or temporal bulbar conjunctiva are the most useful and versatile conjunctival transplant grafts because they generally leave smaller scars to have minimal effects on postoperative vision, allow for postoperative intraocular examination, and do not inhibit drug penetration to the cornea and anterior chamber.[2,5,7]

Conjunctival transplant grafts are usually harvested from adjacent bulbar conjunctiva.[2,5,7] The disadvantage of the palpebral-derived conjunctival graft is that the eyelids are mobile and some tension is applied after surgery during blinking to the sutures of the conjunctival graft, thereby leading to a higher rate of graft dehiscence. The bulbar conjunctival flap moves with the eye, such that little or no eyelid tension is applied to the sutured graft itself. It is also not recommended to use the conjunctiva near the nictitating membrane, because nictitans movement can put tension on the graft sutures to result in premature graft release.[2,5,7] Conjunctival transplant autografts should be thin and should not include Tenon's capsule or the bulbar fascia. The inclusion of Tenon's capsule may contribute to surgical failure by increasing postoperative traction on the transplanted conjunctival tissue.[2,5,7] Conjunctival grafts should have tension-relieving sutures placed at the limbus to prevent the graft from prematurely pulling away from the ulcer bed. With all the conjunctival graft types, it is important that the corneal graft bed and ulcer site be properly and carefully prepared. The recipient bed for the conjunctival graft is prepared by debridement of the epithelium surrounding the ulcer and removal of any necrotic corneal tissues. Great care should be taken to prevent corneal perforation during this debridement.[2,5–7]

Conjunctival transplant autografts are more difficult to perform than nictitating membrane flaps but simpler than operations, such as corneoconjunctival grafts, corneoscleral transpositions, and penetrating keratoplasty (PK).[5] They are also easier to perform in the horse than in other species, because horses have a great deal of mobile bulbar conjunctiva. Temporary tarsorrhaphy is often performed concurrently with conjunctival grafts to minimize blinking movement, prevent excessive lid trauma to the graft and its sutures, and encourage graft adherence to the stroma.[2,5,7]

Technique for pedicle conjunctival transplant graft

The pedicle conjunctival graft should be oriented such that the dissected conjunctival graft tissue is not rotated greater than 45° from its perilimbal conjunctival base of origin. Once the location for mobilizing the graft is determined, the conjunctiva is tented with 0.12-mm Colibri forceps and a small slit is made in the conjunctiva with Westcott scissors 1 to 2 mm from the limbus. This initial conjunctival incision is continued parallel to the limbus. The entire conjunctival flap site is then undermined using blunt dissection with Steven's tenotomy scissors. The underlying fibrous tissue (ie, Tenon's capsule) should be freed from the overlying conjunctiva so that the conjunctiva appears nearly transparent and permits visualization of the scissors' tips underneath the conjunctiva. The second incision is then made perpendicular to the first incision (and to the limbus) at the tip of the graft. The width of the incision should be 1 to 2 mm wider than the size of the corneal lesion to cover. The third and final incision is made parallel to the first, extending to the bulbar attachment of the graft.[2,5,7] The strip of conjunctiva thus created is then rotated to the cornea, such that the graft covers and sits on the corneal defect with no tension or retraction. The angle of rotation should not exceed 45°. The flap is then sutured to the cornea with simple interrupted sutures of 7-0 to 8-0 absorbable suture material positioned 1.0 to 1.5 mm apart. Two interrupted sutures may be placed at the limbus on either side of the graft to decrease the tension applied to the corneal recipient site. To prevent disruption of the blood supply, sutures are not placed within the pedicle portion of the graft or at the proximal portion of the lesion. Conjunctival grafts adhere to the corneal stroma of the lesion, but they do not usually adhere to the epithelium surrounding the flap.

Six to 8 weeks after placement of the flap, the blood supply can be interrupted by cutting the base of the flap at the limbus. The graft transection procedure can usually be performed with the use of topical anesthesia and Steven's tenotomy scissors. Eliminating the blood supply allows the conjunctival graft to recede and lessens the resulting corneal scar. Trimming of the pedicle conjunctival graft should be done carefully in horses, because exacerbation of the ulcer and accompanying episodes of severe uveitis can follow this apparently benign procedure a few days after transection.[2,5,7,10]

Complications

Proper suture placement in a healthy cornea using a thin conjunctival graft concurrent with appropriate medical therapy reduces postoperative complications of conjunctival transplant graft surgery (see **Fig. 10; Figs. 11–17**).[2,5–7] The most common complication from any type of conjunctival grafting procedure is dehiscence and premature retraction of the graft from the corneal lesion. This may occur because the corneal lesion is progressing (worsening), there is excessive tension on the graft, or too much of the fibrous Tenon's capsule was left on the graft.

Graft necrosis from vascular infarction of the conjunctival graft vessels attributable to attempts to make the conjunctival graft too thin causes an initial purple color change followed by graft ischemia manifested by a white discoloration of the flap. Some graft ischemia at the periphery of the flap results from overly tight sutures. Ischemic necrosis or infarction of the graft vessels can result in premature graft retraction and graft failure. Ischemic infarcted conjunctival grafts can still, in some cases, successfully serve a tectonic function but must be observed closely for infection and dehiscence.

Microleaks from a corneal fistula, suture perforation of the cornea, or incisional breakdown can cause graft fibrosis from exposure of the subepithelial conjunctival graft tissue to aqueous humor. Aqueous humor is apparently toxic to conjunctival fibroblasts and results in graft thickening, nonadherence, and graft retraction. Fibrin and increased signs of uveitis may also be seen with microleaks.

Suture abscesses incite a uveitic response. They are generally yellow exudates surrounding a suture and are treated by culture, suture removal, and topical antibiotics. β-hemolytic *Streptococcus* commonly causes this in the horse.

Conjunctival grafts result in various sizes and degrees of corneal scars. Scarring can be minimized, however, by removal of necrotic cornea with a keratectomy before graft placement. Corticosteroids are not recommended, but CsA can be used topically after surgery to reduce postoperative scar tissue formation.[2,5,7]

Transection of the pedicle graft causes acute ischemia to the ulcer site. The whole disease process can thus rapidly begin again, because the acutely ischemic corneal scar can rapidly become infected if microbes are still present on the graft surface.

Amniotic Membrane Grafts

Indications

AM has replaced the use of 360° and 180° conjunctival transplant flaps for melting ulcers involving the entire cornea. AM consists of an epithelium, a thick basement membrane, and an avascular stroma. High concentrations of antiangiogenic, antiprotease, anti-inflammatory, and antifibrotic compounds and cellular growth factors are present in AM.[2,5,11,12] It is a thin but strong biomaterial with a good cell-basement membrane structure that is critical for epithelial proliferation and differentiation.[2,5,11–14] The AM may also function by providing exogenous collagen as a deviant substrate for the

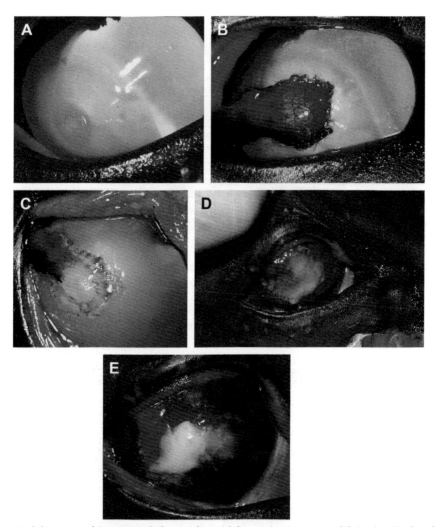

Fig. 11. (*A*) Large melting corneal ulcer with rapid deepening is present. (*B*) Conjunctival pedicle graft was placed over the progressing ulcer. (*C*) Graft is avascular 2 days after surgery. It is still providing some physical support to the cornea. (*D*) Portion of the conjunctival graft covering a melting ulcer in another eye is completely avascular 1 day after surgery. (*E*) Four days later, the conjunctival graft is infiltrated by neutrophils and is revascularizing from the vessels of the remaining vascular part of the conjunctival graft.

tear film proteases and by acting as an alternative attachment site for tear film neutrophils. If the allantoic stromal side of the AM faces the cornea, the corneal epithelial cells migrate along the membrane, the AM graft adheres to the corneal stroma, and the AM is incorporated into the cornea. If the basement membrane of the AM faces the cornea, the AM is expected to slough in 7 to 10 days.

Technique
The AM can be placed focally over an ulcer, or the AM can be placed limbus-to-limbus to cover the complete cornea. Several layers of AM can be placed together to fill in

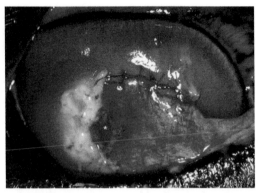

Fig. 12. Sutures infected with β-hemolytic *Streptococcus* cause premature conjunctival graft retraction and exposure of Descemet's membrane (*).

a corneal defect.[14] It is recommended that double AM layering be used in ulcers exhibiting severe melting. One AM is sutured to the diseased cornea, and a second is placed superficial to the first.

The AM is prepared and stored frozen on nitrocellulose paper in antibiotic solution.[11] Before corneal surgery, the AM is naturally thawed and then rinsed with sterile saline.

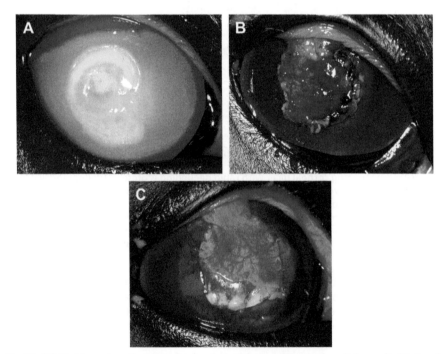

Fig. 13. (*A*) Melting ulcer that is to be treated with a conjunctival pedicle graft. (*B*) Purple discoloration of this conjunctival graft in the eye indicates vascular infarction of the graft vessels. This graft is at risk for retraction. (*C*) Peripheral part of the graft is avascular and ischemic 12 days after surgery of the eye.

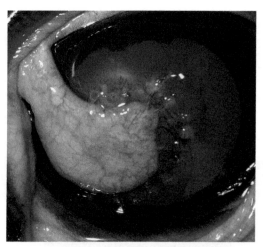

Fig. 14. Graft fibrosis attributable to proliferation of fibroblasts of Tenon's capsule causes graft retraction. Exposure to aqueous humor through a corneal perforation can speed this process of graft thickening and fibrosis.

The recipient corneal site for the AM graft is prepared by removing loose epithelium and necrotic corneal tissues. The AM is cut on the paper according to the size of the corneal defect to be covered and is then slid from the paper to the cornea.[5] AM grafts should cover the corneal defect with little tension present before suture placement to reduce premature graft retraction. The AM is then sutured to the cornea with simple interrupted sutures of 7-0 to 8-0 absorbable suture material.

Complications
Bulging of the AM can occur several days after surgery because of accumulation of debris between the nonattached AM and cornea. It resolves spontaneously. Premature release of the AM to cause exposure of the corneal lesion can occur but is not always a problem if the AM has been there for a week or longer. Suture abscesses

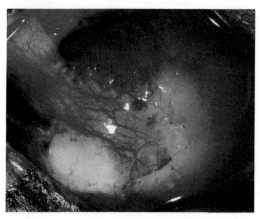

Fig. 15. Conjunctival graft covering a PK site is retracting because of an incisional microleak of aqueous humor. The incision was resutured, and the conjunctival graft was replaced.

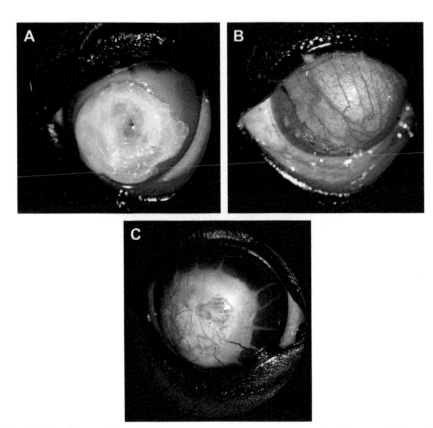

Fig.16. (*A*) Leaking melting corneal ulcer caused by *Staphylococcus* involves nearly the entire cornea. (*B*) Ulcer is covered by a conjunctival transplant graft. (*C*) Large scar allows a minimal amount of peripheral vision in this horse.

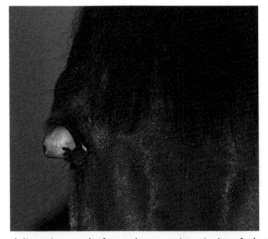

Fig. 17. Severe corneal distortion results from a large conjunctival graft that was used to cover a melting corneal ulcer, although the horse still has light perception. A total corneal transplant graft restored corneal shape to allow normal eyelid function but did not improve vision.

require removal of the suture with topical anesthesia, and the abscess must be evaluated for infection (**Fig. 18**).

Penetrating Keratoplasty

Indications
Corneal transplantation is a viable and successful surgical technique in the horse.[2,15,16] Full-thickness PK may be performed for melting ulcers, iris prolapse or descemetoceles, and full-thickness stromal abscesses. Deep lamellar endothelial keratoplasty (DLEK) and posterior lamellar keratoplasty (PLK) are split-thickness penetrating keratoplasties used for deep stromal abscesses (DSAs) with clear overlying anterior stroma. Corneal transplants in horses are associated with high success rates, good visual outcomes (>88%), and shorter treatment times than medical treatment of these eye problems alone.[2,16] Nevertheless, the corneal transplants in horses do vascularize, have some degree of opacity, and thus exhibit some degree of graft rejection.

Corneal transplantation can be performed for optical, therapeutic, tectonic, and cosmetic reasons.[17] Optical transplants restore or improve vision in cases of corneal edema. Therapeutic grafts attempt to control medically refractory corneal disease by removing necrotic and infected tissue. Tectonic grafts are done to preserve or restore the structural integrity of the eye when corneal tissue is missing, and cosmetic grafts improve the appearance of the eye without necessarily improving vision.[2,15–17]

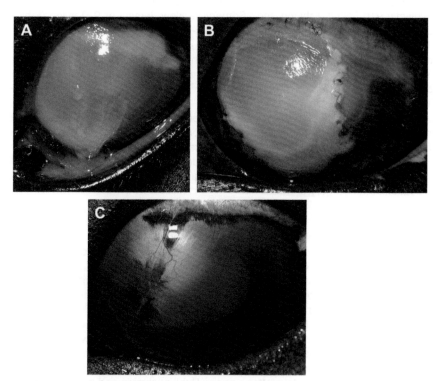

Fig. 18. (A) Entire cornea is melting because of a mixed bacterial and fungal infection in this horse. (B) AM has been sutured over the entire cornea. Some retraction is occurring laterally 2 weeks after surgery. (C) Slight pigmentation is present 6 weeks after surgery in the eye near where the amnion remained adhered to the cornea but is clear where the AM released.

Technique for penetrating keratoplasty

PK involves full-thickness removal and replacement of a portion of the cornea. Donor corneal material is harvested preferentially from fresh or frozen equine cadaver eyes (ie, within 24 hours of death). A full-thickness button of cornea that is 1 mm larger than the recipient bed is trephined from the endothelial side to the epithelial side of the donor cornea. The ideal graft size in horses is 6 to 8 mm in diameter, but larger grafts are possible. The donor button is grasped with fine—toothed forceps, placed on a gauze swab, and kept moistened with LRS. A corneal trephine of appropriate size is centered over the diseased area of the recipient globe and then rotated with minimal downward pressure to obtain a clear—cut round incision with vertical sides to just near the level of Descemet's membrane. A number 65 Beaver blade is used to enter the anterior chamber, being careful to avoid the iris, corpora nigra, and lens, and the button of diseased tissue is then removed with corneal section scissors. Bulging of the iris and the corpora nigra into the incision site may occur. Adhesions or synechia between the corneal lesion and iris may be present. The anterior chamber is reformed by injecting viscoelastic solution (hyaluronate sodium [10 mg/mL], Hylartin V; Pfizer Animal Health, New York, New York) into the anterior chamber. The viscoelastic solution also moves the iris posteriorly and breaks down any adhesions between the cornea and the iris. Iris membranes should be removed with caution because of the risk for hemorrhage. Direct contact with the lens capsule is also avoided by reforming the anterior chamber with the viscoelastic solution. The donor cornea is removed from the moistened swab and placed in the recipient bed, and four cardinal sutures of 8–0 polyglactin 910 (Vicryl; Ethicon, Inc., Somerville, New Jersey) or 9–0 nylon (Ethilon; Ethicon, Inc.) are placed at the 12–, 6–, 9–, and 3–o'clock positions. Simple interrupted sutures are placed to fill in the remaining sectors in each quadrant; alternatively, a simple continuous suture pattern can be placed to hold the graft. Once the donor cornea is sutured into place, viscoelastic solution may again be injected by way of a limbal incision to reform the anterior chamber further.[2,15,16] The incision is checked for leaks with the Seidel's test.

A conjunctival pedicle transplant graft may then be sutured over the keratectomy or graft site in those eyes with evidence of infection or vascularization to achieve more rapid assimilation into the cornea. A temporary tarsorrhaphy is performed to minimize eyelid trauma to the PK. Autogenous serum to decrease tear film proteinases attacking the graft and sutures and CsA to reduce graft rejection are added to the other medications after surgery.

Complications

Suturing in the vascular inflamed corneal environment of the horse is associated with most corneal transplant complications (**Figs. 19–22**). PK suffers from the inherent problem of creating a vertical stromal wound that requires surface corneal sutures.[2,15,16] The incised stroma never develops the structural integrity and strength of normal stroma. The corneal sutures used to heal the vertical stromal PK incision induce some alteration of the topography of the corneal surface.[2,15,16] The PK graft epithelium often sloughs, leaving the graft open to infection and melting. The sutures loosen as stromal edema resolves, and the tissue contracts to allow aqueous leakage.[15,16,18,19] Vertical incisions are less prone to leak at the low intraocular pressure (IOP) levels found after surgery.[20] Vascularization and edema of the grafts, indicating rejection, begins at 5 to 10 days after surgery. Pupil occlusion and anterior synechiation occur in some eyes but are rarely major problems. Excessive anterior chamber fibrin can be cleared with TPA. Suture abscesses can delay healing. Penetrating sutures and incision dehiscence result in microleaks and are common after PK in

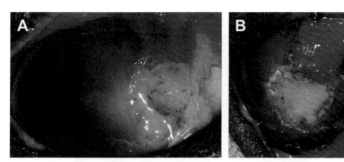

Fig. 19. (A) One day after surgery, a PK site is leaking and the conjunctival graft covering it is avascular to the edge of the corneal transplant site. (B) Corneal graft was replaced, and the avascular portion of the conjunctival graft was covered with amnion in the eye.

horses.[15,16] Leaks around sutures necessitate removal and replacement of the suture. Incisional microleaks require placement of more sutures or repositioning of existing sutures. Microleaks can also be managed with tissue glue and conjunctival or amniotic grafting.

Split-Thickness Penetrating Keratoplasties

Indications
The inherent philosophy of split-thickness or lamellar transplant corneal surgery is to replace only the diseased portion of the cornea, leaving the normal tissue intact—in other words, to do the least amount of tissue resection for the greatest amount of benefit.[2,15,16,18,19] The PLK and DLEK surgical methods are forms of split-thickness PK because they preserve the superficial normal tissue and remove the deep stromal or endothelial abscesses with anterior chamber invasion in horses.[2,15,16,18,19]

Technique for posterior lamellar keratoplasty
PLK is recommended for DSAs in the central cornea that are 8 mm or less in diameter and have a clear overlying normal anterior stroma.[15,16] A rectangular anterior lamellar corneal flap, hinged on one side, is constructed by hand dissection to two thirds of stromal thickness over the stromal abscess.[15,16] A Martinez corneal dissector is

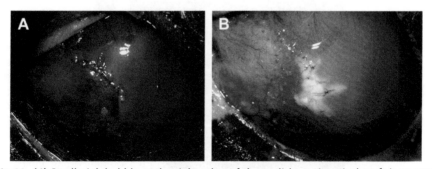

Fig. 20. (A) Small pink bubble at the right edge of the pedicle conjunctival graft is an area leaking aqueous humor from a PK incision beneath the graft. Note the purple discoloration of the conjunctival graft, which indicates vascular infarction of the graft vessels. The corneal graft incision and the conjunctival graft were resutured. (B) Suture abscess is present 3 weeks after surgery in the eye. β-hemolytic *Streptococcus* was cultured from the removed suture.

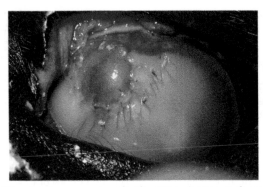

Fig. 21. Swelling of the circular corneal graft after PK indicates graft rejection.

used to undermine and elevate the superficial corneal layers to expose the abscess. The flap is gently elevated, and a trephine, number 65 Beaver blade, and corneal transplant scissors are used to remove the posterior stromal abscess, Descemet's membrane, and endothelium. A retrocorneal posterior collagenous layer with attachment to the iris may be present. The anterior chamber is reformed with viscoelastic solution. A circular graft of posterior stroma, Descemet's membrane, and endothelium 1 mm larger than the defect is cut from donor tissue using a trephine. The graft is placed in the corneal defect and sutured every 2 mm using 8-0 absorbable suture material in a simple interrupted pattern. The three-sided superficial flap is then sutured in place using 8-0 absorbable suture material. The viscoelastic solution can be safely left in the horse's anterior chamber. Partial temporary tarsorrhaphies are placed in both eyes to protect the graft during recovery.

Complications of posterior lamellar keratoplasty
Complications of PLK include superficial suture abscesses, suture microleaks, incision microleaks, and superficial flap ulcers and edema (**Figs. 23** and **24**). The donor

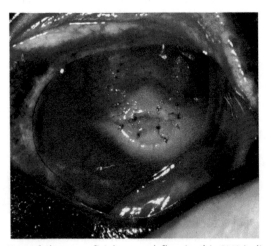

Fig. 22. Vascularization of the superficial corneal flap in this PLK indicates corneal graft rejection. Some dehiscence of the superficial flap is apparent. There was no leakage of aqueous humor, so the site was not surgically repaired but treated medically.

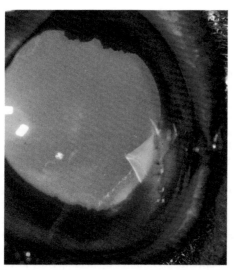

Fig. 23. Clear endothelium of the donor corneal graft is detaching from the stroma into the anterior chamber in this PLK. No therapy was necessary, and it healed satisfactorily.

graft remains transparent for up to 7 days and then opacifies.[15,16] Partial graft rejection and scar formation have been unavoidable for the PLK procedures. The resulting scar is typically vascularized and eventually becomes opaque.[15,16] The retrocorneal and iris membranes can spontaneously resolve in many cases. Pupil occlusion and synechia often occur. Cataract formation from fibrin on the anterior lens capsule and focal lens capsular rupture caused by entering the anterior chamber improperly can occur. Excessive anterior chamber fibrin can be cleared with TPA.

Technique for deep lamellar endothelial keratoplasty
DLEK is recommended for DSAs in the peripheral cornea that are 6 mm or less in diameter and have a clear overlying anterior stroma. It avoids the superficial incisions

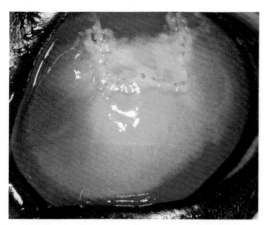

Fig. 24. Superficial corneal flap in this PLK is ulcerated, and the entire cornea is edematous immediately after surgery. Medical therapy resolved the condition.

and suturing of the central cornea. DLEK transfers healthy endothelium while preserving the corneal surface integrity. A fully intact epithelium with no corneal sutures is present after surgery.[15,16]

A two-thirds depth limbal incision up to 23 mm in length is made with a number 64 Beaver blade. A stromal pocket is formed over the DSA with a Martinez corneal dissector. Bleeding from the vascularized cornea is controlled with electrocautery. The superficial corneal flap is gently retracted, and the abscess is removed with a trephine, number 65 Beaver blade, and corneal scissors. The anterior chamber is reformed with viscoelastic solution.

The anterior two thirds of the donor cornea is removed by hand dissection, and a trephine 1 mm larger in diameter than the recipient site is used to obtain the circular donor graft from the remaining split-thickness cornea. The superficial corneal flap is partially sutured with 8-0 polyglactin 910. The donor graft is inserted into place with Utrata forceps, and the limbal incision is closed. The graft self-adheres to the recipient stroma by action of the endothelial pump but may need to be positioned in place by a needle inserted between the flap sutures or at the limbus. The graft is supported by the viscoelastic solution in the anterior chamber. The viscoelastic solution can be safely left in the horse's anterior chamber. Partial temporary tarsorrhaphies are placed in both eyes to protect the surgical site during recovery.

Complications of deep lamellar endothelial keratoplasty

Suturing in the vascular and inflamed corneal environment of the horse is associated with most corneal transplant complications (**Figs. 25–29**). Too few sutures yield incisional compression zones that are not contiguous. Sutures too close or too far from the incision also affect incision strength and water-tightness. Incisional tissue swelling affects water-tightness, because sutures placed in this condition loosen and the incision gapes when the swelling decreases.[15,16,20] Gaping wounds occur at incision angles less than 90° at low IOP. Incision angles in the cornea should be perpendicular to the surface for best closure at the low IOP present after surgery. Suture loops must be circular in the cornea and should not penetrate to the anterior chamber, or wound gaping and aqueous leakage can occur.[15,16,20] Careful technical suturing can minimize wound gaping, which results in microleaks of aqueous humor.

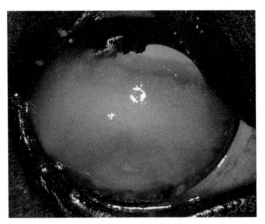

Fig. 25. Cornea is edematous 2 days after surgery in this DLEK for a deep stromal abscess. Medical therapy was continued and resolved the condition.

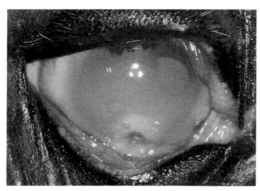

Fig. 26. Suture abscess from β-hemolytic *Streptococcus* is present near the incision of this DLEK. Medical therapy was altered, and the lesion was covered with a conjunctival graft.

Other complications of the DLEK procedure include suture abscesses, incision edema, and graft slippage and misalignment. Infection of the incision and contaminated corneal donor tissue are also associated with incisional microleaks and graft failure and with persistent uveitis, respectively.[15,16,20] Lens capsule rupture and focal cataract formation can occur when dissecting the button of Descemet's membrane and endothelium. Lens removal may be necessary if severe cataract formation results from intraoperative rupture of the lens capsule.

The donor graft remains transparent for up to 7 days and then vascularizes and opacifies.[15,16] Excessive anterior chamber fibrin can be cleared with TPA.

LENS
Cataract Surgery

Indications
The purpose of cataract surgery is visual rehabilitation.[2,21] Recent advances in cataract surgical techniques and equipment have increased the success of equine cataract surgery. Most veterinary ophthalmologists recommend surgical removal of cataracts in foals less than 6 months of age if the foal is healthy, no uveitis or other ocular problems are present, and the foal's personality tolerates aggressive topical

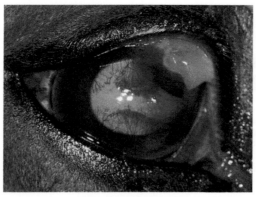

Fig. 27. Donor graft is protruding after incision dehiscence in this DLEK. The incision was resutured and covered with a conjunctival graft.

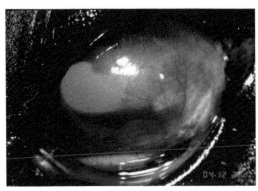

Fig. 28. Orange subendothelial tissue indicates fungal regrowth after DLEK. The infection could not be controlled, and the globe was enucleated.

therapy. Early return of vision is paramount in foals for development of the higher visual centers.[2,21] Foals are easiest to do because the globe size is small enough that the standard cataract surgical equipment is of satisfactory size, general anesthesia is generally less of a risk in foals, and foals heal quickly after cataract surgery.[2,21] Foals should be carefully evaluated for the presence of subclinical infectious systemic diseases, such as *Rhodococcus* and streptococcal pneumonia.[2,21]

Adult horses with visual impairment attributable to cataracts are also candidates for cataract surgery but are more difficult because of the large size of the adult equine eye and the frequent presence of uveitis in adult equine eyes with cataracts.[2,21] If the horse is healthy, has controlled uveitis, and has the personality and temperament to tolerate aggressive postoperative topical therapy and repeat postoperative ophthalmic examinations, the adult horse with uveitic cataracts can be a good candidate for cataract surgery.

Phacoemulsification is the preferred cataract extraction technique for the foal and horse. Immature, mature, and hypermature equine cataracts have been successfully removed with this technique.[2,21] Foals and horses generally begin to see immediately after surgery. Subluxated or partially luxated lenses may also be successfully removed in some horses using phacoemulsification.

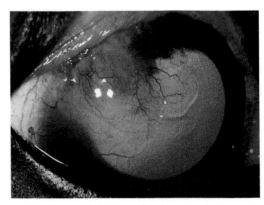

Fig. 29. The circular graft is clear and the superficial cornea is opaque in this common DLEK complication.

Equine phacoemulsification cataract surgery technique

General anesthesia is required for equine cataract surgery. Neuromuscular paralysis is also highly recommended but not essential.[2,21] The horse is positioned in lateral recumbency, and the periocular skin is cleaned with 1:50 povidone—iodine solution and appropriately draped. A Castroviejo eyelid speculum is used to retract the lids. The globe is entered dorsally with a 3.2-mm keratome blade through a scleral tunnel under a limbal-based conjunctival flap. The peripheral anterior chamber of the horse is quite narrow, so care is used not to touch the iris. The keratome blade is entered to one side of the corpora nigra because they can hemorrhage quite severely if touched. The corpora nigra should be cauterized during surgery if they begin to hemorrhage slowly.

Two milliliters of air is injected into the anterior chamber, and trypan blue dye is then injected to stain the anterior lens capsule. Viscoelastic (hyaluronate sodium [10 mg/mL], Hylartin V) is quickly injected into the anterior chamber to remove the trypan blue dye and maintain anterior chamber depth. A 20-gauge cystotome is used to incise the anterior capsule, and a piece of anterior capsule 6 to 10 mm in diameter is removed with Utrata forceps. The thin posterior capsule is generally left intact. Irrigation or aspiration with LRS containing epinephrine (epinephrine [0.5 mL] at a ratio of 1:1000 epinephrine/LRS [500 mL]) and heparin (2 IU/mL) is used to maintain the anterior chamber during phacoemulsification and to remove any remaining cortex after most of the lens has been removed. The 30°, 0.9-mm diameter phacoemulsification needle tip is kept parallel to the iris in the anterior chamber and only carefully angled posteriorly. Viscodissection with viscoelastic solution or a two-handed surgical technique using a second incision and a lens manipulator can be used to move large pieces of the lens closer to the phacoemulsification needle so that they can be emulsified and aspirated. The posterior capsule tears quite easily and can rapidly move anteriorly and posteriorly with the vitreous when the eye is open in horses. Lens cortex that remains attached to the posterior capsule of foals and horses after removal of the cortex and nucleus can be aspirated through a 0.3-mm aspiration needle on an irrigation-aspiration handpiece. Larger cataract pieces may only pass through the larger diameter phacoemulsification needle. An intraocular lens of suitable size can be placed in the capsular bag. The scleral and conjunctival incisions are closed with 8-0 absorbable suture in a simple interrupted pattern. The incisions are carefully checked for leakage with a Seidel's test.[2,21]

Complications and expectations of cataract surgery

Intraoperative complications of cataract surgery in the horse include iris protrusion into the incision, miosis, hyphema or vitreal hemorrhage, corpora nigra hemorrhage, lens nucleus dislocation to the vitreous, vitreous presentation into the anterior chamber, posterior capsular tears, choroidal hemorrhage, and retinal detachment. Opacification of the anterior and posterior capsules may be present during surgery. Retinal swelling and retinal folds may be noted during surgery during the profound hypotony found with the open incision. The retinal folds soon disappear as the IOP returns to near normal after surgery.

Slight corneal edema, especially near the incision, is usually present from 24 to 72 hours after surgery. Flare is generally slight and clears in days. Fibrin in the anterior chamber occurs infrequently. The anterior chamber is shallow because of the posterior capsule bulging forward for 3 to 5 days after surgery. Lens fragments can be noted in the anterior chamber or vitreous but slowly resorb and do not seem to cause serious harm. The vitreous can appear yellow for a week or so after surgery. The tapetal reflection may also be more yellow than that found before surgery. The foal tapetum may appear "granular" during surgery and normal a few days later.

One week after surgery, the pupil should be functional, any fibrin in the anterior chamber should be resorbing, and the fundus should be visible. Postoperative infectious endophthalmitis may result 7 to 10 days after surgery if the subclinical rhodococcal and streptococcal infections are not detected and treated before cataract surgery.[2,21] Three weeks after surgery, the eye should be nonpainful, the patient should have vision, the pupillary movement should be normal, and the ocular media should be clear. Medications should be maintained for at least 2 months after surgery to minimize posterior capsule opacification and suppress subclinical signs of iridocyclitis.

Late-term postoperative complications include persistent iridocyclitis and plasmoid aqueous, hyphema, fibropupillary membranes, synechiae, iris bombé, corneal ulceration, persistent corneal edema attributable to endothelial cell damage, corneal fibrovascular infiltrates, mild to severe anterior and posterior capsular opacification, retained lens cortex, wound leakage, incision dehiscence, vitreous presentation into the anterior chamber, surgical light retinopathy, retinal degeneration, and retinal detachment (**Figs. 30–35**). Topical and systemic nonsteroidal anti-inflammatory drugs are necessary to manage eyes with persistent uveitis. Combined 1% atropine and 2.5% phenylephrine topically can aid in breakdown of adhesions and synechia. TPA can be injected into the anterior chamber to remove large fibrin adhesions and blood clots. Thermatokeratoplasty can aid in persistent corneal edema. The other late complications, such as lens capsular opacification and retinal disease, have no reasonable treatments.

Intracapsular Surgery for Cataract or Luxated Lens

Intracapsular lens removal for luxated lenses and extracapsular cataract removal are no longer recommended for the horse. Both of these operations require a corneal or limbal incision over half of the circumference of the cornea. The equine eye does not tolerate the intraoperative hypotony of such a procedure. Hyphema, incision

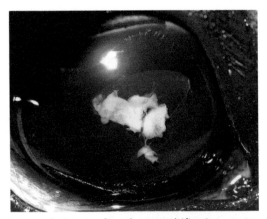

Fig. 30. Lens cortical regrowth 2 years after phacoemulsification was treated by observation but needs surgery again if it continues. The lens material is not interfering with vision at this point.

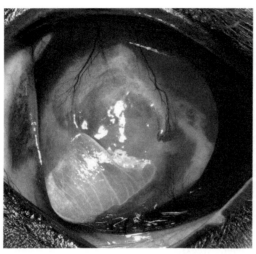

Fig. 31. *Klebsiella* infection of an ulcer after phacoemulsification was treated medically and resolved with a corneal scar.

dehiscence, infectious endophthalmitis, and retinal detachment are common complications (**Fig. 36**).

SURGICAL THERAPY FOR UVEITIS
Sustained-Release Cyclosporine A Delivery Devices

Indications
The use of CsA in patients that have equine recurrent uveitis (ERU) has come into favor as the inflammatory reaction has been further characterized in affected horses. CsA is a cyclic peptide that specifically blocks interleukin-2 (IL-2) production. Decreasing

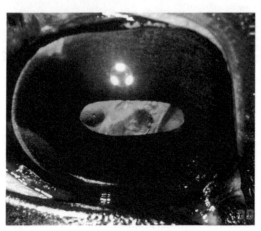

Fig. 32. Posterior cortical opacification 3 years after initially uncomplicated successful phacoemulsification surgery as a foal was so severe that the horse was blind in this eye. The posterior cortical opacification is too thick to break down with a laser or needling. Posterior cortical opacification occurs even before cataract removal in the horse and is a major problem of cataract surgery in horses.

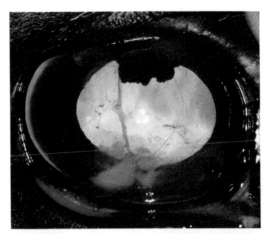

Fig. 33. Pieces of lens cortex lie in the anterior chamber immediately after surgery. They resorbed slowly over several weeks.

IL-2 minimizes T-lymphocyte activation, which is the source of elevated cytokines in the uveitic equine ciliary body.[2,22–24] Topical CsA preparations have been shown to penetrate the cornea poorly, preventing sufficient intraocular concentrations.[22,24] A polyvinyl alcohol–ethylene vinyl acetate–coated CsA delivery device has been

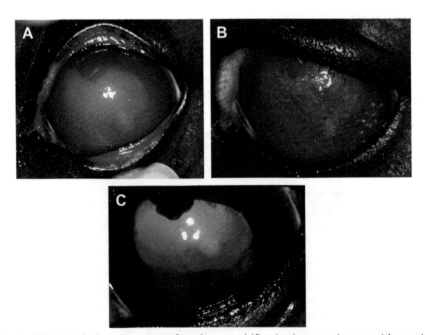

Fig. 34. (*A*) Corneal edema is present after phacoemulsification in an equine eye with a uveitic cataract. The uveitis weakened the corneal endothelium, and the surgery further diminished its ability to keep the cornea clear. (*B*) Eye was treated with thermatokeratoplasty to alter the permeability of the corneal epithelium to water so as to reduce the corneal edema. (*C*) Most of the corneal edema resolved after thermatokeratoplasty in the eye, and the cornea remained clear for several years before the endothelium permanently decompensated.

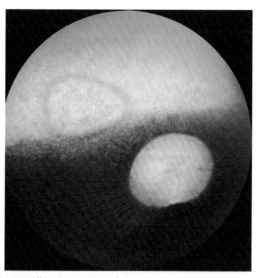

Fig. 35. The round hyperreflective region of chorioretinal degeneration in the tapetum was not present before surgery but was noted immediately after phacoemulsification. It was most likely caused by retinal toxicity from the light of the operating microscope.

used to allow for sustained release of the drug in the horse.[22,24,25] In one study, the recurrence rate decreased to less than 1 uveitic episode per year as compared with the 7.5 episodes per year before surgery.[24]

Technique

For surgical implantation, general anesthesia is essential to minimize intraoperative complications.[22] After sterile preparation of the eye, a conjunctival incision is made parallel to and approximately 10 to 12 mm caudal to the limbus that exposes the anterior insertion of the dorsal rectus muscle. A 7-mm deep scleral flap exposing the underlying uvea is then created. The CsA device is placed under the scleral flap in contact with the pigmented uveal tissue. The scleral flap is closed, followed by

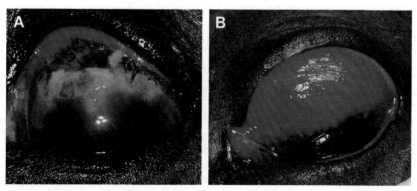

Fig. 36. (A) Dehiscence of the limbal incision after intracapsular lens extraction for a lens luxation occurred several days after surgery. (B) Incision was cultured, debrided, resutured, and covered with a conjunctival flap in the eye.

closure of the conjunctiva overlying the sclerotomy using 7-0 absorbable suture. Horses are treated with systemic antibiotics and nonsteroidal anti-inflammatory drugs and with topical mydriatic, corticosteroid, and antibiotic therapy for 5 to 10 days after surgery.[22,24]

Complications

Intraoperative hemorrhage can be substantial for ophthalmic surgery because of the inflamed conjunctiva and sclera. Care should be taken not to perforate the uvea during the procedure. Complications in the immediate postsurgical period include scleral hemorrhage and mild increases in intraocular vitreal inflammation that seem to resolve within 3 to 5 days with medical therapy. Because levels of cyclosporine do not reach adequate levels until 35 to 40 days after surgery, recurrent episodes of uveitis in this period should be addressed with traditional ERU treatments.[22,24] The progression or development of secondary glaucoma and cataract maturation can occur.[22,24] Vitreal degeneration can progress, despite control of uveitic episodes, to retinal detachment.[22,24] Infectious endophthalmitis that requires implant removal can occur.[22,24]

Pars Plana Vitrectomy for Equine Recurrent Uveitis

Indications

The purpose of the vitrectomy surgical approach for treatment of ERU stems from its ability to remove infectious organisms, vitreal debris, fibrin, toxic metabolites, and vitreal opacities that may affect visual acuity.[22,26] After surgery, horses are reported to have a decreased frequency and severity of the uveitic episodes or to have remained free of clinical signs.[22,26]

Technique

The single-port (described here) or dual-port pars plana vitrectomy is performed under general anesthesia with the horse in lateral recumbency.[22,26] A limbal-based conjunctival flap 10 to 15 mm in length is made to expose the sclera. A penetrating sclerotomy is made approximately 10 mm caudal to the limbus to enter through the pars plana of the ciliary body in an attempt to avoid trauma to the retina and ciliary body. The vitrectomy probe is inserted through the sclerotomy incision. Magnification is required. Care is taken not to contact the posterior lens capsule or retina during the procedure. The vitreal cavity is irrigated during vitrectomy with a balanced salt solution (BSS; Alcon Laboratories, Inc., Fort Worth, Texas) with 0.2 mg/mL of gentamicin added to the fluid. Most of the vitreous should be removed. Closure of the sclerotomy is performed in a continuous pattern with 6-0 polyglactin 910 (Vicryl), followed by closure of the bulbar conjunctival flap.

Complications

Complications of horses having pars plana vitrectomy for ERU are less common and less severe in horses in Europe than in the United States, where the etiology of ERU may be different.[2,22,26]

Most horses experience mild discomfort manifesting as an adverse reaction to ophthalmic examination the first 1 to 3 days after surgery. Anterior chamber fibrin is noted in approximately 60% of cases.[22,26] Mild to moderate vitreal fibrin formation and slight vitreal hemorrhage occur occasionally. More serious complications in the early postoperative period include severe vitreal hemorrhage, hyphema, and retinal detachment, and they have no reasonable therapy. Progression of cataract formation present before vitrectomy can occur and is a major problem after surgery. Cataract surgery would then be necessary to restore sight. Chorioretinal scarring also progresses in some horses.[22,26]

SURGICAL TREATMENT FOR GLAUCOMA
Indications

When medical therapy is inadequate, surgery should be used to control IOP and preserve vision in the horse with glaucoma. The surgical options for a visual eye in a horse include transscleral laser cyclophotoablation and gonioimplant filtration procedures.[2,27–29] Cyclocryoablation, ciliary body ablation, intrascleral prostheses, and enucleation are indicated for blind, chronically painful, and buphthalmic equine eyes.[27–29]

Transscleral Cyclophotocoagulation

Indications

When the IOP cannot be controlled with medical therapy, contact neodymium:yttrium-aluminum-garnet (Nd:YAG) or diode laser transscleral cyclophotocoagulation (TSCPC) may be a viable alternative for long-term IOP control. Lasering the ciliary body damages the ciliary body and supraciliary spaces, and the IOP eventually declines in most equine eyes. The glaucomatous globe of horses responds to laser therapy better in controlling IOP and maintaining vision than that of other species in the author's experience.[2,27–29] Laser cyclophotocoagulation is least efficacious at lowering IOP and maintaining vision in equine eyes that are responsive to atropine, suggesting that these eyes are using their unconventional aqueous humor outflow pathways.

Technique

The author recommends that laser therapy not be performed until any uveitis or corneal edema present is controlled with corticosteroids. Forty to 70 sites 4 to 6 mm posterior to the limbus, except nasally, should be lasered.[29] The settings for the Nd:YAG laser are 10 W and 0.4 seconds.[29] The settings for the diode laser are 1500-mW power and 1500-millisecond duration.[29] A mean drop of 17 mm Hg can be expected for the first few days after Nd:YAG laser TSCPC in the glaucomatous equine eye.[29] The target IOP lowering effects occur 2 to 4 weeks after diode lasering and should be at least 25 mm Hg less than before TSCPC at 20 weeks after laser treatment.[29]

Complications

Uveitis and corneal edema increase initially after TSCPC. The IOP may also spike immediately after lasering. Medical therapy must be maintained until the iridocyclitis is reduced and the IOP is diminished after laser treatment. Paracentesis may be necessary immediately after laser treatment to reduce the IOP. The corneal edema of the horse with glaucoma may become permanent after laser cyclophotocoagulation because of increased uveitic damage to the corneal endothelium.[29] Superficial corneal ulcers may develop as a result of reduced corneal sensation from the TSCPC or corneal exposure during the procedure. Hyphema, retinal detachment, cataract, and corneal ulcers are complications after surgery. Hyphema can be managed with anti-inflammatory therapy and sometimes intracameral TPA injections. Focal cataracts do not require therapy, whereas mature cataracts can be removed surgically. Corneal ulcers are treated according to their cause, degree of melting, presence or absence of infection, and depth. There is no therapy for most retinal detachments in the horse.

Gonioimplants

Gonioimplant filtration surgery to bypass the obstructed iridocorneal angle and direct the outflow of aqueous humor to the subconjunctival space has been successful for only brief periods in horses with glaucoma.[29] The several available gonioimplant types commonly have a tube in the anterior chamber that drains aqueous humor to an attached plate under the conjunctiva. Aqueous humor thus bypasses the blocked drainage angle to drain into a bleb surrounding the footplate. Gonioimplants have a short functional lifespan in the horse because of fibrosis and blockage of the drainage tube or filtration bleb. Implant extrusion can occur.

Cyclocryosurgery

Blind buphthalmic eyes can benefit from cyclocryotherapy, or nitrous oxide—induced cryodestruction of the ciliary body. A cryoprobe 3 mm in diameter is placed on the conjunctiva or sclera 6 mm posterior to the limbus for 1-minute freeze-thaw cycles in six locations. Cyclocryotherapy is associated with severe iridocyclitis after surgery and should only be used in blind eyes.[29] The IOP lowering effects may only last 6 weeks and may need to be repeated. Severe uveitis associated with transient elevations in IOP is a major postoperative complication that is treated with topical and systemic anti-inflammatories.

Ciliary Body Ablation

Intravitreal injection of intravenous gentamicin (25 mg with dexamethasone [1 mg]) can induce phthisis in a painful blind equine eye to result in varying degrees of pain reduction. The gentamicin induces local uveitis, and the dexamethasone minimizes discomfort from the injection.[27,29] A single injection is typically sufficient for pain reduction, but a second may be necessary in some cases.

Technique
After sedation, frontal nerve block, and instillation of topical anesthetic and phenylephrine (2.5% to vasoconstrict conjunctival vessels) and with appropriate restraint, the ciliary body ablation is performed with a 20-gauge needle on a 3-mL syringe. The needle is positioned dorsolaterally approximately 7 mm posterior to the limbus at an angle of 45° (toward the optic nerve and away from the lens).[29] Before injecting the gentamicin and dexamethasone, an equal volume (or greater) of vitreous solution is aspirated. If no vitreous solution can be aspirated, an aqueous paracentesis can be used to decrease the intraocular volume and thereby temporarily decrease IOP. Progressive increases in globe size (buphthalmos) may be prevented.

Complications
Hyphema, cataract formation, retinal detachment, intraocular infection, persistent elevated IOP, and entropion attributable to extreme phthisis can occur after surgery with the ciliary ablation technique. Careful monitoring is required. This salvage technique is reserved for blind eyes only.

GLOBE SURGERY
Exenteration

Indication and surgical technique
Orbital exenteration is a surgical technique used to remove large malignant tumors of the orbit.[30] In this procedure, the entire orbital contents, including the periorbita and globe, are surgically removed. The eyeball or globe is enucleated first. Periosteal elevators may be needed to remove the periorbital fascia. The remaining tissue is excised using scalpel or scissors. Bleeding is controlled with ligation and cautery. A permanent tarsorrhaphy is performed to cover the orbital cavity if the lids were not involved in the

disease process. A skin graft can be used to cover the open socket if excessive eyelid skin must be removed, or the socket can be left to granulate in rare cases.

Complications

Postoperative care should include pressure dressings on the head to reduce swelling and tamponade bleeding if hemorrhage was severe. Systemic antibiotics and nonsteroidal anti-inflammatories are indicated to prevent infection. Inadvertent entry into a paranasal sinus may require trephination of the sinus, with sinus lavage and drainage.[30]

Evisceration and Intrascleral Prosthesis Implantation

Indications

Evisceration refers to the surgical removal of the iris, lens, ciliary body, choroid, vitreous, and retina. The cornea, sclera, and their extraocular muscle attachments are left intact.[30] This is performed before placement of an intrascleral silicone implant or prosthesis. Evisceration is not generally recommended in an eye suspected of having an intraocular tumor or infection or in eyes with severe corneal disease. Horses beginning to undergo globe atrophy or phthisis bulbi are good candidates for evisceration and intrascleral prosthesis placement.

The intrascleral or intraocular silicone prosthesis has been used in horses as a cosmetic alternative to enucleation.[30] The intrascleral silicone prosthesis replaces the intraocular contents, which are removed by evisceration. Implants of 34 to 44 mm in diameter are recommended for adult horses but should not be placed in eyes with severe corneal disease, intraocular neoplasia, or infectious endophthalmitis. The intrascleral silicone prosthesis provides a cosmetically acceptable nonpainful eye that has normal lid movements, normal tear function, and normal globe motility.[30]

Technique

A 180° limbal peritomy is performed with tenotomy scissors. A number 15 blade is used to make a 180° full-thickness scleral incision 4 to 5 mm from the limbus. Suction and cautery are used to control hemorrhage and visualize the incision. A lens loop or evisceration spoon is used to remove all the intraocular contents. Care is taken to avoid scraping the corneal endothelium. A silicone implant of suitable size is inserted through the scleral incision into the globe so that suturing the sclera can be accomplished without undue tension. Preoperative ultrasound measurement of the normal eye can aid in selection of the proper sized implant.[30] Simple interrupted sutures of 7-0 absorbable suture are placed in the sclera, and a simple continuous pattern of 7-0 absorbable suture is placed in the conjunctiva. A temporary tarsorrhaphy can be used to protect the cornea while postoperative eyelid swelling subsides. Healing time of intrascleral implants is typically 6 to 8 weeks.

Complications

The main complications of evisceration and intrascleral implants are extrusion of the implant and corneal ulcers. Protective eyecups help to prevent irritation from head rubbing. The scleral incision can dehisce to reveal the prosthesis and necessitate implant removal.[30] The silicone implant can be rejected because of intrascleral infection and necessitates removal of the globe. Corneal ulcers can occur because of reduced corneal sensation.

Placement of too small an implant results in a cosmetically unacceptable eye. Owners should also be warned that corneal opacification and vascularization occur in some animals, such that cosmesis is not completely normal. Corneal opacification in show horses can be masked for short times with tinted contact lenses.

Enucleation

Indication and types

Enucleation refers to surgical removal of the globe, conjunctiva, and nictitating membrane because of severe corneal infection and endophthalmitis, severe iris prolapse, corneal or adnexal neoplasia, orbital neoplasia, or severe ocular trauma causing a painful blind eye.[30] This procedure does not necessarily indicate a failure of ophthalmic care but may be a necessary and planned treatment for specific conditions. There are two basic approaches to enucleation in the horse: the transpalpebral and subconjunctival techniques.[30] Orbital silicone implants may be placed with either method to reduce the profound postenucleation eyelid skin "pitting" in horses.[30]

Transpalpebral enucleation technique

The transpalpebral technique is most useful for cases of severe corneal infection, endophthalmitis, and widespread neoplasia of the conjunctiva, nictitating membrane, cornea, or orbit. It does leave a large orbital soft tissue defect.[30] In this approach, dissection into the orbit is made external to the extraocular muscles. All the secreting tissues of the conjunctiva, globe, and nictitating membrane are completely removed en masse.

The eyelids are sutured together with a simple continuous suture and the ends held with hemostatic forceps. An incision 5 mm from the eyelid margin (where the skin hair begins) is made with a number 15 blade. The angularis oculi vein located near the medial canthus should be avoided. Blunt subcutaneous dissection with Metzenbaum scissors is performed posteriorly, taking care to avoid breaking into the conjunctival sac. The medial and lateral canthal ligaments are transected with the blade. A large curved Rochester-Carmalt hemostat (8–10 inches) or Satinsky vascular clamp (27.3 mm) is used to crush the optic nerve, and curved scissors are used to transect the optic nerve between the globe and clamp. The optic nerve is best approached from the nasal side of the orbit. Care should be taken not to pull on the optic nerve, because tension at the optic chiasm can result in damage to the contralateral eye. A ligature may be placed on the transected optic nerve stump, and the nerve tissue is cauterized. Soft tissues of the orbit are closed in a simple continuous pattern with 3-0 absorbable suture to minimize postoperative pitting of the eyelids. A silicone prosthesis can be inserted before closure of the muscle, fascial, and eyelid skin layers to reduce the postenucleation orbital tissue defect. Simple interrupted sutures of 4-0 nylon or silk are used to close the skin incision permanently.

Subconjunctival enucleation technique

The subconjunctival approach is quicker and associated with less hemorrhage, but some secreting tissue may be left inadvertently.[30] This approach should be used when a cosmetic shell is to be placed to maintain the integrity of the lid margin. A lateral canthotomy may be necessary to increase exposure. A 360° limbal peritomy is performed using sharp scissors. All four quadrants are undermined posteriorly with tenotomy or Metzenbaum scissors. Extraocular muscles are isolated and transected. The medial and lateral canthal ligaments are transected with a blade. Cautery is used to control bleeding.

A large curved Rochester-Carmalt hemostat (8–10 inches) or Satinsky vascular clamp (27.3 mm) is used to crush the optic nerve, and curved scissors are used to transect the optic nerve between the globe and clamp. The optic nerve is best approached from the nasal side of the orbit. Care should be taken not to pull on the optic nerve, because tension at the optic chiasm can result in damage to the contralateral eye. A ligature may be placed on the transected optic nerve stump, and the nerve

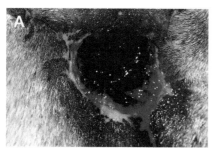
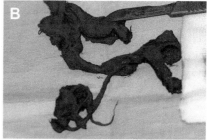

Fig. 37. (*A*) Skin incision has broken down after enucleation for a suspected orbital tumor. (*B*) Gauze had been mistakenly left in the orbit and caused severe cellulitis and incision dehiscence. Removal and placement of a drain allowed for successful orbital granulation.

tissue is cauterized. The nictitating membrane and its gland are carefully removed with scissors. Three to 5 mm of the lid margin is excised with scissors. The conjunctiva is stripped from the remaining lid, and the subcutaneous fascia and orbital septum are closed with a simple continuous suture pattern of 3-0 absorbable suture material to produce a tissue bridge across the front of the orbit. This minimizes postoperative eyelid pitting. The lid incision is permanently closed with simple interrupted sutures of 4-0 nylon or silk. A silicone prosthesis can be inserted before closure of the muscle, fascia, and skin layers to reduce the orbital pitting defect.[30]

Complications

Complications of enucleation include intraoperative rupture of the globe causing orbital contamination with microbes or tumor cells into the orbit and circulation, severe intraoperative and postoperative hemorrhage, orbital cyst formation as a result of failing to remove all secreting orbital and ocular tissues, and blindness as a result of stretching the contralateral optic nerve from intraoperative pulling on the optic nerve. The contaminated orbit should be irrigated with povidone-iodine solution, and intraoperative cultures should be obtained.[30] Broad-spectrum systemic antibiotics should also be administered, and the regimen should be modified according to the sensitivities of the organism isolated. A drain can be placed if contamination is severe. Surgical transection of the optic nerve vessels can result in severe intraoperative hemorrhaging. Wet field cautery or careful ligation should result in hemostasis. Metal

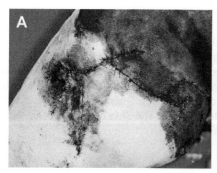
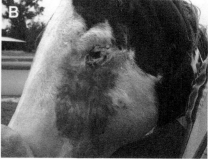

Fig. 38. (*A*) Squamous cell carcinoma of the eyelids and cornea necessitated enucleation and extensive blepharoplasty in an attempt to save the horse's life. (*B*) Six months later, the tumor has returned to cause massive facial deformity, such that euthanasia was necessary.

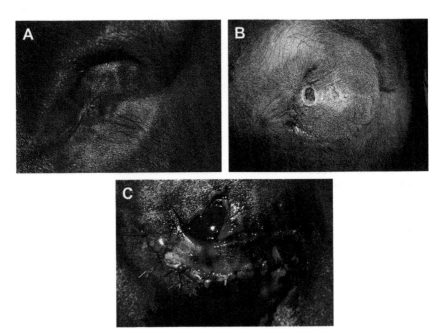

Fig. 39. (*A*) Pitting over the orbit is common after enucleation in a horse. Some owners consider the appearance to be a major disfigurement. Orbital prostheses can be used to minimize this appearance. (*B*) Orbital prosthesis has partially eroded through the skin to cause cutaneous scabs. (*C*) Orbital prosthesis in this eye is exposed after implantation and was removed, and the eyelids were permanently sutured closed.

hemoclips can also be used to control bleeding of the optic nerve and other orbital tissues. Epistaxis is generally slight but may occur after surgery for a few days. Eyelid tamponade and head bandaging suppress slight postoperative orbital swelling and hemorrhaging. An orbital silicone implant should not be placed if infection or a tumor is found in the orbit at enucleation. Failure to remove gauze can incite a terrible reaction. Cyst formation can occur days to months after surgery because of failure to remove all secreting tissues, such as the conjunctiva and the nictitans. The skin incision can dehisce after surgery to reveal the granulating orbital tissues or the implanted prosthesis (**Figs. 37** and **38**).

Intraorbital prostheses
Intraorbital prostheses are used to prevent severe pitting of the skin over the orbital cavity after exenteration or enucleation.[30] The use of intraorbital implants with orbital neoplasia or infection is controversial. Implants for horses are available from Jardon Eye Prosthetics, Inc. (Southfield, Michigan). A silicone orbital implant specifically designed to reduce postenucleation eyelid skin pitting in horses is now available from Veterinary Ophthalmic Specialties (Moscow, Idaho). Despite being biologically inert, these can be rejected and necessitate removal. The skin incision can dehisce to reveal the granulating orbit and prosthesis (**Fig. 39**).

REFERENCES

1. Plummer CE. Equine eyelid disease. Current Techniques in Equine Practice 2005; 4(1):95–105.

2. Brooks DE, Matthews AG. Equine ophthalmology. In: Gelatt KN, editor. Veterinary ophthalmology. 4th edition. Ames (IA): Blackwell Pub; 2007. p. 1165–274.
3. Brooks DE. Ocular emergencies and trauma. In: Auer JA, Stick JA, editors. Equine surgery. 3rd edition. St. Louis (MO): W.B. Saunders; 2006. p. 767–74.
4. Severin GA. Principles of ocular surgery. In: Severin GA, editor. Severin's veterinary ophthalmology notes. 3rd edition. Fort Collins (CO); 1996. p. 139–150.
5. Ollivier FJ. Medical and surgical management of melting corneal ulcers exhibiting hyperproteinase activity in the horse. Current Techniques in Equine Practice 2005;4(1):50–71.
6. Denis HM. Equine corneal surgery and transplantation. Vet Clin North Am Equine Pract 2004;20:361–80.
7. Brooks DE. Equine ophthalmology—made easy. Jackson Hole (WY): Teton New-Media; 2002.
8. Ollivier FJ. The precorneal tear film in horses: its importance and disorders. Vet Clin North Am Equine Pract 2004;20:301–18.
9. Brooks DE, Andrew SE, Biros DJ, et al. Ulcerative keratitis caused by beta-hemolytic Streptococcus equi in 11 horses. Vet Ophthalmol 2000;3:121–5.
10. Nasisse MP, Nelms S. Equine ulcerative keratitis. Vet Clin North Am Equine Pract 1992;8(3):537–55.
11. Ollivier FJ, Kallberg ME, Plummer CE, et al. Amniotic membrane transplantation for corneal surface reconstruction after excision of corneolimbal squamous cell carcinoma in nine horses. Vet Ophthalmol 2006;9(6):404–13.
12. Tseng SC, Prabhasawat P, Lee SH. Amniotic membrane transplantation for conjunctival surface reconstruction. Am J Ophthalmol 1997;124:765–74.
13. Azuara BA, Pillai CT, Dua HS. Amniotic membrane transplantation for ocular surface reconstruction. Br J Ophthalmol 1999;83:399–402.
14. Kruse FE, Rohrschneider K, Volcker HE. Multilayer amniotic membrane transplantation for reconstruction of deep corneal ulcers. Ophthalmol 1999;106:1504–10.
15. Brooks DE. Penetrating keratoplasty, deep lamellar endothelial keratoplasty, and posterior lamellar keratoplasty in the horse. Current Techniques in Equine Practice 2005;4(1):37–49.
16. Brooks DE, Plummer CE, Kallberg ME, et al. Corneal transplantation for inflammatory keratopathies in the horse: visual outcome in 206 cases (1993–2007). Vet Ophthalmol 2008;11(2):123–33.
17. Whittaker CJG, Smith PJ, Brooks DE, et al. Therapeutic penetrating keratoplasty for deep corneal stromal abscesses in eight horses. Vet Comp Ophthalmol 1997; 7(1):19–28.
18. Terry MA. Endothelial replacement: the limbal pocket approach. Ophthalmol Clin North Am 2003;16(1):103–12.
19. Terry MA, Ousely PJ. Replacing the endothelium without corneal surface incisions or sutures. Ophthalmol 2003;110(4):755–64.
20. Taban M, Rao B, Reznik J, et al. Dynamic morphology of sutureless cataract wounds—effect of incision angle and location. Surv Ophthalmol 2004;49(Suppl 2): S62–72.
21. Brooks DE. Phacoemulsification cataract surgery in the horse. Current Techniques in Equine Practice 2005;4(1):11–20.
22. Keller RL, Hendrix DVH. New surgical therapies for the treatment of equine recurrent uveitis. Current Techniques in Equine Practice 2005;4(1):81–6.
23. Gilger BC, Malok E, Cutter KV, et al. Characterization of T-lymphocytes in the anterior uvea of eyes with chronic equine recurrent uveitis. Vet Immunol Immunopathol 1999;71:17–28.

24. Gilger BC, Wilkie DA, Davidson MG, et al. Use of an intravitreal sustained-release cyclosporine delivery device for treatment of equine recurrent uveitis. Am J Vet Res 2001;62:1892–6.
25. Gilger BC, Michau TM. Equine recurrent uveitis: new methods of management. Vet Clin North Am Equine Pract 2004;20:417–27.
26. Werry H, Gerhards H. Surgical treatment of equine recurrent uveitis (ERU). Tierarztl Prax 1992;20:178–86.
27. Lassaline ME, Brooks DE. The enigma of equine glaucoma. In: Gilger B, editor. Equine ophthalmology. St. Louis (MO): Elsevier; 2005. p. 323–40.
28. Brooks DE. Equine glaucoma. In: Robinson NE, editor. Current therapy in equine medicine. 5th edition. Philadelphia: W.B. Saunders; 2003. p. 486–8.
29. Brooks DE. Hypertensive uveitis and glaucoma of horses. Current Techniques in Equine Practice 2005;4(1):72–80.
30. Brooks DE. Orbit. In: Auer JA, Stick JA, editors. Equine surgery. 3rd edition. St. Louis (MO): W.B. Saunders; 2006. p. 755–66.

Complications in Equine Anesthesia

Ann E. Wagner, DVM, MS

KEYWORDS

- Equine anesthesia • Complication
- Morbidity • Hypotension • Postanesthetic myopathy

General anesthesia of horses entails considerable risk of morbidity and mortality. The perianesthetic mortality rate for horses is higher than that for people, which is reported to be 0.0075% to 0.0079% (approximately 1 death per 12,000 to 13,000 anesthetics),[1] and that for dogs, which is approximately 0.11% (1 death per 909 anesthetics).[2] A large-scale, multicenter study reported that the death rate from non–colic-related anesthetics in horses was 0.9% (1 death per 111 anesthetics),[3] while the perianesthetic mortality rate at a single, busy equine surgical practice was somewhat more favorable, at 0.12% (1 death per 833 anesthetics).[4] Considering that, except for colics, equine surgical patients tend to be relatively healthy systemically, it is apparent that equine anesthesia is fraught with risk.

While any perianesthetic death is devastating, mortality figures alone do not reflect the overall morbidity of equine anesthesia in terms of nonterminal events, such as hemorrhage, extreme alterations in heart rate or blood pressure, postanesthetic myopathy or neuropathy, or in terms of injuries related to recovery, such as lacerations, breakdown of surgical incisions, or destruction of bandages or casts. In some circumstances, recognition of perianesthetic complications may serve as a guide to appropriate intervention to prevent the complication from worsening or progressing to mortality. This article describes some of the complications that may occur during and after general anesthesia of horses, and suggests ways to prevent or mitigate them.

INTRAOPERATIVE COMPLICATIONS
Hypotension

The most common complication that occurs during inhalation anesthesia in horses is low arterial blood pressure, or hypotension. Hypotension is not typically a problem during injectable anesthesia or total intravenous anesthesia.[5,6] For reasons not well understood, horses as a species are particularly susceptible to the negative inotropic and vasodilatory effects of the inhaled anesthetics.[7] In the late 1980s and early 1990s,

Department of Clinical Sciences, Colorado State University, Fort Collins, CO 80523, USA
E-mail address: ann.wagner@colostate.edu

Vet Clin Equine 24 (2009) 735–752
doi:10.1016/j.cveq.2008.10.002
0749-0739/08/$ – see front matter © 2009 Elsevier Inc. All rights reserved.

the relationship of intraoperative hypotension to postanesthetic myopathy was documented.[8,9] Since that time, monitoring of arterial blood pressure and prompt treatment of hypotension have been considered mandatory in equine anesthesia.

Mean arterial blood pressure (MAP) of 60 mm Hg or less during anesthesia has been shown to increase the risk of postanesthetic myopathy.[8] The effect of hypotension on other organs is not as well documented, but is presumed to be potentially detrimental. Therefore most anesthesiologists strive to maintain MAP of 70 mm Hg or more in anesthetized equine patients. There are several options to increase MAP in hypotensive animals: (1) Decrease delivery of inhaled anesthetic or other potentially hypotensive agents; (2) increase intravenous fluid administration; (3) administer inotropic drugs; and (4) administer vasopressors.

Decrease delivery of inhaled anesthetic or other potentially hypotensive agents
In many species, hypotension occurs mainly when the individual is simply too deeply anesthetized. However, horses appear to be particularly sensitive to the negative cardiovascular effects of inhaled anesthetics, such that even healthy horses that are lightly anesthetized and moving can be hypotensive. Certainly anesthetic depth should be evaluated and adjusted if appropriate. However, frequently, turning down the vaporizer is not an option, or is an option only if adjunct anesthetics, such as alpha-2 agonists, ketamine, or lidocaine, are administered to augment a surgical plane of anesthesia.

Increase intravenous fluid administration
One goal of routine intravenous fluid administration during inhalation anesthesia is to maintain sufficient vascular volume and venous return to the heart despite anesthetic-related vasodilation. An especially low diastolic blood pressure (<45 mm Hg) may be an indication of too little blood volume for the current size of the vascular space, either because of absolute hypovolemia from hemorrhage or dehydration, or because of relative hypovolemia resulting from excessive vasodilation. Unless the horse is dehydrated or hypovolemic from blood loss, a maintenance fluid administration rate of 10 mL/kg/h of balanced electrolyte solution during anesthesia is usually sufficient. If the horse is dehydrated, the required volume of intravenous replacement fluids can be calculated (percent dehydration times body weight [kg] equals number of liters of fluid required). Many equine colic cases require 25 to 30 L of intravenous replacement fluids, in addition to their normal maintenance fluids. Additional intravenous fluids can be administered to any hypotensive horse, but delivering fluids quickly may entail placing more than one intravenous catheter, or the use of pressure bags or a fluid pump. Management of hemorrhage is further discussed later in this article.

Administer inotropic drugs
Because horses are so susceptible to inhalant anesthetic–induced depression of myocardial contractility, typically more than half of horses undergoing gas anesthesia require inotropic support.[10] Dobutamine (1–4 μg/kg/min) is commonly the inotrope of choice because it is usually very efficacious and has few side effects. Ephedrine (0.06–0.12 mg/kg) is another alternative and may be simpler, more convenient, and more economical for practices where horses are anesthetized infrequently and where setting up a dobutamine constant rate infusion is troublesome or wasteful.[11,12]

Administer vasopressors
Although vasopressors, such as phenylephrine, can be used to increase MAP, vasoconstriction of vascular beds may decrease tissue perfusion and potentially result in muscle damage.[13] Therefore, phenylephrine should be used to treat hypotension

only when excessive vasodilation is suspected (eg, in cases of endotoxemia evidenced by hyperemic mucous membranes) and only when other treatments (fluids, dobutamine) have failed to restore MAP to at least 60 mm Hg. If indicated, phenylephrine should be dosed at 1 to 2 µg/kg intravenously; it can be repeated if needed.

Hypercapnia

Horses are very susceptible to the respiratory depressant effects of inhalant anesthetics,[7,14–17] which, combined with muscle relaxation and recumbency, frequently lead to hypoventilation, with increased arterial P_{CO_2} (hypercapnia). As long as oxygen is supplemented and arterial P_{O_2} is acceptable, most horses tolerate moderate hypercapnia (P_{CO_2} between 45 and 65 mm Hg) without detriment and in fact may benefit from the resulting increase in endogenous catecholamines that support cardiac function and MAP.[18] However, because newer inhalants, such as isoflurane and sevoflurane, are even more profound respiratory depressants than is halothane, few horses breathing spontaneously at a surgical plane of isoflurane or sevoflurane anesthesia can maintain acceptable P_{CO_2}. Potential effects of severe hypercapnia may include acidemia, cardiac arrhythmias, increased intracranial pressure, and a "vicious cycle" whereby rising P_{CO_2} worsens respiratory depression and exacerbates hypercapnia. Although extreme hypercapnia should be avoided, the author has seen P_{CO_2} values as high as 125 mm Hg in a few horses, all of which were breathing oxygen and recovered uneventfully once normocapnia was restored by mechanical ventilation. However, in general, mechanical ventilation is recommended whenever isoflurane or sevoflurane is used to maintain anesthesia in horses.

Hypoxemia

Absolute hypoxemia is somewhat arbitrarily defined as an arterial P_{O_2} of less than 60 mm Hg. In many species, such as humans and dogs, hemoglobin is 90% saturated at a P_{O_2} of approximately 57 to 58 mm Hg.[19] However, equine hemoglobin has greater affinity for oxygen, such that 90% saturation is typically achieved at a P_{O_2} of only 54 mm Hg. This means that horses are somewhat more tolerant of low P_{O_2} values.[20] Absolute hypoxemia is most likely to occur in horses anesthetized with injectable drugs and breathing ambient air without supplemental oxygen, when arterial P_{O_2} values of less than 60 mm Hg are not unusual.[6,21–25] During inhalation anesthesia, oxygen is almost always used as the carrier gas, making absolute hypoxemia much less common. However, even in an oxygen-supplemented anesthetized horse, mild to moderate decreases in arterial P_{O_2}, or relative hypoxemia, may occur in association with mismatching of ventilation and perfusion in the lungs, leading to physiologic shunt. Dorsal recumbency and abdominal distension, a common issue for colic cases, increase the likelihood of hypoxemia.[26–29] Methods that may improve Pa_{O_2} include using intermittent positive-pressure ventilation, increasing peak inspiratory pressure and tidal volume, employing positive end-expiratory pressure, and administering inhaled albuterol.[30,31] Fortunately, as long as cardiovascular function is reasonably normal, oxygen delivery to vital organs and tissues can often be maintained despite hypoxemia by ensuring adequate cardiac output (blood flow), and many horses with P_{O_2} values in the 50s (mm Hg) have apparently recovered from anesthesia with only minor sequellae.[28,32] Oxygen insufflation (at 15 L/min for a full-size horse) in recovery is always recommended, but is especially important for horses that have been hypoxemic during anesthesia.

Alterations in Heart Rate or Rhythm

Bradycardia

Unlike in many species, heart rate in anesthetized horses tends not to vary much with plane of anesthesia or with surgical stimulation, making it unreliable as an indicator of appropriate depth.[14,17,33] When bradycardia (heart rate <25 beats per minute) occurs, it is often associated with administration of specific drugs, such as alpha-2 agonists or dobutamine. The bradycardic effects of alpha-2 agonists are well-known.[34] Dobutamine is thought to cause reflex bradycardia occasionally because of an inappropriate baroreceptor mechanism during inhalation anesthesia that results in a decrease in heart rate as MAP increases. This inappropriate bradycardic response seems to be more common with halothane than with the newer inhaled anesthetics.[35] If heart rate remains greater than 20 beats per minute and MAP equal to or greater than 70 mm Hg, specific treatment for bradycardia is generally not required. However, if heart rate is less than 20 beats per minute, a small dose of atropine (0.002–0.003 mg/kg intravenously) is usually sufficient to restore heart rate of at least 25 beats per minute, without causing appreciable effects on gastrointestinal motility. One such dose is typically enough to improve heart rate and does not need to be repeated.

Tachycardia

As previously suggested, tachycardia (heart rate > 50 beats per minute) is rather unusual in anesthetized horses, and does not typically signal an insufficient depth of anesthesia. In fact, heart rate tends to increase slightly, though not significantly, with deeper planes of sevoflurane anesthesia.[17] Even severe hypercapnia or severe blood loss in anesthetized horses is not associated with increased heart rate.[18,36] Tachycardia during general anesthesia may result from preexisting sympathetic stimulation, as occurs in some colic cases, or may develop intraoperatively from hypoxemia or tourniquet use.[37] Inotropes, such as dobutamine or dopamine, may occasionally cause or exacerbate tachycardia in some horses, so terminating or reducing the inotrope infusion rate may correct tachycardia in some horses. An effort should be made to rule out or correct abnormalities in vascular volume and blood gases (P_{CO_2}, P_{O_2}) as well as to assess anesthetic depth. If tachycardia persists despite correction of abnormalities, a small dose of alpha-2 agonist (0.1–0.2 mg/kg of xylazine) may help bring the heart rate down.

Second degree atrioventricular block

Second-degree atrioventricular block is a common arrhythmia in awake, nonsedated horses, and can be expected to occur or be exacerbated after alpha-2 agonist administration.[34] Typically, even if a preanesthetic dose of alpha-2 agonist causes second-degree atrioventricular block, induction with ketamine or thiopental increases heart rate and abolishes atrioventricular block. Horses that have received high doses of alpha-2 agonists, are on a constant rate infusion of alpha-2 agonists, or are receiving dobutamine during inhalation anesthesia, are more likely to experience second-degree atrioventricular block. Generally, second-degree atrioventricular block itself is not problematic, as long as the overall ventricular rate is not too low (<20 beats per minute). The same guidelines suggested for treatment of bradycardia apply.

Atrial premature contractions

Atrial premature contractions sometimes occur in anesthetized horses. They do not generally impact MAP very profoundly, and therefore do not usually warrant treatment.

Ventricular premature contractions

In contrast to dogs, horses rarely experience ventricular premature contractions during anesthesia. When ventricular premature contractions do occur in an anesthetized horse, there is greater cause for concern because ventricular premature contractions in horses may progress to ventricular tachycardia or ventricular fibrillation with less warning than in other species.[38] If halothane is being used, switching to isoflurane or sevoflurane may reduce frequency of ventricular premature contractions. Appropriate ventilation (P_{CO_2}), oxygenation (P_{O_2}), and depth of anesthesia should be ensured. Lidocaine (0.5–1.5 mg/kg bolus for immediate control, or 25–50 µg/kg/min constant rate infusion) can be administered if ventricular premature contractions continue.[39]

Atrial fibrillation

A horse with spontaneous atrial fibrillation, or atrial fibrillation induced by colic, may require anesthesia. In addition, atrial fibrillation has reportedly been induced by general anesthesia in a horse that had normal cardiac rhythm when not anesthetized.[40] Most horses with atrial fibrillation tolerate anesthesia reasonably well; they may be somewhat more hypotensive than horses with normal rhythm, but atrial fibrillation is not necessarily a contraindication for anesthesia. Indeed, general anesthesia is required for some types of electrocardioversion of atrial fibrillation.[41] Minimizing use of alpha-2 agonists, by using acepromazine for sedation, and avoiding thiopental and halothane is recommended.[40]

Hypertension

As previously stated, hypotension is extremely common during inhalation anesthesia in horses. The opposite extreme, hypertension, is uncommon, but may occur with especially painful procedures, such as neurectomy or enucleation, with tourniquet use, or during hypoxemia or severe hypercapnia. The same issues mentioned in association with tachycardia should be investigated and corrected if necessary.

Hemorrhage

Whenever possible, appropriate vascular volume, packed cell volume (PCV), and plasma total protein (TP) should be ensured before anesthesia. Volume deficits should be corrected using balanced crystalloid fluids, such as lactated Ringer's solution or Normosol-R, with the caution that PCV and TP should be maintained to at least 20% and at least 3.5 g/dL, respectively, to ensure sufficient oxygen-carrying capacity and oncotic pressure. Transfusions of whole blood, packed red blood cells, or plasma should be used if indicated.

If a surgical procedure is anticipated to cause significant blood loss, the horse should be cross-matched before surgery to identify an appropriate blood donor or donors. Pretreating the horse with 30 to 40 mL/kg of balanced electrolyte solution before the onset of bleeding may help maintain vascular volume and dilute PCV and TP concentration, resulting in reduced mass of red blood cells and protein lost per unit of blood loss. Intraoperative blood loss should be measured as accurately as possible by, for example, placing a bucket under the surgical area to catch blood running off drapes, observing suction containers, and counting or weighing laparotomy sponges.[42] Blood volume of horses is reported to be approximately 8% to 10% of body weight. Therefore, a 500-kg horse normally has about 40 to 50 L of blood. While extreme blood loss is not recommended, a previously healthy horse with normal PCV and TP and good cardiovascular function could theoretically lose nearly 50% of its blood volume (~20 L) as long as volume replacement and cardiovascular support are appropriate. In general, when replacing blood loss, crystalloid fluid should be administered at a volume three times that of the blood lost, since approximately two thirds of the crystalloid fluid will redistribute to the interstitial fluid space and only one third will remain in the vascular space. If PCV drops to less than 20%, enough whole blood or packed red blood cells should be administered to restore PCV to 20% to 25%. The formula:

$$\frac{PCV_{patient\ (desired)} - PCV_{patient\ (actual)}}{PCV_{donated\ blood}} \times patient\ blood\ volume$$

can be used to calculate the appropriate amount of whole blood or packed red blood cells to administer. The lifespan of appropriately cross-matched red blood cells transfused into a horse is only about 2 to 4 days, however, so blood transfusion provides only a temporary benefit.[43]

Hypoproteinemia becomes problematic if there is insufficient albumin to maintain adequate plasma oncotic pressure, leading to pulmonary edema or edema of other tissues. Generally, albumin of less than 1.5 g/dL is a concern; if the albumin/globulin ratio is 1:1, then TP of less than 3.0 g/dL is too low. Plasma transfusions can be quite expensive, but a formula similar to the one above can be used to calculate an appropriate dose of equine plasma to transfuse:

$$\frac{TP_{patient\ (desired)} - TP_{patient\ (actual)}}{TP_{donated\ plasma}} \times patient\ plasma\ volume$$

(Note: Plasma volume is approximately 5% of body weight; therefore a 500-kg horse would normally have a plasma volume of about 25 L.) Synthetic colloids, such as hydroxyethyl starch, can also be used to augment oncotic pressure. Hydroxyethyl starch can be administered at 5 to 20 mL/kg.

Severe nasal hemorrhage has been reported in a horse anesthetized for colic surgery, during which time a nasogastric tube was in place.[44] The hemorrhage began immediately after the tube was removed near the end of surgery, and continued until the nasal passage was packed with gauze; a tracheostomy was performed to provide an airway. Estimated blood loss in this horse was 24 L, representing between 37% and 65% of its total blood volume. The investigators speculated that the hemorrhage resulted from drying and subsequent tearing of the nasal mucosa adjacent to the tube.[44] Although this was an extreme case, this author has observed similar, but less profuse, hemorrhage in several horses after removal of nasogastric tubes at the end of colic surgery. During dorsal recumbency, the horse's heart is generally higher than its head, so that gravity enhances blood flow from the nose. Therefore, we recommend that nasogastric tubes be well lubricated before insertion, and be removed only after the horse is placed in lateral recumbency at the end of surgery.

Reactions to Administration of Intravenous Antibiotics During Anesthesia

Because hypotension is a potential side effect of intravenous antibiotic administration, antibiotics administered intravenously during anesthesia should be given slowly, and arterial blood pressure should be closely monitored during and after administration. Sodium penicillin has been documented to decrease blood pressure for 5 to 10 minutes in both awake and anesthetized horses, while sodium cefazolin did not affect blood pressure.[45] Potassium penicillin is even more likely to cause cardiac depression or hypotension because of the effect of potassium ions on electrophysiology.[46] Aminoglycoside antibiotics, such as gentamycin, have the potential to potentiate neuromuscular blockade through their effect on calcium.[47]

Allergic Responses

Very occasionally an anesthetized horse shows evidence of some type of allergic or hypersensitivity reaction, presumably to a drug or blood product. Skin wheals or hives are a common manifestation of such reactions. Hypotension is a concern, but seems to be rare. If local or systemic reaction to any foreign substance is suspected, terminate delivery of the substance. Depending on the severity of the reaction and the suspected cause, administration of an intravenous steroid, such as dexaamethasone sodium phosphate at 0.02 to 0.04 mg/kg intravenously, or an antihistamine, such as diphenhydramine at 0.5 to 1 mg/kg intravenously, may be appropriate. Generally a single dose of one or both is sufficient to reduce clinical signs. Arterial blood pressure should be closely monitored until the reaction subsides.

IMMEDIATE POSTOPERATIVE COMPLICATIONS
Fractures or Soft Tissue Injuries

Fractures that occur during recovery, while not common, are one of the most devastating complications of equine anesthesia. Retrospective studies report that fractured bones occur in approximately 0.2% of anesthetized horses (2 of every 1000).[3,48] Clinical impression suggests that such fractures often occur at or near the site of a preexisting injury, such as a stress fracture, or adjacent to an orthopedic implant, such as a bone plate or transfixation pins. Very old horses may also be at higher risk. In many cases, observers have reported that, surprisingly, the affected horse did not seem to be having a particularly rough or difficult recovery at the time the fracture occurred. However, for horses with major orthopedic repairs, or horses that are very old or debilitated, it is recommended that recovery be assisted or controlled to minimize the risk of fracture. Furthermore, if a long-term cast will not be used, a cast or bandage cast may be used only for the recovery process to minimize strain and torque on the fracture repair.

Soft tissue injuries, such as lacerations of the lips, tongue, or limbs occur fairly commonly during recovery, but are rarely serious. Anesthetized horses are also at risk for corneal abrasions during anesthesia and recovery, so special care should be taken to protect the eyes from drying or trauma during surgery, and especially anytime the horse's head is moved.

Myopathy

Postanesthetic myopathy was once a fairly common complication of general anesthesia in horses. By the late 1980s, however, there was evidence that the occurrence of myopathy was directly related to hypotension that occurred during inhalation (halothane) anesthesia.[8,9] Since that time, monitoring of arterial blood pressure and prompt treatment of hypotension have drastically reduced the incidence of postanesthetic myopathy in horses. Occasionally, especially after long procedures or instances of prolonged recumbency with insufficient padding, localized areas of muscle may become swollen and painful. Typical locations for local myositis are the masseter, triceps, gluteals, and over the ribs (**Fig. 1**). Careful attention to padding of these areas may reduce the problem. If local or generalized myopathy occurs after anesthesia, recommended treatments generally include nonsteroidal anti-inflammatory drugs, such as phenylbutazone (4 mg/kg intravenously), intravenous fluid therapy to promote diuresis and elimination of myoglobin, and sometimes acepromazine (0.02 to 0.03 mg/kg intravenously) to promote vasodilation and improve muscle perfusion. Furthermore, if the horse has difficulty supporting weight on a limb, such as in a triceps

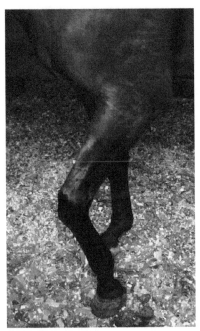

Fig. 1. An example of the forelimb stance of a triceps myopathy. The elbow has a classic "dropped" appearance and the horse cannot bear weight on the affected limb. A radial nerve paralysis or a fractured ulna would have a similar appearance.

myopathy, splinting the affected limb may be necessary until the myopathy resolves (**Fig. 2**).

Neuropathy

Superficial nerves, such as the facial and radial nerves, are subject to pressure damage during anesthesia and recumbency. Special attention should be paid to padding and protecting these nerves from such pressure damage. The facial nerve is particularly at risk during surgeries involving the head or eye, when surgical manipulations may subject the head to extra weight or pressure (**Fig. 3**). The radial nerve is most at risk during lateral recumbency; a common problem is insufficient padding, or pads that do not completely support the entire shoulder and elbow region but instead end somewhere in between, with the edge of the pad pushing into the area where the nerve lies. Because the dropped-elbow appearance of a horse with radial nerve paresis is similar to that of a horse with triceps myopathy or a fractured olecranon, careful physical examination and perhaps radiographs may be required to differentiate these injuries. Another problem is excessive stretching or tension of a nerve, such as during traction to reduce or repair a limb fracture. Whenever possible, such extremes of positioning should be avoided. Clinical signs of nerve damage indicate which nerve is involved. For the facial nerve, one side of the face may be partially paralyzed; for the radial nerve, the classic "dropped elbow" stance and inability to extend the foreleg are seen. Symptomatic treatment, such as anti-inflammatories including steroids in the acute stage and nonsteroidals as resolution of the neuropathy occurs and support with a splint if indicated, may result in a successful outcome within several days if the nerve damage is not severe.

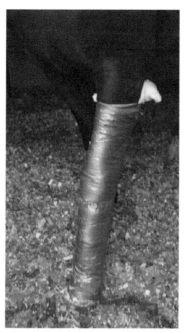

Fig. 2. The horse from **Fig. 1** with the limb splinted from the point of the elbow to the floor. With the limb splinted, forcing the knee into extension, the horse can support weight on the affected limb. It is important that the splint extend from the point of the elbow to the floor and the splint be positioned on the caudal aspect of the limb.

Myelopathy

There are occasional reports in the literature of horses developing a postanesthetic hemorrhagic myelopathy or myelomalacia following inhalation (halothane) anesthesia.[49,50] Affected horses were typically young (1 to 2 years) and rapidly growing, positioned in dorsal recumbency, and not necessarily anesthetized for long periods. Signs observed in recovery included inability to stand or move the pelvic limbs, while tail tone and anal tone were normal or hypertonic. All horses were euthanized because of deteriorating neurologic condition. Necropsy indicated myelomalacia, sometimes with hemorrhage, anywhere from the caudal cervical to the lumbar spinal cord. The etiology is uncertain, but is speculated to involve poorly developed blood supply or poor venous drainage in combination with reduced arterial blood pressure during anesthesia. Because the exact cause is unknown, the only recommendation for prevention is to avoid deep anesthesia and low arterial blood pressure.[49]

Upper Airway Obstruction

Upper airway obstruction may occur in horses when an endotracheal tube becomes kinked by extreme positioning or is otherwise occluded. Upper airway obstruction can also occur after extubation if the nasal passages are blocked by secretions or swelling; the soft palate remains dorsally displaced above the epiglottis; the horse has laryngeal dysfunction, such as laryngeal hemiplegia; or the horse falls during anesthetic recovery with its head or neck twisted under its body. Complete upper airway obstruction is a true emergency, as the extreme negative intrathoracic pressures

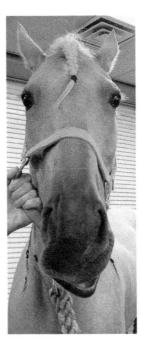

Fig. 3. An example of facial nerve paralysis caused by inappropriate pressure, causing neuropraxia.

resulting from inspiratory efforts against a closed airway quickly lead to pulmonary edema, which can be fatal even if the initial airway obstruction is resolved.

Factors that are thought to predispose the upper airway to obstruction after extubation include preexisting laryngeal hemiplegia;[51] laryngeal dysfunction induced by intraoperative trauma or hyperextension of the neck;[52] relative hypoxemia (Pao$_2$ <100 mm Hg) during anesthesia;[53] prolonged duration of recumbency,[53] especially dorsal recumbency (resulting in marked congestion of nasal passages); and any procedure that involves significant nasal or laryngeal hemorrhage or swelling, or packing of the region. A report of nine horses that suffered severe postanesthetic upper respiratory tract obstruction stated that five had preexisting laryngeal hemiplegia, three were draft breeds, two were relatively hypoxemic (Pao$_2$ <100 mm Hg), all nine were in dorsal recumbency, and eight were under anesthesia for at least 90 minutes.[51] Note that certain draft breeds are highly susceptible to laryngeal hemiplegia,[54] so a careful history and physical examination of the airway should be obtained on all draft horses, even if the presenting complaint or procedure is not related to the airway.

Management procedures that may reduce the risk of upper airway obstruction include instilling phenylephrine (10 mg diluted in 10 to 20 mL saline, divided between the two nasal passages) before extubation,[55] elevating the head in recovery to promote venous drainage of the nasal passages, maintaining the endotracheal tube until the horse is completely recovered and standing,[53] replacing the orotracheal tube with a nasotracheal tube, and insufflating oxygen (15 L/min) into the endotracheal tube for several minutes before extubation. Excited or agitated horses may benefit from sedation at the time of extubation. A preemptive tracheostomy should be performed if the upper airway is likely to be seriously compromised by blood clots, swelling, packing material, or other factors.

Pulmonary Edema

Postanesthetic pulmonary edema has been reported in horses in association with transient airway obstruction[56–58] or re-expansion of atelectatic lung during anesthesia.[59] Even if airway obstruction lasts less than a minute, within a few minutes after relieving the obstruction, pink or white frothy fluid may be expelled from the endotracheal tube (if still intubated) or nasal passages (if extubated). Tachypnea, tachycardia, hypoxemia, and hypercapnia typically accompany the onset of pulmonary edema. Oxygen insufflation should be provided, and a diuretic, such as furosemide (0.5 to 1 mg/kg intravenously) should be administered. Nonsteroidal anti-inflammatory drugs (phenylbutazone, 4 mg/kg intravenously) or steroids (dexamethasone, 0.02–0.04 mg/kg intravenously) have also been recommended, to decrease any potential airway swelling.[56] Some affected horses have recovered, but several deteriorated and either died or were euthanized.[56–58]

The proposed mechanism for pulmonary edema after transient airway obstruction is thought to be the extremely high negative intrathoracic pressure gradients created by inspiratory efforts against the obstructed airway, leading to decreased interstitial hydrostatic pressure and increased fluid flux into the pulmonary interstitium. Hypoxemia during or after obstruction may also contribute by increasing pulmonary vascular resistance.[56] The methods above, suggested to prevent airway obstruction, apply to the prevention of post–airway obstruction pulmonary edema.

Prolonged Recovery

Recoveries from inhalation anesthesia generally take less than 1 hour. Inhalation anesthetics, and particularly the newer agents, isoflurane and sevoflurane, are removed rather quickly from the brain to the blood and then to the lungs, where they are exhaled. Nonsurgical horses recovering from isoflurane or sevoflurane without postanesthetic sedation frequently stand in less than 20 minutes.[7,17] If other drugs, such as alpha-2 agonists, have been administered shortly before the end of anesthesia, or throughout anesthesia, recovery is likely to be prolonged in a dose-dependent fashion.[60,61]

Recoveries from total intravenous anesthesia tend to be much longer than those associated with inhalation anesthesia. A general rule of thumb is that every minute of total intravenous anesthesia requires at least a minute of recovery time. Thus, an hour-long total intravenous anesthesia procedure might be expected to result in an hour or more of recovery time, depending on the specific drugs used. Note that propofol, an injectable anesthetic known for its rapid and smooth recovery characteristics in many species, is associated with smooth, but not necessarily rapid, recoveries in horses. After 75 minutes of either xylazine-ketamine or xylazine-propofol infusion, horses receiving the propofol combination had slightly better quality of recovery to standing, but required an average of 80 to 90 minutes to stand, compared with 45 minutes for the horses in the ketamine group.[62] However, the combination of medetomidine and propofol has been associated with relatively rapid recoveries, requiring only about 42 minutes to stand after 112 minutes of total intravenous anesthesia.[5]

A horse that is taking longer than expected to recover should be assessed for mentation; musculoskeletal injury, such as fracture or myopathy; and metabolic abnormalities, such as hypoglycemia or hypocalcemia.

METHODS FOR ASSISTING RECOVERY

Because recovery from general anesthesia incurs risk of injury, a variety of methods have been used to assist or modify recoveries. These include both physical and pharmacologic methods.

Deep Mattress, Padding, or Bedding

Horses should be allowed to recover from general anesthesia in an area that is safe and free from sharp objects, with a surface that provides sufficient padding to avoid muscle or nerve damage during recumbency, and good, nonslip footing when the horse attempts to stand. This may be an open grassy area, part of an indoor arena, or a designated recovery stall. If a stall, the walls should also be padded. If an open area, the horse should be controlled in some way to prevent it from developing excessive momentum in its efforts to stand. Extra padding, such as a thick (12 in) mattress or deep straw or shavings, may be used to impede the horse's standing so that the horse is unable to attain sternal recumbency or stand until it has regained sufficient awareness and muscle control to make a coordinated effort.

Head-and-Tail Ropes

Ropes attached to the halter and tail are frequently used to control or influence the horse's movements during recovery without requiring direct contact with the horse, thereby minimizing the risk of injury to personnel.[63] Mechanical advantage is gained by running the ropes through rings placed high (~6 ft) on the walls, or over a partial wall. Additional mechanical advantage can be obtained by use of a block-and-tackle or pulley system to facilitate traction on the horse's tail (**Fig. 4**). The object of head-and-tail ropes is not to lift the horse, but to provide some stability and support when the horse attempts to stand, as well as to prevent it from careening from wall to wall in an uncoordinated fashion.

Sling

Sling recoveries have been described and seem to reduce the risk of injury in recovery, particularly in horses with existing musculoskeletal injuries. Successful use of a sling requires more personnel, as well as experience in placing and fitting the sling on a recumbent horse. Sedation is typically required, and some horses may fight the sling or refuse to cooperate. Ideally, a horse should have the sling fitted and become accustomed to it before undergoing anesthesia and surgery. Use of a sling for anesthesia recovery has been described in detail elsewhere.[64]

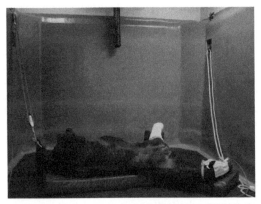

Fig. 4. A block-and-tackle system for rope-assisted recoveries. The block and tackle provides a mechanical advantage so only one or two people can provide the support the horse needs to get to its feet. The head rope is used only to guide the head during recovery.

Pool-Raft or Hydropool System

Only a few equine hospitals have facilities that enable horses to recover in water.[65,66] Therefore, this specialized recovery technique will not be discussed here.

Inflatable Air Cushion

A relatively new technique that appears to promote safe recoveries is the use of a rapidly inflating and deflating air cushion developed at Kansas State University (**Fig. 5**). The inflated air cushion inhibits the horse's attempts to roll into sternal recumbency while protecting the horse from injury during potentially violent movements. Once the horse is judged to be awake enough to stand, the pillow can be rapidly deflated, and most horses then successfully stand with fewer attempts compared with horses recovering on a normal padded floor.[67]

Comparison of Recoveries from Various Inhalation Anesthetics and from Total Intravenous Anesthesia

Recovery quality and duration may vary among various inhalation anesthetics, and between inhalation anesthesia and injectable anesthesia. Sevoflurane in horses is typically associated with shorter and better recoveries than isoflurane,[68,69] while isoflurane recoveries, though generally slightly shorter than halothane recoveries, are not significantly better than halothane recoveries[70] and subjectively appear to be worse, with isoflurane-anesthetized horses requiring more attempts to stand.[61]

Recoveries of horses from short-term injectable anesthesia, such as xylazine and ketamine, are generally smooth and controlled. Historically, maintenance of anesthesia by injectable drugs, or total intravenous anesthesia, has been limited to short procedures (less than or equal to 1 hour) because of concerns about excessive drug accumulation and about saturation of tissue redistribution sites and metabolic pathways, potentially leading to prolonged and stormy recoveries. However, there is renewed interest in total intravenous anesthesia, mainly combinations incorporating an alpha-2 agonist and either ketamine or propofol, which are typically associated with smooth and safe recoveries.[6,21–23,62] It is not yet clear exactly how long general anesthesia in horses can safely be maintained by total intravenous anesthesia.

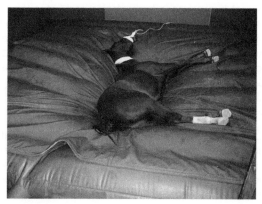

Fig. 5. The pillow support system developed at Kansas State University. (*Courtesy of* David S. Hodgson, DVM, Manhattan, KS.)

Sedative use During Recoveries from Inhalation Anesthesia

Clinical impression and a limited amount of research suggest that equine recoveries after inhalation anesthesia can be modified and improved by administration of sedatives just before or during recovery. Because of their rapid onset and profound sedative properties, alpha-2 agonists administered intravenously have been widely used for this purpose.[60,68,71] A 1998 study reported that administering xylazine (0.1 mg/kg intravenously) at the end of sevoflurane anesthesia did not significantly improve recovery quality compared with sevoflurane alone.[68] However, a study comparing xylazine (0.2 mg/kg intravenously) to romifidine (0.02 mg/kg intravenously) for postanesthesia sedation found that either drug improved recoveries compared with isoflurane alone.[71] Another study compared xylazine (0.1 mg/kg intravenously), detomidine (2 µg/kg intravenously), and romifidine (8 µg/kg intravenously) administered at the end of 120 minutes of isoflurane anesthesia, and reported that recoveries were longer, but smoother and free of excitement and ataxia, with any of the three sedatives, compared with recoveries from isoflurane alone.[60] The administration of medetomidine for both premedication (7 µg/kg intravenously) and as a continuous infusion (3.5 µg/kg/h) during isoflurane anesthesia, was reportedly associated with excellent recoveries in 299 of 300 horses. Therefore this technique is gaining popularity in equine inhalation anesthesia.[72]

Injectable Anesthetic use During Recoveries from Inhalation Anesthesia

Because of better recoveries associated with injectable anesthesia, but concern about accumulation of injectable drugs during prolonged anesthetic procedures, combinations of inhalation and injectable drugs are being studied. One option is to administer both injectable anesthetics and inhalation anesthesia simultaneously, combining reduced doses of each. When guaifenesin, ketamine, and medetomidine were infused continuously during sevoflurane anesthesia, horses required fewer attempts to stand[73] or required less time to stand[74] than when sevoflurane alone was administered.

Another option is to use inhalation anesthesia but follow it with a short period of injectable anesthesia, allowing time for the inhalation agent to be eliminated before recovery. In a recent study, single boluses of xylazine (0.15 mg/kg) and ketamine (0.3 mg/kg) were administered to seven horses 5 minutes after the termination of isoflurane anesthesia, followed by continuous infusions at 20 µg/kg/min and 60 µg/kg/min, respectively, for 30 minutes. Although that study could not document any statistically significant improvement in recovery when xylazine and ketamine were infused after the end of isoflurane anesthesia, recovery-quality scores tended to be slightly better with the infusions.[75] The author's own clinical experience with several horses recovering after major orthopedic surgeries suggests that use of either xylazine and ketamine together or propofol alone to delay recovery from inhalation anesthesia usually results in calmer, more controlled recoveries.

SUMMARY

General anesthesia of horses entails considerable risk of complications during both the anesthetic period and recovery. With appropriate monitoring and support, many intra-anesthetic complications, such as hypotension and hypercapnia, can be recognized and corrected, and hemorrhage can be appropriately managed. This article has described means to prevent postanesthetic complications, such as fractures and myopathies, and has suggested methods, physical and pharmacologic, for improving the quality of recovery.

REFERENCES

1. Lagasse RS. Anesthesia safety: model or myth? A review of the published literature and analysis of current original data. Anesthesiology 2002;97:1609–17.
2. Dyson DH, Maxie MG, Schnurr D. Morbidity and mortality associated with anaesthetic management in small animal veterinary practice in Ontario. J Am Anim Hosp Assoc 1998;34:325–35.
3. Johnston GM, Eastment JK, Wood JLN, et al. The confidential enquiry in perioperative equine fatalities (CEPEF); mortality results of phases 1 and 2. Vet Anaesth Analg 2002;29:159–70.
4. Bidwell LA, Bramlage LR, Rood WA. Equine preoperative fatalities associated with general anaesthesia at a private practice—a retrospective case series. Vet Anaesth Analg 2007;34:23–30.
5. Bettschart-Wolfensberger R, Kalchofner K, Neges K, et al. Total intravenous anaesthesia in horses using medetomidine and propofol. Vet Anaesth Analg 2005;32:348–54.
6. Mama KR, Wagner AE, Steffey EP, et al. Evaluation of xylazine and ketamine for total intravenous anesthesia in horses. Am J Vet Res 2005;66:1002–7.
7. Grosenbaugh DA, Muir WW. Cardiorespiratory effects of sevoflurane, isoflurane, and halothane anesthesia in horses. Am J Vet Res 1998;59:101–6.
8. Grandy JL, Steffey EP, Hodgson DS, et al. Arterial hypotension and the development of postanesthetic myopathy in halothane-anesthetized horses. Am J Vet Res 1987;48:192–7.
9. Richey MT, Holland MS, McGrath CJ, et al. Equine postanesthetic lameness—a retrospective study. Vet Surg 1990;19:392–7.
10. Donaldson LL. Retrospective assessment of dobutamine therapy for hypotension in anesthetized horses. Vet Surg 1988;17:53–75.
11. Grandy JL, Hodgson DS, Dunlop CI, et al. Cardiopulmonary effects of ephedrine in halothane-anesthetized horses. J Vet Pharmacol Ther 1989;12:389–96.
12. Lee YHL, Clarke KW, Ablibbai HIK, et al. The effects of ephedrine on intramuscular blood flow and other cardiopulmonary parameters in halothane-anesthetized ponies. Vet Anaesth Analg 2002;29:171–81.
13. Lee YL, Clarke KW, Alibhai HIK, et al. Effects of dopamine, dobutamine, dopexamine, phenylephrine, and saline solution on intramuscular blood flow and other cardiopulmonary variables in halothane-anesthetized ponies. Am J Vet Res 1998;59:1463–72.
14. Steffey EP, Dunlop CI, Farver TB, et al. Cardiovascular and respiratory measurements in awake and isoflurane-anesthetized horses. Am J Vet Res 1987;48:7–12.
15. Steffey EP, Kelly AB, Woliner MJ. Time-related responses of spontaneously breathing, laterally recumbent horses to prolonged anesthesia with halothane. Am J Vet Res 1987;48:952–7.
16. Steffey EP, Hodgson DS, Dunlop CI, et al. Cardiopulmonary function during 5 hours of constant-dose isoflurane in laterally recumbent, spontaneously breathing horses. J Vet Pharmacol Ther 1987;10:290–7.
17. Steffey EP, Mama KR, Galey FD, et al. Effects of sevoflurane dose and mode of ventilation on cardiopulmonary function and blood biochemical variables in horses. Am J Vet Res 2005;66:606–14.
18. Wagner AE, Bednarski RM, Muir WW. Hemodynamic effects of carbon dioxide during intermittent positive-pressure ventilation in horses. Am J Vet Res 1990;51:1922–9.
19. Bartels H, Harms H. Sauerstoffdissoziationskurven des blutes von saugetieren. Pfligers Archiv 1959;268:334–65.

20. Clerbaux T, Serteyn D, Willems E, et al. Determination de la courbe de dissociation standard de l'oxyhemoglobine du cheval et influence, sur cette courbe, de la temperature, du pH et du diphosphoglycerate. Can J Vet Res 1986;50:188–92.
21. Wan PL, Trim CM, Mueller POE. Xylazine-ketamine and detomidine-tiletamine-zolazepam anesthesia in horses. Vet Surg 1992;21:312–8.
22. Matthews NS, Hartsfield SM, Hague B, et al. Detomidine-propofol anesthesia for abdominal surgery in horses. Vet Surg 1999;28:196–201.
23. Yamashita K, Wijayathilaka TP, Kushiro T, et al. Anesthetic and cardiopulmonary effects of total intravenous anesthesia using a midazolam, ketamine and medetomidine drug combination in horses. J Vet Med Sci 2007;69:7–13.
24. Bettschart-Wolfensberger R, Freeman SL, Jaggin-Schmucker N, et al. Infusion of a combination of propofol and medetomidine for long-term anesthesia in ponies. Am J Vet Res 2001;62:500–7.
25. Bettschart-Wolfensberger R, Bowen MI, Freeman SL, et al. Cardiopulmonary effects of prolonged anesthesia via propofol-medetomidine infusion in ponies. Am J Vet Res 2001;62:1428–35.
26. Hubbell JAE, Muir WW, Casey MF. Retrospective study of horses with low arterial oxygen tensions. [abstract]. Proc Ann Mtg Am Coll Vet Anes 1986;15.
27. Gleed RD, Dobson A. Improvement in arterial oxygen tension with change in posture in anaesthetized horses. Res Vet Sci 1988;44:255–9.
28. Trim CM, Wan PY. Hypoxaemia during anaesthesia in seven horses with colic. J Assoc Vet Anaesth 1990;17:45–9.
29. Whitehair KJ, Willits NH. Predictors of arterial oxygen tension in anesthetized horses: 1,610 cases (1992–1994). J Am Vet Med Assoc 1999;215:978–81.
30. Moens Y, Lagerweij E, Gootjes P, et al. Influence of tidal volume and positive end-expiratory pressure on inspiratory gas distribution and gas exchange during mechanical ventilation in horses positioned in lateral recumbency. Am J Vet Res 1998;59:307–12.
31. Robertson SA, Bailey JE. Aerosolized salbutamol (albuterol) improves Pao_2 in hypoxaemic anaesthetized horses—a prospective clinical trial in 81 horses. Vet Anaesth Analg 2002;29:212–8.
32. Whitehair KJ, Steffey EP, Woliner MJ, et al. Effects of inhalation anesthetic agents on response of horses to three hours of hypoxemia. Am J Vet Res 1996;57:351–60.
33. Wagner AE, Dunlop CI, Heath RB, et al. Hemodynamic function during neurectomy in halothane-anesthetized horses with or without constant dose detomidine infusion. Vet Surg 1992;21:248–55.
34. Wagner AE, Muir WW, Hinchcliff KW. Cardiovascular effects of xylazine and detomidine in horses. Am J Vet Res 1991;52:651–7.
35. Hellyer PW, Dodam JR, Light GS. Dynamic baroreflex sensitivity in anesthetized horses, maintained at 1.25 to 1.3 minimal alveolar concentration of halothane. Am J Vet Res 1991;52:1672–5.
36. Wilson DV, Rondenay Y, Shance PU. The cardiopulmonary effects of severe blood loss in anesthetized horses. Vet Anaesth Analg 2003;30:80–6.
37. Abrahamsen E, Hellyer PW, Bednarski RM, et al. Tourniquet-induced hypertension in a horse. J Am Vet Med Assoc 1989;194:386–8.
38. Gaynor JS, Bednarski RM, Muir WW. Effect of xylazine on the arrhythmogenic dose of epinephrine in thiamylal halothane-anesthetized horses. Am J Vet Res 1992;53:2350–4.
39. Doherty T, Valverde A. Manual of equine anesthesia and analgesia. Ames (IA): Blackwell Publishing; 2006.

40. Hubbell JAE, Muir WW, Bednarski RM. Atrial fibrillation associated with anesthesia in a Standardbred gelding. Vet Surg 1986;15:450–2.

41. Frye A, Selders CG, Mama KR, et al. Use of biphasic electrical cardioversion for treatment of idiopathic atrial fibrillation in two horses. J Am Vet Med Assoc 2002; 220:1039–45.

42. Wagner AE, Dunlop CI. Anesthetic and medical management of acute hemorrhage during surgery. J Am Vet Med Assoc 1993;203:40–5.

43. Kallfelz FA, Whitlock RH, Schultz RD. Survival of ^{59}Fe-labeled erythrocytes in cross-transfused equine blood. Am J Vet Res 1978;39:617–20.

44. Trim CM, Eaton SA, Parks AH. Severe nasal hemorrhage in an anesthetized horse. J Am Vet Med Assoc 1997;210:1324–7.

45. Hubbell JAE, Muir WW, Robertson JT. Cardiovascular effects of intravenous sodium penicillin, sodium cefazolin, and sodium citrate in awake and anesthetized horses. Vet Surg 1987;16:245–50.

46. Swain HH, Kiplinger GF, Brody TM. Actions of certain antibiotics on the isolated dog heart. J Pharmacol Exp Ther 1956;117:151–9.

47. Hildebrand SV, Hill T. Interaction of gentamycin and atracurium in anesthetized horses. Equine Vet J 1994;26:209–11.

48. Young SS, Taylor PM. Factors influencing the outcome of equine anaesthesia: a review of 1,314 cases. Equine Vet J 1993;25:147–51.

49. Yovich JV, Lecouteur RA, Stashak TS, et al. Postanesthetic hemorrhagic myelopathy in a horse. J Am Vet Med Assoc 1986;188:300–1.

50. Joubert KE, Duncan N, Murray SE. Post-anaesthetic myelomalacia in a horse. J S Afr Vet Assoc 2005;76:36–9.

51. Southwood LL, Baxter GM, Wagner AE. Postanesthetic upper respiratory tract obstruction in horses. [abstract]. Vet Surg 2003;32:602.

52. Abrahamsen EJ, Bohanon TC, Bednarski RM, et al. Bilateral arytenoids cartilage paralysis after inhalation anesthesia in a horse. J Am Vet Med Assoc 1990;197:1363–5.

53. Thomas SJ, Corbett WT, Meyer RE. Risk factors and comparative prevalence rates of equine postanesthetic respiratory obstruction at NCSU. [abstract]. Vet Surg 1987;16:324.

54. Brakenhoff JE, Holcombe SJ, Hauptman JG, et al. The prevalence of laryngeal disease in a large population of competition draft horses. Vet Surg 2006;35: 579–83.

55. Lukasik VM, Gleed RD, Scarlett JM, et al. Intranasal phenylephrine reduces post anaesthetic upper airway obstruction in horses. Equine Vet J 1997;29:236–8.

56. Kollias-Baker CA, Pipers FS, Heard D, et al. Pulmonary edema associated with transient airway obstruction in three horses. J Am Vet Med Assoc 1993;202: 1116–8.

57. Ball MA, Trim CM. Post anaesthetic pulmonary oedema in two horses. Equine Vet Educ 1996;8:13–6.

58. Tute AS, Wilkins PA, Gleed RD, et al. Negative pressure pulmonary edema as a post-anesthetic complication associated with upper airway obstruction in a horse. Vet Surg 1996;25:519–23.

59. Day TK, Holcombe S, Muir WW. Postanesthetic pulmonary edema in an Arab stallion. Vet Emerg Crit Care 1993;3:90–5.

60. Santos M, Fuente M, Garcia-Iturralde P, et al. Effects of alpha-2 adrenoceptor agonists during recovery from isoflurane anaesthesia in horses. Equine Vet J 2003;35:170–5.

61. Durongphongtorn S, McDonell WN, Kerr CL, et al. Comparison of hemodynamic, clinicopathologic, and gastrointestinal motility effects and recovery characteristics

of anesthesia with isoflurane and halothane in horses undergoing arthroscopic surgery. Am J Vet Res 2006;67:32–42.

62. Mama KR, Pascoe PJ, Steffey EP, et al. Comparison of two techniques for total intravenous anesthesia in horses. Am J Vet Res 1998;59:1292–8.

63. Castillo S, Matthews NS. How to assemble, apply, and use a head-and-tail rope system for the recovery of the equine anesthetic patient. Proc Am Assoc Eq Pract 2005;51:490–3.

64. Taylor EL, Galuppo LD, Steffey EP, et al. Use of the Anderson sling suspension system for recovery of horses from general anesthesia. Vet Surg 2005;34:559–64.

65. Sullivan EK, Klein LV, Richardson DW, et al. Use of a pool-raft system for recovery of horses from general anesthesia: 393 horses (1984–2000). J Am Vet Med Assoc 2002;221:1014–8.

66. Tidwell SA, Schneider RK, Ragle CA, et al. Use of a hydro-pool system to recover horses after general anesthesia: 60 cases. Vet Surg 2002;31:455–61.

67. Ray-Miller WM, Hodgson DS, McMurphy RM, et al. Comparison of recoveries from anesthesia of horses placed on a rapidly inflating-deflating air pillow or the floor of a padded stall. J Am Vet Med Assoc 2006;229:711–6.

68. Matthews NS, Hartsfield SM, Mercer D, et al. Recovery from sevoflurane anesthesia in horses: comparison to isoflurane and effect of postmedication with xylazine. Vet Surg 1998;27:480–5.

69. Matthews NS, Mercer D, Beleau MH, et al. A comparison of recoveries from sevoflurane and isoflurane anesthesia in 9 Arabian horses. [abstract]. Proc Ann Mtg Am Coll Vet Anes 1996;29.

70. Matthews NS, Miller SM, Hartsfield SM, et al. Comparison of recoveries from halothane vs isoflurane anesthesia in horses. J Am Vet Med Assoc 1992;201: 559–63.

71. Bienert A, Bartmann CP, Von Oppen T, et al. Recovery phase of horses after inhalant anaesthesia with isofluorane (Isoflo[R]) and postanaesthetic sedation with romifidine (Sedivet[R]) or xylazine (Rompun[R]). Dtsch Tierarztl Woschenschr 2003;110:244–8.

72. Kalchofner KS, Ringer SK, Boller J, et al. Clinical assessment of anesthesia with isoflurane and medetomidine in 300 equidae. Pferdeheilkunde 2006;22:301–8.

73. Yamashita K, Muir WW, Tsubakishita S, et al. Infusion of guaifenesin, ketamine, and medetomidine in combination with inhalation of sevoflurane versus inhalation of sevoflurane alone for anesthesia of horses. J Am Vet Med Assoc 2002;221: 1150–5.

74. Yamashita K, Satoh M, Unikawa A, et al. Combination of continuous intravenous infusion using a mixture of guaifenesin-ketamine-medetomidine and sevoflurane anesthesia in horses. J Vet Med Sci 2000;62:229–35.

75. Wagner AE, Mama KR, Steffey EP, et al. A comparison of equine recovery characteristics after isoflurane or isoflurane followed by a xylazine-ketamine infusion. Vet Anaesth Analg 2008;35:154–60.

Index

Note: Page numbers of article titles are in **boldface** type.

Vet Clin Equine 24 (2009) 753–768
doi:10.1016/S0749-0739(08)00079-5
0749-0739/08/$ – see front matter © 2009 Elsevier Inc. All rights reserved.

vetequine.theclinics.com

Printed and bound by CPI Group (UK) Ltd, Croydon, CR0 4YY

03/10/2024

01040453-0011